D0944486

Developmental Psychoacoustics

Developmental Psychoacoustics

Edited by Lynne A. Werner and Edwin W Rubel

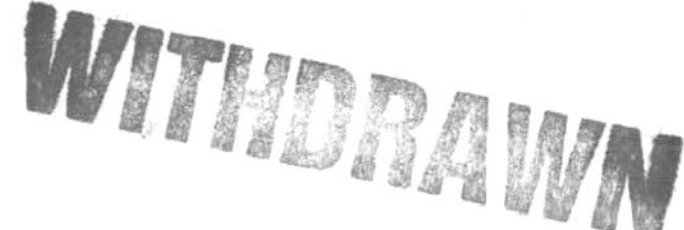

American Psychological Association • Washington, DC

Published by the
American Psychological Association
750 First Street, NE
Washington, DC 20002

Copies may be ordered from
APA Order Department
P.O. Box 2710
Hyattsville, MD 20784

Typeset in Century Light Condensed by Techna Type, Inc., York, PA

Printer: BookCrafters, Chelsea, MI
Cover and Jacket Designer: Berg Design, Albany, NY
Technical/Production Editor: Valerie Montenegro

Library of Congress Cataloging-in-Publication Data

Developmental psychoacoustics / edited by Lynne A. Werner and Edwin W Rubel.
p. cm.
Includes bibliographical references and index.
ISBN 1-55796-159-0 (acid-free paper)
1. Auditory perception in children—Congresses.
2. Psychoacoustics—Congresses. I. Werner, Lynne A. II. Rubel, Edwin W.
[DNLM: 1. Psychoacoustics—in infancy & childhood—congresses.
WV 270 D489]
BF723.A77D49 1992
152.1′5—dc20
DNLM/DLC
for Library of Congress 92-49922
CIP

Printed in the United States of America
First Edition

APA Science Volumes

Best Methods for the Analysis of Change: Recent Advances, Unanswered Questions, Future Directions

Cognition: Conceptual and Methodological Issues

Cognitive Bases of Musical Communication

Conceptualization and Measurement of Organism–Environment Interaction

Developmental Psychoacoustics

Hostility, Coping, and Health

Organ Donation and Transplantation: Psychological and Behavioral Factors

The Perception of Structure

Perspectives on Socially Shared Cognition

Psychological Testing of Hispanics

Researching Community Psychology: Issues of Theory and Methods

Sleep and Cognition

The Suggestibility of Children's Recollections: Implications for Eyewitness Testimony

Taste, Experience, and Feeding

Through the Looking Glass: Issues of Psychological Well-Being in Captive Nonhuman Primates

APA expects to publish volumes on the following conference topics:

Cardiovascular Reactivity to Psychological Stress and Cardiovascular Disease
The Contributions of Psychology to Mathematics and Science Education
Emotion and Culture
Lives Through Time: Assessment and Theory in Personality Psychology From a Longitudinal Perspective
Maintaining and Promoting Integrity in Behavioral Science Research
Stereotypes: Brain–Behavior Relationships
Temperament: Individual Differences in Biology and Behavior

As part of its continuing and expanding commitment to enhance the dissemination of scientific psychological knowledge, the Science Directorate of the APA established a Scientific Conferences Program. A series of volumes resulting from these conferences is jointly produced by the Science Directorate and the Office of Communications. A call for proposals is issued several times annually by the Science Directorate, which, collaboratively with the APA Board of Scientific Affairs, evaluates the proposals and selects several conferences for funding. This important effort has resulted in an exceptional series of meetings and scholarly volumes, each of which individually has contributed to the dissemination of research and dialogue in these topical areas.

The APA Science Directorate's conferences funding program has supported 22 conferences since its inception in 1988. To date, 15 volumes resulting from conferences have been published.

William C. Howell, PhD
Executive Director

Virginia E. Holt
Scientific Conferences Manager

Contents

Contributors

Prudence Allen, Department of Communication Disorders, University of Western Ontario

Martin S. Banks, School of Optometry, University of California, Berkeley

Arlene Earley Carney, Boys Town National Institute, Omaha, NE

Marsha G. Clarkson, Department of Psychology, Georgia State University

Rachel K. Clifton, Department of Psychology, University of Massachusetts

Lincoln Gray, Department of Otolaryngology, University of Texas Medical School, Houston

Patricia K. Kuhl, Department of Speech and Hearing Sciences, University of Washington

Corinne Mar, Department of Psychology, Ohio State University

Karen L. Preston, Department of Psychology, University of Washington

Dan H. Sanes, Center for Neuroscience, New York University

Robert S. Schlauch, Department of Communication Disorders, University of Minnesota

Bruce A. Schneider, Center for Research in Human Development, University of Toronto

Davida Y. Teller, Department of Psychology, University of Washington

Constantine Trahiotis, Department of Otolaryngology, University of Connecticut Health Center

Sandra E. Trehub, Center for Research in Human Development, University of Toronto

Neal F. Viemeister, Department of Psychology, University of Minnesota

Lynne A. Werner, Department of Speech and Hearing Sciences, University of Washington

Frederic Wightman, Department of Psychology, University of Wisconsin–Madison

Preface

Why do things appear as they do? The nature of perception has been an important issue since the time of Aristotle, and as long as the question has been asked, the development of perception has been at the crux of the matter. Is it the innate properties of the nervous system or the learned associations between sensory cues and physical events that form the bases of perception? Long before anyone thought to observe infants and children directly, philosophers, physiologists, and psychologists argued over events that occurred during development to account for the characteristics of perception in adults.

Every model of perception must include a consideration of the properties of sensory systems. Psychophysics is distinguished from other approaches to studying perception in that it involves varying well-defined stimuli to establish sensory capacity and measurement of thresholds, using one of several well-characterized procedures. Psychophysics has always held a central position in psychology. In fact, Boring credited Fechner, the inventor of psychophysics, with founding the field of experimental psychology:

> We come at last to the formal beginning of experimental psychology, and we start with Fechner ... who was not a great philosopher nor at all a physiologist, but who performed with scientific rigor those first experiments which laid the foundation for the new psychology and still lie at the basis of its methodology.... The embryo had been maturing and had already assumed, in all great essentials, its later form. With Fechner it was born, quite as old, and also quite as young, as a baby.[1]

Despite Boring's developmental metaphor and the ever-present issue of perceptual development, psychophysical studies of development were not conducted until some 75 years after Fechner's death. Largely as a result of tremendous increases in interest in the capacities of human infants and in developmental neu-

[1]From *A History of Experimental Psychology* (2nd ed.) by E. G. Boring, 1950, New York: Appleton-Century-Crofts.

roscience, developmental psychophysics was finally established as a field of study in the early 1970s. Only rigorous studies of perceptual behavior could determine what information about the world was available to the infant during development or establish the functional implications of sensory system maturation.

Developmental psychoacoustics deals with the application of psychophysical methods to the study of auditory development. The field has grown exponentially in the past 15 years, but it is not difficult to summarize this now rather extensive body of literature in 25 words or less: Psychoacoustical performance of infants and children is generally not mature. Even in the simplest psychoacoustical tasks, such as detection of a sound in quiet, infants and children exhibit what might be interpreted as auditory deficits compared to normally hearing adults. At this time, developmental papers have been published on absolute sensitivity, differential sensitivity, frequency and temporal resolution, binaural processing, and complex sound processing. In each area, age-related changes in performance have been identified during the first years after birth. One purpose of this volume is to summarize these findings and to begin to offer explanations for them.

Progress in any scientific field is rarely without setbacks, and it is often the case that the limitations of a method or an approach are not recognized until it has been in use for some time. Developmental psychoacoustics is no exception: It was only after many reports of age-related differences in psychoacoustical performance had been published that doubts about the degree to which such measures reflect the optimal sensory capacities of infants and children began to be voiced. The interpretation of age effects in psychoacoustical performance is a major issue in this field today, and one on which there is currently no consensus. A second motivation for preparing this volume is to discuss the variety of ways that we may interpret psychoacoustical data on immature listeners.

The findings of developmental psychoacoustics have relevance for many related fields, including perceptual development, particularly the development of speech perception; auditory nervous system development; psychoacoustics; and pediatric audiology. The growth of knowledge in these fields, in turn, should have relevance for developmental psychoacoustics. To date, the extent of interaction among these fields has been limited. The reasons range from the fact that scientists in some of these related fields generally do not have training in psychology to a certain degree of defensiveness on the part of developmental psychoacousticians about the psychophysical methods they use. A strong case can be made, however, that interactions with related fields will be important to continued progress in developmental psychoacoustics. It is doubtful, for example, that we will be able to understand age-related change in psychoacoustic performance without reference to the underlying neural structure and function. One might also note that while developmental psychoacousticians have been busy demonstrating that infants and children perform poorly in psychoacoustic tasks, others have shown that at the same ages, the ability to categorize and discriminate speech is remarkably well developed. Certainly there is a need to reconcile these findings. Finally, it is ironic that while the most commonly used method in assessing infants' psychoacoustic skills was developed by pediatric audiologists as a clinical measure of hearing, developmental psychoacoustics has had very little contact with pediatric audiology, either in terms of further methodological developments or in the substance of our discoveries concerning normally hearing infants and children. Thus, a final purpose of this volume is to encourage increased dialogue between developmental psychoacoustics and related fields.

This book has three parts, reflecting the three purposes already outlined. Part One, "Developmental Psychoacoustics: Current Progress," contains summaries of recent findings from six laboratories. The first four chapters examine basic auditory capacities in infants and children. Schneider and Trehub discuss their work on the development of auditory sensitivity; Werner summarizes studies of absolute sensitivity, frequency discrimination, and detection in noise in human infants; Gray presents information about the ontogeny of a variety of auditory processes in newborn chicks; and Wightman and Allen report on temporal, frequency, and spectral resolution in children. The last two chapters discuss more complex processes. Clifton summarizes the results of her program of research on spatial hearing in infants and children, and Clarkson describes the results of her studies on pitch perception in infants.

Throughout the chapters included in Part One, the reader will observe the following theme: How do nonsensory factors contribute to age-related changes in psychophysical performance? Schneider takes the position that as long as a bias-free measure of sensitivity is used, nonsensory variables, such as motivation or attention, have little effect on thresholds of infants and children. Both Gray and Werner, on the other hand, take the position that although thresholds obtained from human and avian infants do reflect sensory processes, they are also affected by nonsensory variables. Finally, Wightman and Allen present a model of performance that includes attentional and memory effects that essentially account for all of the threshold differences seen between preschool children and adults.

The question of nonsensory effects and the general issue of interpretation of developmental psychophysical data are taken up directly in Part Two, "Interpretative Issues in Developmental Psychoacoustics." Viemeister and Schlauch offer a series of simulations of infant psychometric functions that take into account criterial and attentional effects and suggest a procedure for "correcting for attention" that seems to produce stable threshold estimates. Teller presents an impressive study of the characteristics of the infant psychometric function in visual acuity measurements. The section ends with Banks's discussion of interpretive issues in the context of visual development that incorporates the "ideal observer" approach to trying to account for infant–adult differences in visual acuity.

The third part of the volume, "Developmental Psychoacoustics in the Context of Hearing Science," addresses the relationship between developmental psychoacoustics and related fields. Sanes's chapter describes his work on the development of structure and function in the auditory nervous system, suggesting ways that changes in the nervous system with age might be reflected in behavior. Trahiotis outlines some key points with respect to binaural hearing in adults that may have important implications for studies of development in this area and describes a recent model of mature spatial hearing. Kuhl's chapter gives a historical perspective on the interactions that have occurred between psychoacoustics and speech perception research as well as a detailed account of her recent work on the development of speech prototypes in human infants. Carney's chapter ends the book with a discussion of the potential and the limitations of developmental psychoacoustical approaches in the clinic and ways that developmental psychoacoustics can provide information that would be useful to the pediatric audiologist.

It is our hope that this volume will stimulate additional research in developmental psychoacoustics, promote an appreciation for the importance of understanding the sensory capacities of infants and children during development, and encourage mutually beneficial interactions across disciplines.

This volume grew out of a conference held in August 1991 at the University of Washington. The conference was supported by the American Psychological Association, the National Institute of Deafness and Communication Disorders, the Virginia Merrill Bloedel Hearing Research Center, and several divisions of the

University of Washington: the Center for Advanced Studies in the School of Medicine, the College of Arts and Sciences, the Graduate School, and the Center for Child Development and Mental Retardation. The American Psychological Association also provided support for the preparation of this book. The authors, coeditor, and I would like to thank, in addition to those who provided financial support, several individuals who were instrumental in the organization of the conference and the preparation of this volume: Jo Ann Chavira-Bash, Lisa Rickard Mancl, Janelle Constantino, Jill Bargones, Cam Marean, Beth Kopyar, Andrea Ernst, Lisa Rubel, and Nevada Smith. Finally, our thanks go to a number of colleagues who provided critical reviews of the chapters included in this volume, including Dan Ashmead, Kathy Arehart, Ed Burns, Rachel Clifton, Rich Folsom, Lincoln Gray, Rick Hyson, Cam Marean, Davida Teller, and Neal Viemeister.

Lynne A. Werner

PART ONE

Developmental Psychoacoustics: Current Progress

CHAPTER 1

Sources of Developmental Change in Auditory Sensitivity

Bruce A. Schneider and Sandra E. Trehub

A sensible first step in studying the development of any perceptual system is to determine how its basic operating characteristics change with age and the implications of such changes. In vision, any pattern can be decomposed into sinusoidal gratings of different spatial frequencies and orientations. Because infants are unable to resolve high spatial frequencies (see Banks & Bennett, 1988, for a review of issues), information carried by the high-frequency components of a visual pattern will be unavailable to them. This will impose severe limitations on their ability to perceive objects in space. Because complex sounds can also be decomposed into sets of sine waves, infants' ability to perceive complex sounds will be limited by their sensitivity to sounds of different frequencies. Therefore, complete characterization of auditory development depends on knowledge of age-related changes in sensitivity to sound and other basic operating characteristics

This research was supported by grants from the Medical Research Council of Canada and the University of Toronto. *Correspondence concerning this chapter should be sent to Bruce A. Schneider, Centre for Research in Human Development, University of Toronto, Erindale Campus, Mississauga, Ontario, Canada L5L 1C6.*

of the auditory system. The specification of such changes in operating characteristics is one of the primary goals of developmental psychoacoustics.

In studying age-related changes in sensitivity to sound, developmental psychoacousticians have had to overcome two major obstacles. The first was methodological—finding or developing a technique to determine absolute and masked thresholds, with the minimal requirements for such a technique being sensitivity, efficiency of administration, and applicability over a wide age range. The second was the identification of factors responsible for any observed developmental changes. With respect to the methodological obstacle, it quickly became clear that infant psychophysical methods could be based on the head-turning component of the orienting response to sound (Sokolov, 1963; see Schneider, Trehub, & Bull, 1979; Schneider & Trehub, 1985 for a discussion of issues). In the first part of this chapter, we will compare and contrast different psychophysical methods that use a head-turn response, demonstrating that they meet the criteria of sensitivity, efficiency, and applicability. In the second part, we will present a model of auditory threshold to identify factors responsible for the developmental changes revealed by conditioned head-turning techniques.

Psychophysical Methods

Over the past 2 decades, visual reinforcement of the orienting response to a sound (visual reinforcement audiometry [VRA]) has become the method of choice in most developmental studies of basic auditory processes. A central feature of this technique is the presentation of a visual reinforcer, usually a mechanically activated toy, following the head-turning component of an orienting response to sound. The head-turning or localization response can be elicited reliably by 5 or 6 months of age (Chun, Pawsat, & Forster, 1960), and reinforcement can maintain it at high levels for 30 to 40 trials within a single session (Moore, Thompson, & Thompson, 1975; Suzuki & Ogiba, 1961; Trehub, Schneider, & Bull, 1981). Currently, two versions of this technique are used to determine absolute and masked thresholds in infants.

Go/No-Go Signal Detection

In the go/no-go detection (G/NG-D) version of VRA (Moore et al., 1975), the infant sits on the parent's lap with a single loudspeaker located to one side. The experimenter sits facing the infant and initiates a trial when the infant is looking directly ahead. A signal is presented for a limited duration on some trials and no signal is presented on others. On both signal and no-signal trials, the experimenter indicates the presence of a turn toward the loudspeaker by pressing a button. In signal-detection terms, a head turn (go response) within a fixed time following signal onset (the trial duration) is considered a hit; a head turn on a no-signal trial is a false alarm; no turn (no-go) on a signal trial is a miss; and no turn on a no-signal trial is a correct rejection. Adaptive procedures are typically used, and infants who turn on "too many" no-signal trials are often eliminated, although the number of such false alarms and other exclusion criteria vary considerably across studies (Berg & Smith, 1983, greater than .33 false-alarm rate; Sinnott, Pisoni, & Aslin, 1983, 2 or more false alarms). Furthermore, threshold is usually computed from hits alone.

An examination of the infant G/NG-D task indicates that it is not ideally designed from the perspective of signal-detection theory. In signal-detection theory, it is assumed that on no-signal or noise trials, there is residual random activity in the auditory system that gives rise to a distribution of events along a decision axis, referred to as the noise (N) distribution. On signal trials, the signal is added to the background noise, thereby providing a boost in activity on that trial. This distribution of activity on signal trials is referred to as the signal-plus-noise (SN) distribution. Figure 1 depicts a plot of these two hypothetical distributions. It is assumed that the listener is presented with a sample from the N distribution on no-signal trials and from the SN distribution on signal trials. The listener's task is to decide which distribution generated the observation. The listener presumably accomplishes this task by locating a criterion along the decision axis depicted in Figure 1, responding that a signal is present (head turn) if the observation falls to the right of the criterion, or absent (failure to turn) if it falls to the left. The location of the criterion will depend on instructional variables, on the relative frequency of signal and no-signal trials, and on the payoff structure for hits and misses.

The first problem to surface in the G/NG-D task concerns the location of the infant's criterion along the decision axis. Note that turning to the left on signal trials is rewarded whereas turning on no-signal or catch trials is not. Because there is no penalty for responding on no-signal trials (for an exception, see Sinnott et al., 1983), infants who attempt to maximize the number of rewards would locate their criterion far to the left. Adults placed in this situation are

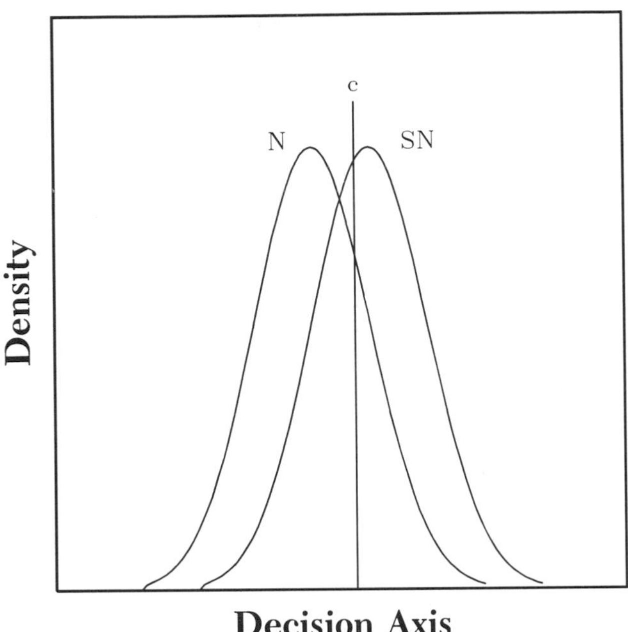

FIGURE 1 Hypothetical distributions of events associated with no-signal (noise) trials and signal-plus-noise trials. The observer's criterion is indicated by the vertical line at *c*.

unlikely to adopt such an extreme strategy because of explicit or implicit expectations or instructions. Rather, they are more likely to locate their criterion midway between the two distributions, so that performance would more accurately discriminate between the two types of trials. In G/NG-D tasks, however, it is assumed that the infant will behave like an adult in this respect, and not locate the criterion far to the left. As a result, infants with high false-alarm rates are typically excluded from the study, presumably because they are not under procedural control. It is theoretically possible, however, that such infants are "listening" but have simply adopted a strong bias to respond "Yes."

Thus, infants, children, and adults may adopt different strategies for determining criterion location, which may result in different threshold estimates, especially if psychometric functions (see next section) are constructed from hit rates alone. Thus, even if infant and adult sensitivity are equivalent (i.e., the same degree of separation between the N and SN distributions), different response-bias strategies (i.e., different criterion locations) will produce different threshold estimates in adaptive G/NG-D tasks. Of course, this difficulty can be overcome when appropriate estimates of false-alarm rates are available. For example, if the intensity of a signal is held constant on signal trials, and "catch" trials are used to calculate a false-alarm rate, d' scores can be computed (Schneider, Trehub, & Thorpe, 1991), where d' measures the separation between the means of the N and SN distributions scaled in normal deviate units. Thus, d' is independent of criterion location. However, the typical practice of using adaptive techniques in conjunction with the G/NG-D task precludes the possibility of estimating false-alarm rates. To understand why this is the case, note that at the beginning of an adaptive run, with N and SN distributions widely separated, listeners still have to select a criterion location along the decision axis. Consider the following two strategies: In the first strategy, the listener locates the criterion at a fixed point along the decision axis with respect to the noise distribution, keeping this unchanged throughout the session. This strategy yields a constant false-alarm rate throughout the session, which can be calculated by means of the percentage of head turns on catch trials. The listener who adopts the second strategy locates the criterion at the intersection of the N and SN distributions. As trials progress, and the separation between the two distributions decreases, the false-alarm rate will increase. This strategy precludes the computation of d', because the false-alarm rate changes over a session, and there are too few catch trials that are temporally proximal to specific stimulus levels. In fact, Trehub, Schneider, Thorpe, and Judge (1991) have shown that the two strategies can generate quite different threshold estimates when these are computed from psychometric functions based on hit rates. In short, different response-bias strategies will affect threshold estimates in adaptive G/NG-D techniques.

It is apparent, then, that adult–infant threshold differences in the G/NG-D task could be affected by response-bias factors that have little to do with sensitivity. Such differences can emerge even when "attentional" variables are identical for both infants and adults. In our laboratories, we have avoided response-bias problems inherent in adaptive G/NG-D procedures by using a two-alternative, forced-choice localization procedure to determine absolute and masked sensitivity.

Two-Alternative, Forced-Choice Localization

In the two-alternative, forced-choice localization task (2AFC-L), loudspeakers are located to the infant's left and right. As in the G/NG-D task, the experimenter faces the infant and initiates a trial only when the infant is looking directly ahead. A signal is presented on every trial, sometimes on the infant's left and sometimes on the right, remaining on until the infant turns 45° to either side. Correct responses (i.e., turns toward the loudspeaker producing the signal) are also reinforced by a toy near the loudspeaker; incorrect responses result in a short intertrial delay before the next trial. (For further details, see Schneider, Trehub, & Bull, 1980; Schneider, Trehub, Morrongiello, & Thorpe, 1986, 1989; Trehub, Schneider, & Endman, 1980; Trehub, Schneider, Morrongiello, & Thorpe, 1988, 1989.)

The 2AFC-L procedure enjoys several advantages over the Go/No-Go procedure. First, in 2AFC-L, correct responses are always rewarded, whereas incorrect responses produce a time-out period. Payoff structures of this sort favor unbiased responding, increasing the likelihood of greater consistency in criterion location both within and across age groups. As a result, psychometric functions (i.e., percentage correct as a function of stimulus intensity) should be relatively unaffected by response-bias factors in all age groups. Second, because rewards are given for both kinds of correct responses (i.e., turns to one side or the other), reinforcement is available on every trial in the 2AFC-L procedure as opposed to signal trials only in the G/NG-D procedure. If no-signal trials promote boredom in infant listeners, we might expect them to be less attentive in the G/NG-D than in the 2AFC-L task. Third, returning to midline after responding (i.e., readiness for the next trial) results in a .5 or greater probability of signal presentation and associated potential for reinforcement in G/NG-D, compared with a 1.0 probability of signal presentation and potential reinforcement in 2AFC-L. Finally, the 2AFC-L procedure may pose fewer cognitive demands than the G/NG-D procedure for infant listeners. In G/NG-D, infants must withhold responding on no-signal trials. Although verbal instruction in this regard is successful with older children, infants, for whom this is obviously precluded, might require more visual entertainment or distraction, which might decrease the likelihood of responding toward the reinforcer on signal trials (see Schneider et al., 1991). It would seem then, that G/NG-D, as typically applied with infants, might function as a divided-attention task, potentially degrading performance.

Although 2AFC-L has several advantages over G/NG-D, it also has the distinct disadvantage of being a localization rather than a detection task. Clearly, failure to localize a sound does not preclude its detectability. With adult listeners and selected auditory stimuli, thresholds for lateralization (i.e., detecting the ear of presentation in an earphone experiment) are considerably higher than those for detection (Egan & Benson, 1966). If the extent of such dissociation is age-related, then the developmental course for lateralization thresholds need not parallel that for detection thresholds. However, locating the source in a sound field differs in many ways from identifying the side of presentation in an earphone experiment. Furthermore, the octave and one-third octave stimuli used in the 2AFC-L task (see Schneider et al., 1980, 1986; Schneider, Trehub, Morrongiello, & Thorpe, 1989; Trehub et al., 1980, 1988, 1989) are considerably easier to localize than the pure tones used in the typical lateralization task (Egan & Benson, 1966). In any case, the extent of dissociation between detection and localization measures of threshold at any particular age is a question amenable to empirical resolution.

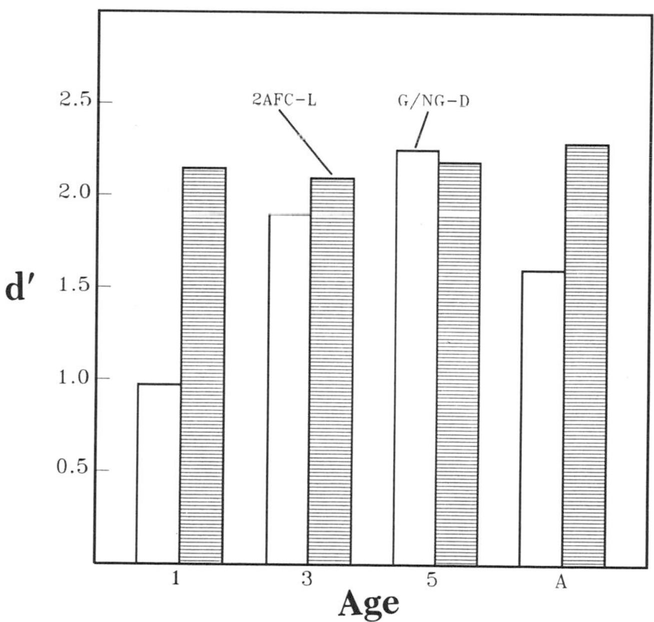

FIGURE 2 Performance differences in a quiet background, measured in *d′* units between 2AFC-L (two-alternative, forced-choice localization) and G/NG-D (go/no-go detection) tasks at four different ages. From Schneider, Trehub, and Thorpe (1991). Copyright 1991 by the Psychonomic Society. Reprinted by permission.

Schneider et al. (1991) have compared the detection (G/NG-D) and localization (2AFC-L) of high- and low-frequency signals in quiet and in masking noise. In both tasks, a single stimulus (0.4 or 10 kHz) was used throughout the test session, and d' scores were computed. Performance differences between the tasks were similar at high and low frequencies, indicating that signal frequency did not exert differential effects. Figure 2 presents the average d' scores obtained in quiet for each task as a function of age. Figure 3 presents comparable data for signals in a background of broadband noise. The figures reveal no evidence that performance is superior in detection procedures for infant, child, and adult listeners. In fact, localization yielded better performance than detection for the youngest group tested (1-year-olds). Schneider et al. attributed this performance difference to the greater cognitive demands associated with the G/NG-D procedure. Adults' slight advantage on 2AFC-L may result from their ability to capital-

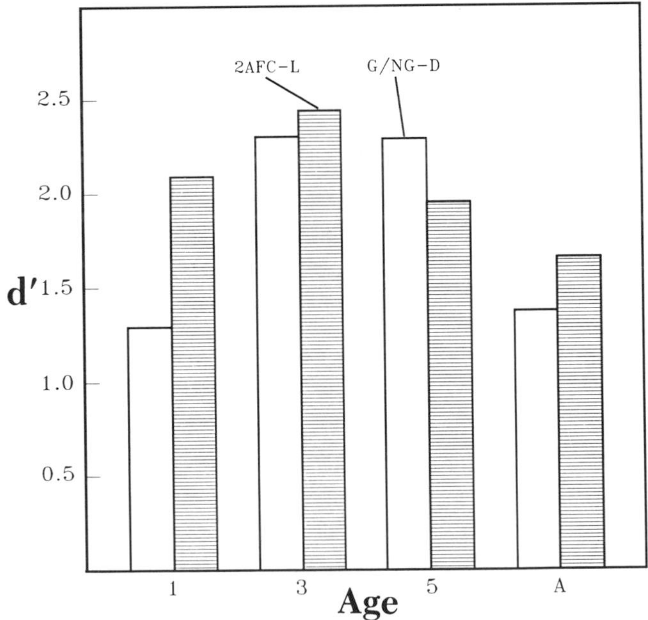

FIGURE 3 Performance differences in a noisy background, measured in d' units between 2AFC-L (two-alternative, forced-choice localization) and G/NG-D (go/no-go detection) tasks at four different ages. From Schneider, Trehub, and Thorpe (1991). Copyright 1991 by the Psychonomic Society. Reprinted by permission.

ize on ear asymmetries (i.e., guessing the poorer ear when the signal is inaudible; see Schneider et al., 1991). We conclude, therefore, that the two variants of VRA, when evaluated within a signal-detection framework, produce nearly equivalent measures of sensitivity over the entire age range.

Adult–Infant Differences

If there are minimal performance differences between G/NG-D and 2AFC-L tasks at different ages, we would expect adult–infant differences obtained with G/NG-D to be equivalent to those obtained with 2AFC-L. Figure 4 plots adult–infant abso-

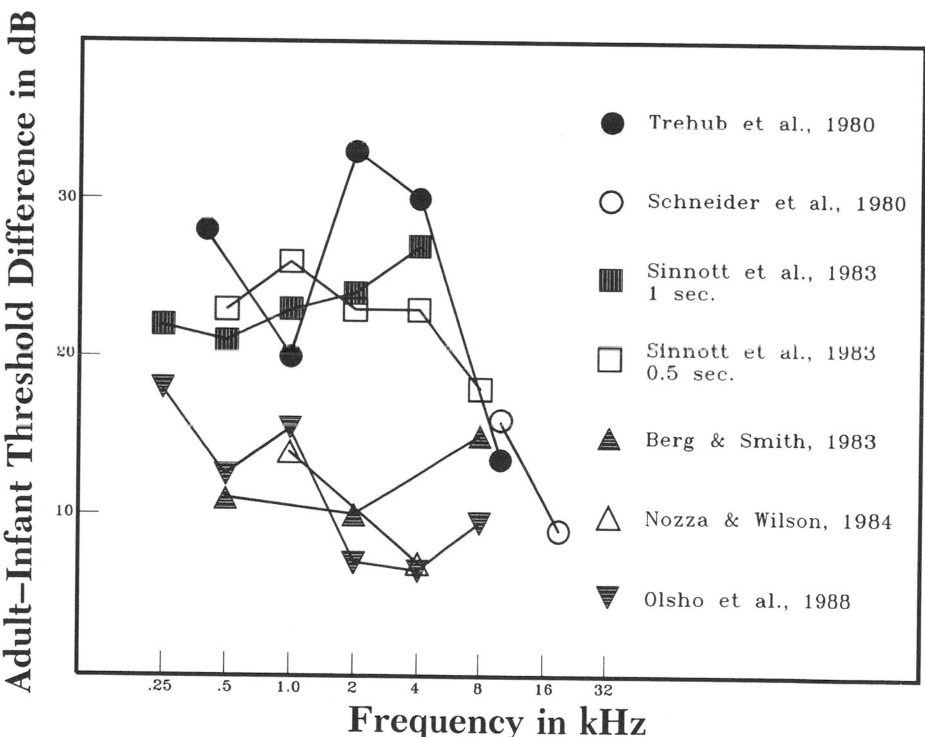

FIGURE 4 Adult–infant differences in absolute threshold (measured in decibels) in six different studies. Infant thresholds in Trehub et al. (1980) were compared to adult thresholds in Schneider et al. (1986). All other adult–infant comparisons were from the same investigations. Data derived from Berg and Smith (1983); Nozza and Wilson (1984); Olsho, Koch, Carter, Halpin, and Spetner (1988); Schneider, Trehub, and Bull (1980); Sinnott, Pisoni, and Aslin (1983); and Trehub, Schneider, and Endman (1980). All material adapted by permission.

lute threshold differences obtained from several studies for 6- to 8-month-old infants. The studies can be grouped into two sets: Adult–infant differences obtained by Schneider et al. (1980), Sinnott et al. (1983), and Trehub et al. (1980) are larger than those obtained by Berg and Smith (1983), Nozza and Wilson (1984), and Olsho, Koch, Carter, Halpin, and Spetner (1988). It is interesting to note that the studies with relatively large adult–infant differences were conducted in the sound field, whereas those with smaller adult–infant differences used earphone presentation. Some of the adult–infant differences obtained in the sound field may be attributable to differences in resonance properties of the ear canals of infants and adults. Because of resonance in the ear canal, the sound pressure level at the eardrum is not the same as that measured when the listener is absent. Thus, an infant and an adult listening to the same sound might experience different eardrum sound pressures because of differences in ear canal shape and mechanics. If, for example, adults develop higher eardrum sound pressures than infants, this could account for some of the adult–infant differences obtained in the sound field. At least one study has indicated that there are no substantial adult–infant differences in ear canal sound pressure when earphones are involved (Hesketh, 1983, cited in Nozza & Wilson, 1984). Thus, adult–infant differences in ear canal sound pressure may account, in part, for the larger adult–infant differences with sound-field presentation than with earphone presentation. Indeed, it is interesting to note that the magnitude of the difference between sound-field and earphone thresholds decreases substantially by 1 year of age (see Olsho et al., 1988, Figure 1). Such a decline would be expected as the dimensions of the infant ear approach those of the adult ear.

When considering only those studies involving the G/NG-D task, an interesting fact emerges. Berg and Smith (1983), Nozza and Wilson (1984), and Olsho et al. (1988) reported false-alarm rates that were considerably higher for infants than adults, together with smaller adult–infant differences than those obtained with 2AFC-L. In the one G/NG-D study in which infant and adult false-alarm rates were roughly comparable (Sinnott et al., 1983), adult–infant differences were as large as those obtained with 2AFC-L. It is reasonable, therefore, to consider the impact of different false-alarm rates in infants and adults on adult–infant threshold differences derived from adaptive G/NG-D tasks.

To understand how a change in the false-alarm rate would alter the threshold estimates in G/NG-D tasks, consider the effect of criterion location on the

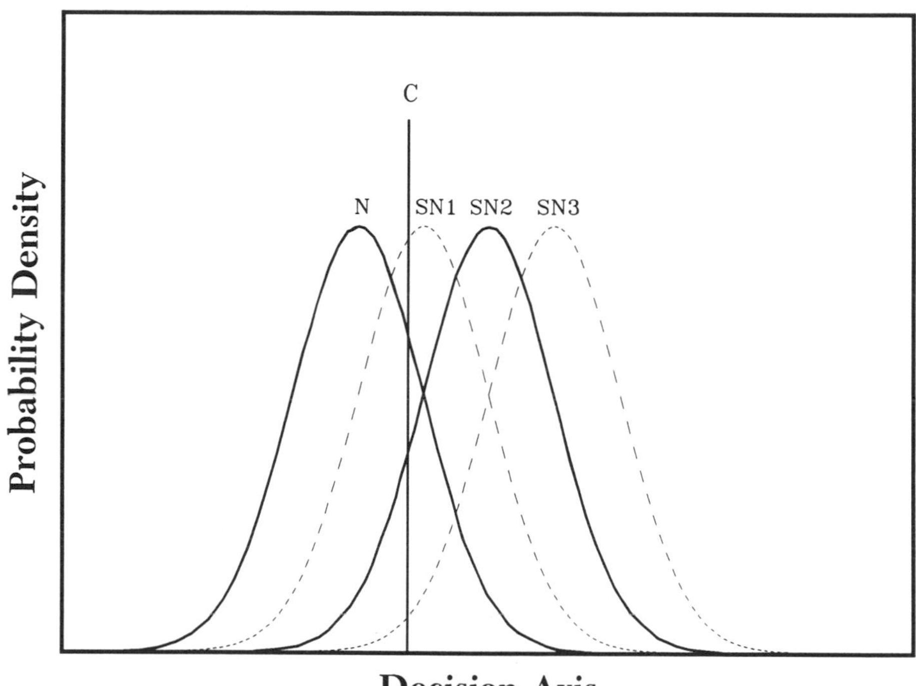

FIGURE 5 Three hypothetical signal-plus-noise distributions are shown along with the noise distribution. The vertical line represents the criterion location.

shape of the psychometric function. Figure 5 shows the noise (N) distribution and three signal-plus-noise (SN) distributions. Recall that a "Yes" response occurs for any observation to the right of the criterion. Clearly, changing the criterion location will change the probability of a hit for each of the SN distributions. Because the psychometric function relates the probability of a hit to stimulus intensity, changing the criterion location (i.e., changing the false-alarm rate) will shift the location of the psychometric function. To determine the extent of the shift in decibels, it is necessary to know how d', the separation between the SN and N distributions, changes with sound pressure level in infants. Jeffress (1967) has shown that d' is very nearly a power function of the signal-to-noise ratio in a detection experiment, that is,

$$d' = a + b(I/I_0)^n, \tag{1}$$

where I is signal intensity, I_0 is the spectrum level of the background noise, and a, b, and n are constants. To estimate this relation for infants, we used the psychometric functions obtained from a masked threshold experiment with 6-month-old listeners (Schneider et al., 1989; masker level = 10 dB/cycle). Psychometric functions from a masking experiment were used instead of the equivalent functions from an absolute threshold experiment because the former functions would be unaffected by (a) differences in ear-canal resonance, and/or (b) the presence of undetected otitis media in a subset of infants. (Both of these conditions would affect signal and noise to the same extent, leaving the signal-to-noise ratio unchanged.) Figure 6 plots percentage correct in the 2AFC-L task as a function of signal-to-noise ratio at five different frequencies. Note that percentage correct never quite reaches 100 in 6-month-olds but appears to asymptote at around 93. An asymptote of 93% would correspond to an inattention rate of about 14%. Assuming an inattention rate of 14%, these data points were used to find values of a, b, and n in Equation 1 that minimized the sum of squared differences between the obtained and predicted d' scores.[1] The smooth curves drawn through the data points were constructed by using Formula 1 to find the d' value corresponding to a particular intensity, converting that d' to a probability of being correct on trials in which a listener was attending, and then correcting for inattention. The resulting psychometric functions provide a good description of the data.

[1]The psychometric functions fit to the data were determined in the following way. First, based on performance at the highest of five intensity levels in Schneider et al. (1989), it was estimated that infants were inattentive on approximately 14% of the trials. Second, it was assumed that inattentive trials were randomly distributed across the session. Third, the percentage correct for the four lowest stimulus intensities was corrected for inattention. If p_c is the observed proportion of correct responses at a given intensity, the proportion after correcting for inattention (p_{ci}) is given by $p_{ci} = (p_c - .5x)/(1 - x)$, where x is the probability of being inattentive on a trial. Corrected probabilities of less than 50% (2 cases) were changed to 50%. These corrected probabilities were converted to d' scores, assuming an unbiased observer. (Recall that locating the criterion midway between the means of the N and SN distribution maximizes rewards in 2AFC-L.) Thus, if $p_c = .7$ and $x = .14$, then $p_{ci} = .733$, and $d' = 1.24$. Values of a, b, and n were simultaneously sought to minimize the sum of squared deviations between the predicted d' values (using Equation 1) and the obtained d' values, for the 10 dB/cycle masking functions (0.4 to 4 kHz) from Schneider et al. (1989). The values of a, b, and n that minimized the sum of squares for the frequencies 0.4 to 4 kHz were $a = -0.847$, $b = 0.127$, and $n = 0.323$. To obtain the predicted psychometric functions for 0.4 to 4 kHz, signal-to-noise ratio was converted to d' using equation 1, d' was converted to p_{ci} in the 2AFC-L task, and p_{ci} was converted to p_c assuming a 14% inattention rate. To fit this psychometric function to the 10-kHz, masked threshold data, and to all frequencies for the absolute threshold data, this psychometric function was shifted along the abscissa until a point was found at which the sum of squared deviations of the data points from the function was minimized. These are the functions shown in Figure 7.

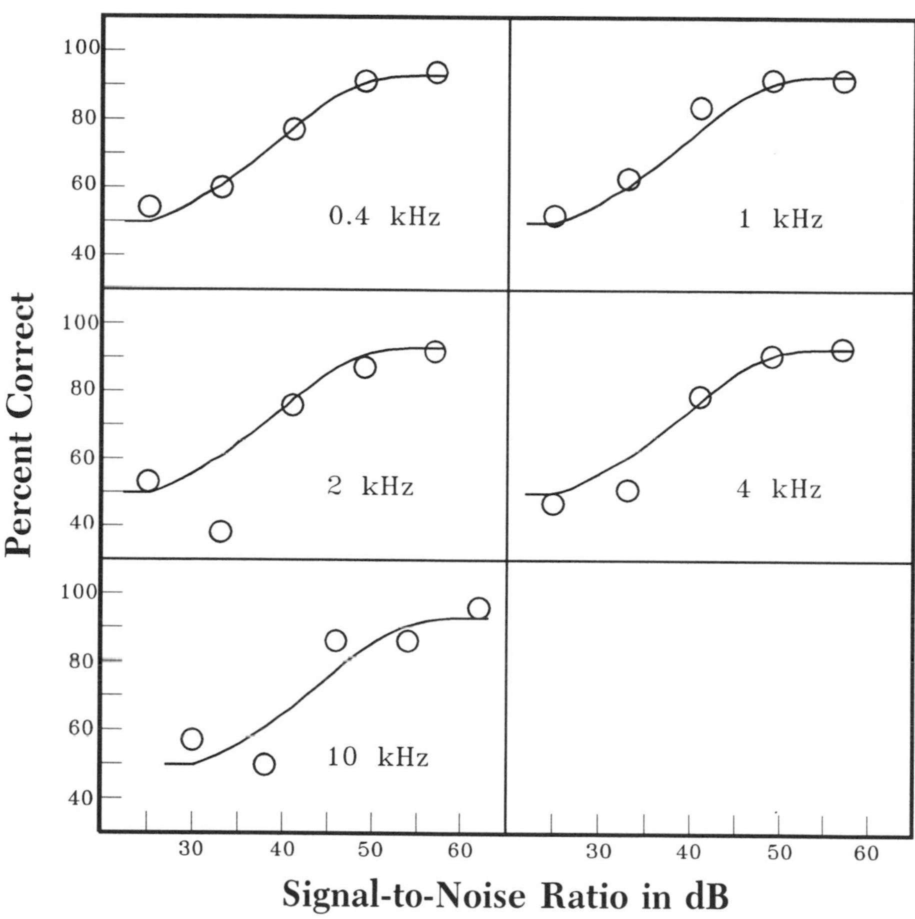

FIGURE 6 Percentage of correct responses in a 2AFC-L task as a function of signal-to-noise ratio (in dB) for octave-band noises masked by a broadband noise (spectrum level = 10 dB/cycle). The same psychometric function (see text) is fit to the data points at all frequencies. Psychometric functions are based on a minimum of 100 trials per stimulus level from 6-month-old infants. From Schneider, Trehub, Morrongiello, and Thorpe (1989). Copyright 1989 by the Acoustical Society of America. Reprinted by permission.

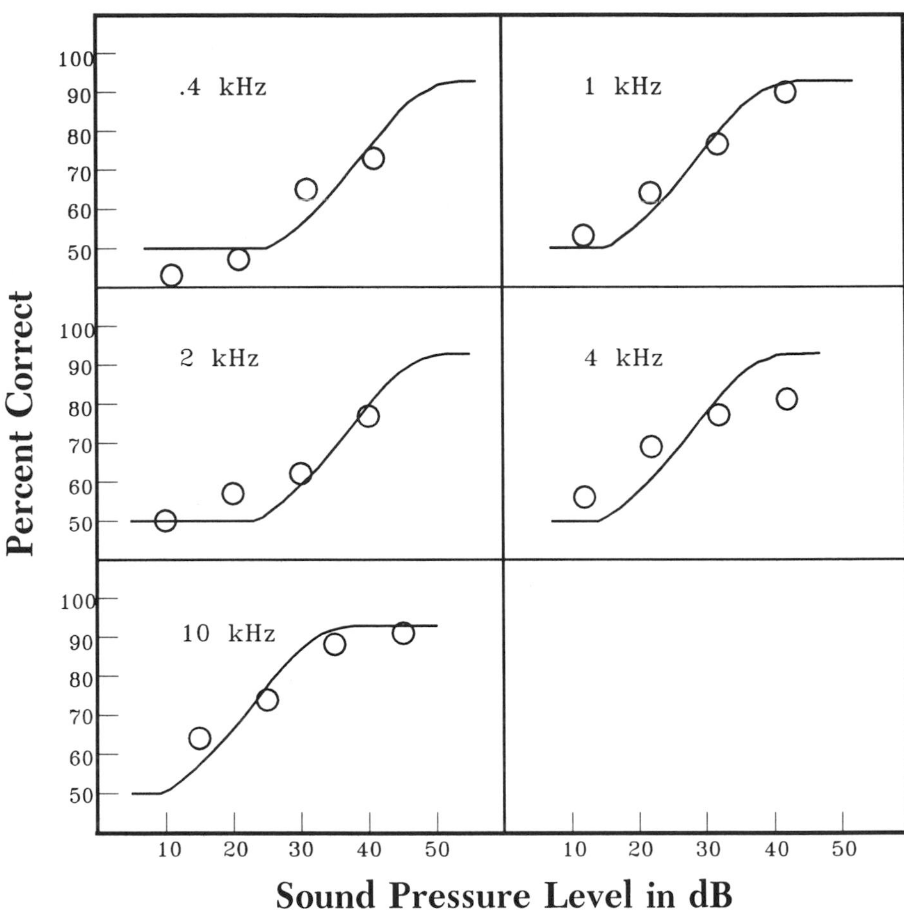

FIGURE 7 Percentage of correct responses in 2AFC-L as a function of decibels of sound pressure for octave-band noises presented in a quiet background. The same psychometric function (see text) is fit to the data points at all frequencies. Psychometric functions are based on a minimum of 100 trials per stimulus level from 6-month-old infants. From Trehub, Schneider, and Endman (1980). Copyright 1980 by Academic Press. Adapted by permission.

These same psychometric functions were used to fit the data from an absolute threshold experiment (see Figure 7) with 6-month-old listeners (Trehub et al., 1980). The psychometric functions in Figure 7 have the same slopes as those shown in Figure 6 but are simply shifted along the abscissa to provide a good fit to the data points. Note that the same psychometric function provides a good fit

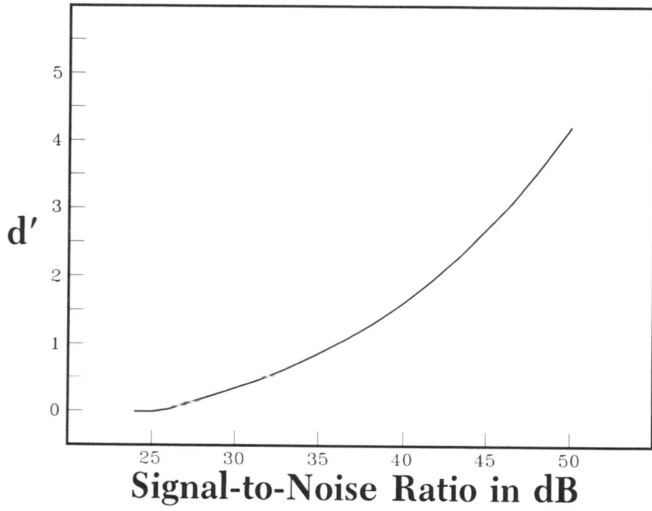

FIGURE 8 The best fitting power function relating *d′* to signal-to-noise ratio in 6-month-old infants. To fit this function, *d′* values were computed from the data points in Figure 6. Values of *a*, *b*, and *n* were found that minimized the sum of squared differences between these *d′* values and the predicted values from Equation 1 (see footnote 1).

to both the masked and unmasked threshold data over the frequency range from 0.4 to 10 kHz.

Figure 8 shows how d' varies as a function of the signal-to-noise ratio in dB for masked octave-band noises over the frequency range 0.4-4 kHz. (This function is the one that simultaneously minimized the sum of squared deviations between the predicted and obtained d's for frequencies of 0.4, 1, 2, and 4 kHz. All other infant psychometric functions are shifted versions of this one.) Note that for d' values between 0.1 and 3, a 1-dB step results in a change of approximately 0.15 in d' value. Olsho et al. (1988) reported that the average slope of the psychometric function for 6-month-olds was approximately .13 z-units per decibel. Thus, the slope of the psychometric function estimated from the masked threshold data in the 2AFC-L task is approximately equal to the average value of the slopes of individual psychometric functions found in G/NG-D tasks, and to the slopes of the group psychometric functions found in absolute and masked threshold experiments. It is encouraging that the same form of the psychometric function appears to characterize data gathered with different techniques in several laboratories.

To examine the effect of a change in criterion location on infant psychometric functions in the G/NG-D task, we constructed hypothetical infant psychometric functions for false-alarm rates of 12.5% and 3%. In doing so, we assumed that the relationship between d' and signal-to-noise ratio was the same as that shown in Figure 8 and that the inattention rate was 14% (i.e., the inattention rate estimated from the 2AFC-L masked threshold experiment). An examination of psychometric functions in Olsho et al. (1988) reveals that they asymptote between 80% and 90%, lending credence to an inattention rate of 14%. We chose a false-alarm rate of 12.5%, which falls between the 11.5% false-alarm rate observed for 6-month-old infants by Nozza and Wilson (1984) and the 13.7% rate found by Olsho et al. (1988) for the equivalent age group. We chose to compare this with a false-alarm rate of 3%, which was close to the 2.5% false-alarm rate of adult listeners in Nozza and Wilson (1984). The two psychometric functions are shown in Figure 9. Note that changing the false-alarm rate from 3% to 12.5% shifts the psychometric function to the left, and that increasing the false-alarm rate even further would increase the extent of the shift. In short, as the separation between adult and infant false-alarm rates increases, the resulting adult–infant threshold differences would be expected to decrease.

The adaptive psychophysical procedure used by Nozza and Wilson (1984) to determine masked thresholds was designed to estimate the 50% point on the psychometric function. If it did so accurately, and if the relationship between d' and signal-to-noise ratio was as specified in Figure 8, then Nozza and Wilson's (1984) estimate of adult–infant differences would be about 4.5 dB too low (i.e., the separation of the 50% points on the two psychometric functions in Figure 9). In fact, they found adult–infant masked threshold differences of 8 dB at 1 and 4 kHz. By contrast, Schneider et al. (1989) found adult–infant differences (averaged over two levels of masking noise) of 11.5 and 14 dB for the same two frequencies. The discrepancy in adult–infant differences between the two studies is about 4–5 dB, which would be expected from the adult–infant differences in false-alarm rate. Assuming that the inattention rate and the relation between d' and signal-to-noise ratio were the same for both studies, the discrepancy in estimated adult–infant threshold differences can be attributed entirely to the differences in false-alarm rates between infants and adults.

Applying this logic to measures of absolute thresholds, whenever infant false-alarm rates exceed those of adults, G/NG-D tasks will underestimate adult–

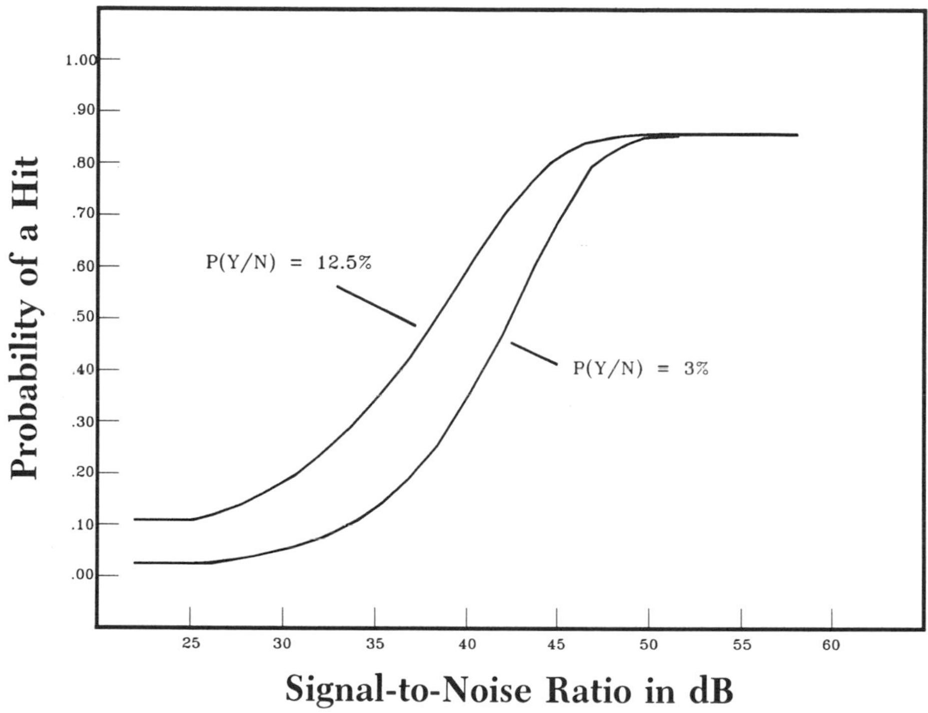

FIGURE 9 Hypothetical psychometric functions (probability of a hit as a function of signal-to-noise ratio) for masked thresholds in a G/NG-D task. In constructing these functions, it was assumed that the relation between *d'* and signal-to-noise ratio was the same as that shown in Figure 8, and that inattention rate was 14%. The parameter differentiating the two functions is the false-alarm rate. False-alarm rates of about 12.5% are typical of 6-month-old infants, whereas false-alarm rates of 3% or less are typical of adults.

infant differences. Consequently, the "real" adult–infant differences in threshold would be larger than the estimated differences shown in Figure 4 for all of the G/NG-D studies except Sinnott et al. (1983). We conclude, then, that most, if not all, of the variation among studies shown in Figure 4 is attributable to (a) differences in infant and adult false-alarm rates or to (b) differences between sound-field and earphone test conditions.

It is important to reiterate that adult–infant ear resonance differences should not affect masked thresholds because such resonances do not change the signal-to-noise ratio. Also, the inadvertent inclusion of any infants with otitis media (and associated conductive hearing loss) would not change the signal-to-noise ratio. As a result, adult–infant masked-threshold differences in Schneider et al. (1989) and in Nozza and Wilson (1984) should be comparable when corrected for the effect of false-alarm rate on psychometric functions in G/NG-D tasks. Indeed, we have shown (above) that once such a correction is made, the two studies yield virtually identical adult–infant differences. The foregoing analysis indicates that performance differences between the two methods are minimal, even in the context of stimulus (pure tone vs. narrow-band noise) and presentation (earphone vs. sound field) differences. Another window on the reliability of the method was provided by Schneider et al. (1991), who superimposed their data (obtained by presenting a single stimulus intensity in a session) on psychometric functions obtained under a variety of conditions (see Figure 10). It can be seen that the individual points fall close to the expected location on the psychometric functions obtained from other experiments. The obvious conclusion is that VRA produces reliable and replicable masked thresholds, and that, aside from the effect of false-alarm rate on threshold estimates, there are no substantial differences between 2AFC-L and G/NG-D. Because 2AFC-L (a) yields an unbiased estimate of adult–infant threshold differences, and (b) has been used to study masked and absolute thresholds over a broader age and frequency range than G/NG-D, we can use the data gathered with 2AFC-L to ascertain the potential factors contributing to the observed developmental changes. It is encouraging to find that different methods yield very similar adult–infant differences in masked threshold across diverse laboratories, once G/NG-D threshold estimates are corrected for adult–infant differences in false-alarm rate. In short, VRA is efficient, effective, and reliable.

Otitis Media and Infant Absolute Thresholds

Before proceeding to examine the factors that might contribute to age-related changes in sensitivity, it is necessary to consider a potentially confounding influence on absolute thresholds in infancy—the undetected presence of otitis media. Teele, Klein, and Rosner (1980), in a prospective study of 2,500 children in the Boston area, found that 25% of the sample had experienced at least one acute episode of otitis media by 6 months of age. Although great care was taken in the threshold studies reported here to exclude children with middle-ear problems at the time of test, such screening procedures did not include an otoscopic exami-

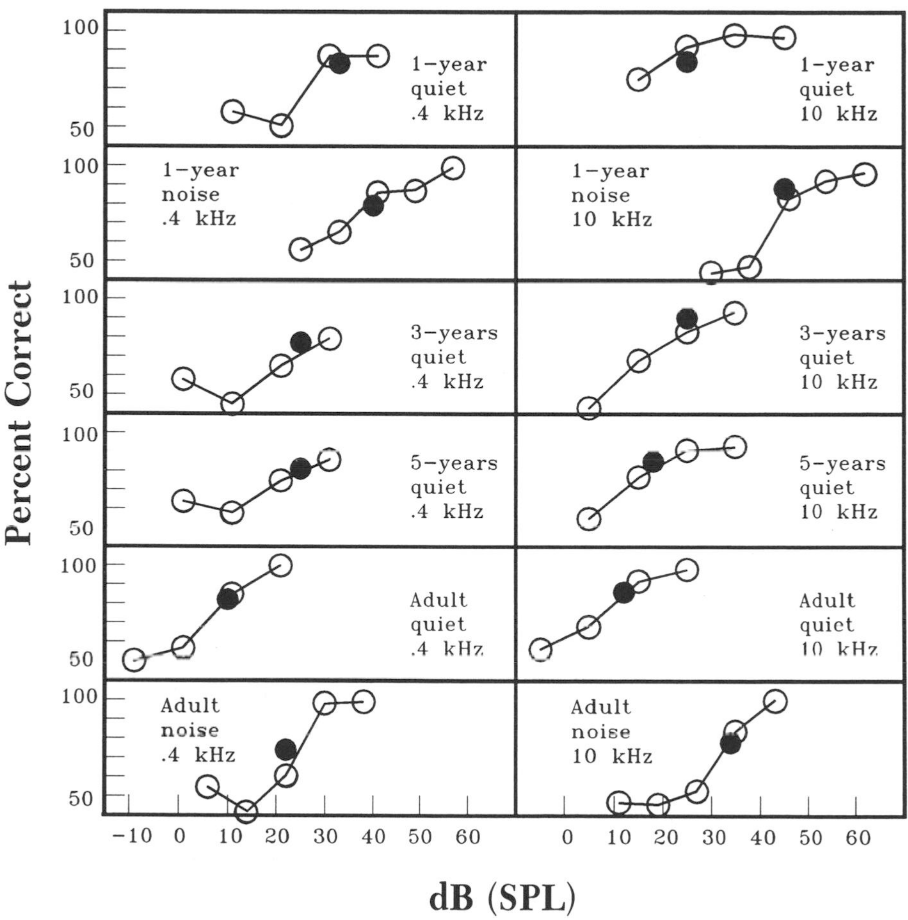

FIGURE 10 Percentage of correct head turns in 2AFC-L as a function of sound pressure level (SPL) for infants, children, and adults in quiet and in noise. Open circles are data from Schneider, Trehub, Morrongiello, and Thorpe (1986, 1989), copyright 1986 and 1989, respectively, by the Acoustical Society of America; and Trehub, Schneider, and Endman (1980), copyright 1980 by Academic Press. Filled circles are for single-stimulus presentations from Schneider, Trehub, and Thorpe (1991). Copyright 1991 by the Psychonomic Society. All material reprinted by permission.

nation or ear-impedance measurements. Unfortunately, asymptomatic otitis media can occur in infants and children (e.g., Marchant et al., 1984) so that some of the infants included in the absolute threshold studies may have had a conductive hearing loss at the time of testing. The number of such infants is likely to be small because of the exclusion from the sample of infants who (a) were born prematurely; (b) had recently experienced an earache, cold, or congestion; (c) had any documented hearing loss; (d) had frequent or recurrent ear infections; (e) had been fitted with ventilation tubes; or (f) had a family history of hearing loss. Furthermore, the population from which our sample was drawn consisted largely of middle-class families who were caring for their infants in their own home, a group that is considered at low risk for otitis media (see Klein, 1986). Nevertheless, we have tried to consider the implications of a worst-case scenario on our absolute threshold estimates.

In the worst-case scenario, we assume the incidence of undetected otitis media in our studies to be 15%. Recall that 25% of an unselected sample of infants would have experienced one or more episodes of otitis media between birth and 6 months of age. At any specific time, such as the test day, the incidence would be considerably lower. Because otitis media can lead to a threshold shift of as much as 20 to 30 dB, we can assume, for discussion purposes, a 30-dB shift in the psychometric function for the subset of infants with asymptomatic otitis media. This is likely an overestimate because undetected otitis media is unlikely to be associated with a severe pressure buildup in the middle ear and a substantial conductive loss. Moreover, in the single study with tympanometric screening (Nozza & Wilson, 1984), infants with abnormal tympanograms had absolute thresholds that were only 10 dB higher than infants with normal tympanograms.

In this worst-case scenario, we assumed that the group psychometric function for 85% of our infants was that specified by the functions in Figure 6. We assumed, further, that the psychometric function for the remaining 15% of the infants was shifted 30 dB to the right. We then calculated the average psychometric function after combining the two groups, assuming a 14% inattention rate. Figure 11 plots the psychometric function for this worst-case scenario, along with the psychometric function associated with a 0% incidence of otitis media. The worst-case psychometric function is shifted slightly to the right and has a lower asymptote (87% vs. 93%). In all of our masked and absolute threshold studies, we have defined threshold as the point on the psychometric function corresponding

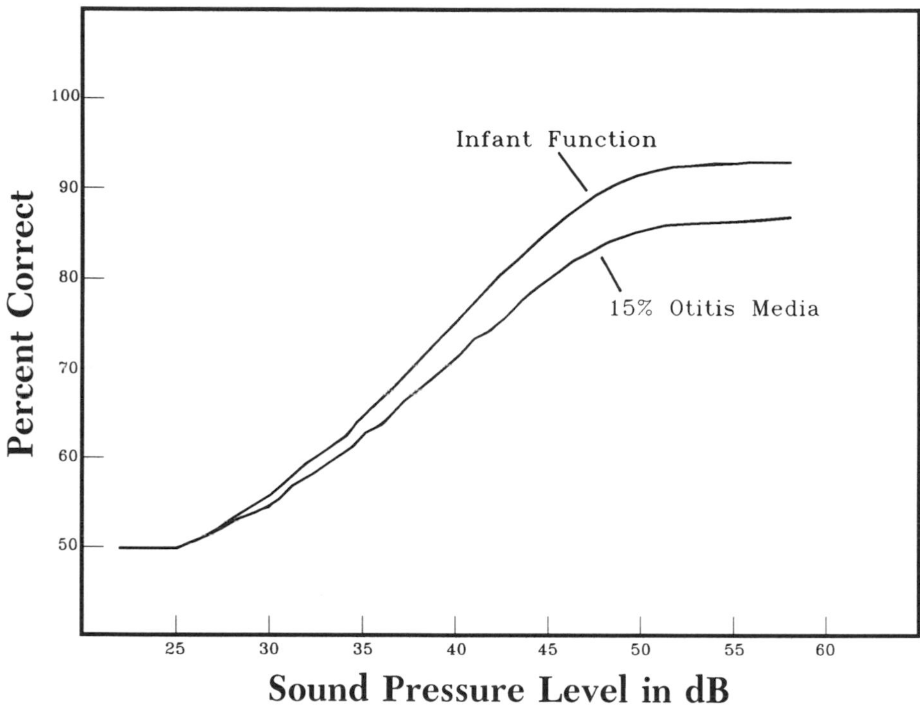

FIGURE 11 Hypothetical psychometric functions for infants in 2AFC-L. Two functions are shown. The one designated "infant function" is the psychometric function fit to the data in Figure 7. The other would be expected if the group psychometric function for 85% of the population was the same as in Figure 7, with the remaining 15% having a 30-dB hearing loss from otitis media. With 15% of the population suffering from asymptomatic otitis media, the worst-case scenario produces only a modest threshold shift (see text).

to 65% correct. The expected threshold shift produced by the assumption that 15% of our sample had acute otitis media is on the order of 1.5 dB. Because this is the worst case that can reasonably be expected, we can assume that undetected, middle-ear fluid in some of our 6-month-old listeners would shift group thresholds by much less than 1.5 dB. For older infants and young children, for whom the incidence of otitis media is declining, and who have steeper psychometric functions and lower rates of inattention, it is extremely unlikely that otitis media would have any effect on group threshold estimates.

Inattention and Infant Thresholds

Another factor that may affect threshold estimates is the rate of inattention. If our infant psychometric functions were corrected for an inattention rate of 14%, the estimate of the average 6-month-old infant's threshold drops by 1.1 dB. Because inattention rate clearly declines with age, it is unlikely that a small number of randomly dispersed trials on which the older infant or child is inattentive will have any measurable effect on threshold. In any case, it is unlikely to exceed 1 or 2 dB at even the youngest ages. Indeed, simulations by Wightman and Allen (chapter 4 in this volume) indicate that inattention has a rather negligible effect on thresholds. We conclude, then, that VRA yields efficient and reliable estimates of masked and absolute thresholds at all ages.

A Model of Developmental Changes in Sensitivity

Having demonstrated that there are substantial differences in absolute and masked sensitivity between infants and adults, we have attempted to specify how absolute and masked thresholds change from 6 months to 20 years of age (Schneider et al., 1986, 1989; Trehub et al., 1980, 1988). The observed developmental changes in sensitivity could be attributed to many different factors. To identify what these factors may be and to isolate the contribution of each factor to the development of auditory sensitivity, we propose a threshold model that reflects the contributions of these factors.

Factors Affecting Auditory Sensitivity

Assume, for the moment, that the signal to be detected is either a pure tone or a narrow-band noise so that its energy is confined to a relatively narrow portion of the spectrum. We know that the detectability of such a signal is affected by the presence of other sound sources. The degree to which other sounds mask the signal depends on the amplitude of the masker and on its spectral composition. If, for example, the signal is a 2-kHz, narrow-band noise, maskers with spectral distributions well above or well below 2 kHz will not affect its detectability. Only maskers that produce energy in the 2-kHz region will be effective in elevating signal threshold. To account for phenomena such as these, psychoacousticians assume that the auditory system can impose a filter on the incoming signal (Green, 1976). In the example given, an auditory filter or critical band centered on 2 kHz would explain why maskers with spectral compositions remote from 2 kHz would be ineffective. On the other hand, when the distribution of energy in the noise overlaps that of the critical band, the masker should affect the detection of the signal. A general finding in adult psychophysics (e.g., Zwislocki, 1978), for signal presentations longer than 0.25 seconds, is that when the ratio of power in the signal to power in the filtered noise reaches a certain criterial value, the signal reaches threshold. This general principle is illustrated in the following equation

$$\frac{\int_0^\infty F_{cf}(f) * S(f)df}{\int_0^\infty F_{cf}(f) * N_e(f)df} = C(cf), \tag{2}$$

where f is frequency; cf is the center frequency of the signal; $F_{cf}(f)$ is the transfer function of the auditory filter at cf; $N_e(f)$ is the spectral power density function of the external noise, $n_e(t)$; $S(f)$ is the spectral power density function of the signal, $s(t)$; and $C(cf)$ is the signal-to-noise ratio required for a threshold response at the center frequency of the signal. Equation 2 indicates that the ratio of the power in the filtered signal to the power in the filtered noise is a constant at threshold. Note that both the transfer function of the auditory filter and the criterion ratio for detection can vary as a function of the center frequency of the signal.

Equation 2 requires that if the spectrum level of the masker is decreased by x dB, the spectrum level of the signal required for threshold also decreases by x dB. Clearly, however, the signal intensity required for threshold cannot continue to decrease indefinitely with decreases in masker intensity, because the masked threshold function is bounded by the absolute threshold function. This lower boundary can be incorporated into Equation 2 by hypothesizing that there is a certain level of internal background noise in the auditory system. This internal noise, which we will represent by $n_i(t)$, has its own spectral density function, $N_i(f)$, and is assumed to be independent of the external noise, $n_e(t)$. Therefore, Equation 2 can be generalized to incorporate absolute thresholds by assuming that threshold is reached when the ratio of signal power to the power of the combined internal and external noises is a constant, that is,

$$\frac{\int_0^\infty F_{cf}(f) * S(f)df}{\int_0^\infty F_{cf}(f) * N_e(f)df + \int_0^\infty F_{cf}(f) * N_i(f)df} = C(cf). \tag{3}$$

Equation 3 is capable of accounting for a number of findings on masked and unmasked monaural sensitivity (see Zwislocki, 1978). This theoretical framework for absolute and masked thresholds in adults can provide a basis for considering how sensitivity changes with age. This can be done by specifying the different factors within the model that might change with age. The bandwidth of the auditory filter is one such factor. The signal-to-noise ratio required for threshold is another. The spectrum level and distribution of internal noise might also change with age. Finally, the mechanical efficiency with which sound energy is delivered to the hair cells might also show age-related changes. That these four factors might affect performance is indicated in Equation 4,

$$\frac{\int_0^\infty F_{cf}(f,a) * M(f,a) * S(f)df}{\int_0^\infty F_{cf}(f,a) * M(f,a) * N_e(f)df + \int_0^\infty F_{cf}(f,a) * N_i(f,a)df} = C(cf,a), \qquad (4)$$

where a is age in years, and $M(f,a)$ is the mechanical advantage at f. Equation 4 illustrates that the task of determining how auditory sensitivity changes with age is not as simple as it seems at first glance. How can we isolate and specify all of these factors?

The first step is to show that Equation 4 does indeed describe the performance of infants. To do this, we first note that when the spectrum level of $n_e(t) \gg n_i(t)$, Equation 4 reduces to

$$\frac{\int_0^\infty F_{cf}(f,a) * S(f)df}{\int_0^\infty F_{cf}(f,a) * N_e(f)df} = C(cf,a). \qquad (5)$$

Therefore, at all ages and frequencies, an x-dB increase in masker level should produce an x-dB increase in threshold, providing that the masker is sufficiently intense. In each of the three studies that varied masker level in infants and children (Bull, Schneider, & Trehub, 1981; Schneider et al., 1989; Trehub, Bull, & Schneider, 1981), threshold signal-to-noise ratio was found to be independent of masker level. We conclude, then, that threshold is reached when the signal-to-noise level reaches a certain criterion value for infants, children, and adults.

The next question to ask is whether the bandwidth of the auditory filter changes with age. Examination of Equation 5 indicates that if age is held constant, and the bandwidth of the external noise is increased (spectrum level held constant), then the amount of power in the filtered noise increases until the bandwidth of the filter is reached. If signal-to-noise ratio is to remain constant, then threshold must increase with bandwidth until the bandwidth of the filter is exceeded. After that point, further increases in the bandwidth of the noise should not produce any further increases in threshold. In a recent study (Schneider, Morrongiello, & Trehub, 1990), we confirmed this prediction for infants, children, and adults using the 2AFC-L technique with one-third-octave-band signals at 0.8 and 4 kHz. Figure 12 shows how threshold changes for a 0.8-kHz, one-third-octave-band signal as masker bandwidth is increased. The listeners were 6 months, 2 years, 5 years, and approximately 20 years old. Note that when bandwidth reaches a certain width, further increases do not produce an increase in threshold. Furthermore, the point at which bandwidth ceases to have an effect on threshold is the same for all ages.[2] Olsho (1985) obtained comparable findings when measuring the tuning curve of the auditory filter for infants and adults. Irwin, Stillman, and Schade (1986) found that the size of the critical band was only marginally larger for 6-year-olds than for adults. More recent work by Allen, Wightman, Kistler, and Dolan (1989), Veloso, Hall, and Grose (1990), and Hall and Grose (1991) suggests that auditory filter width in 6-year-olds is equivalent to that of adults. Although Allen et al. (1990) found that frequency selectivity in preschool children was poorer than that of adults, a recent study by Hall and Grose (1991) showed that the frequency selectivity of preschool children was probably equivalent to that of adults when the children and adults were tested at the same sensation levels. Thus, there is no evidence that the bandwidth of the auditory filter changes with age. To reflect this, we have modified Equation 4 to indicate that the auditory filter is no longer dependent on age. Thus, Equation 4

[2]In Figure 12, the bandwidth at which there are no further increases in threshold is larger than that typically found in a critical band experiment. It is, however, the bandwidth to be expected given a signal bandwidth of one-third octave (see Schneider et al., 1990).

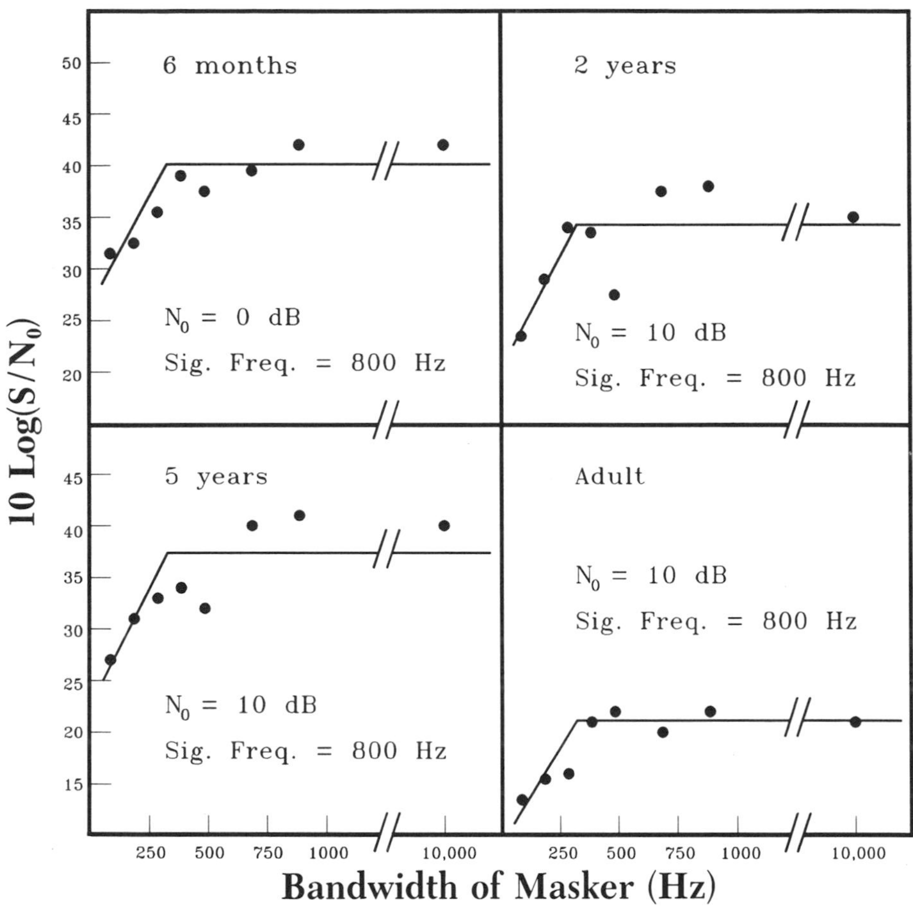

FIGURE 12 Thresholds at four different ages for a 0.8-kHz, one-third-octave signal as a function of the bandwidth of the masker. Thresholds should increase with masker bandwidth until the masker bandwidth equals the critical band (the point of intersection between the rising and horizontal straight lines). Beyond this point, thresholds should be independent of bandwidth. The same value of the critical band was used to fit the two straight lines in each panel, with the value of the critical band representing the upper limit to be expected for a one-third-octave, 0.8-kHz signal. From Schneider, Morrongiello, and Trehub (1990). Copyright 1990 by American Psychological Association. Reprinted by permission.

becomes

$$\frac{\int_0^\infty F_{cf}(f) * M(f,a) * S(f)df}{\int_0^\infty F_{cf}(f) * M(f,a) * N_e(f)df + \int_0^\infty F_{cf}(f) * N_i(f,a)df} = C(cf,a). \quad (6)$$

Equation 6 indicates that the criterion signal-to-noise ratio might vary as a function of age. To assess whether this is true or not, we note that when $n_e(t) \gg n_i(t)$, Equation 6 becomes

$$\frac{\int_0^\infty F_{cf}(f) * S(f)df}{\int_0^\infty F_{cf}(f) * N_e(f)df} = C(cf,a). \quad (7)$$

Equation 7 indicates that if there are no changes in the criterion with age, then masked thresholds should be equivalent at all ages. To evaluate this, we examined masked thresholds at two levels of masking noise for several center frequencies of an octave-band signal (Schneider et al., 1989). The results are shown in Figure 13. Masked thresholds decline exponentially as a function of age at all frequencies. Furthermore, the rate of decline in threshold (the time constant of the exponential decay function) is essentially independent of frequency. Therefore, we can rewrite Equation 7 as

$$\frac{\int_0^\infty F_{cf}(f) * S(f)df}{\int_0^\infty F_{cf}(f) * N_e(f)df} = C(cf) * (1 + 20.7 \exp[-a/3.2]). \quad (8)$$

Equation 8 specifies how the infant's masked threshold changes with age over the entire frequency region from 0.4 to 10 kHz for octave-band noises. Masked thresholds are 12 to 13 dB higher at 6 months of age and decline rapidly so that, by 10 to 12 years of age, they are at or near adult levels. Recall that once Nozza and Wilson's (1984) masked thresholds for pure tones (earphone experiment) were corrected for false-alarm rate, their infant thresholds agreed quite closely with ours. Irwin et al. (1986) also found that masked thresholds for their 6-year-

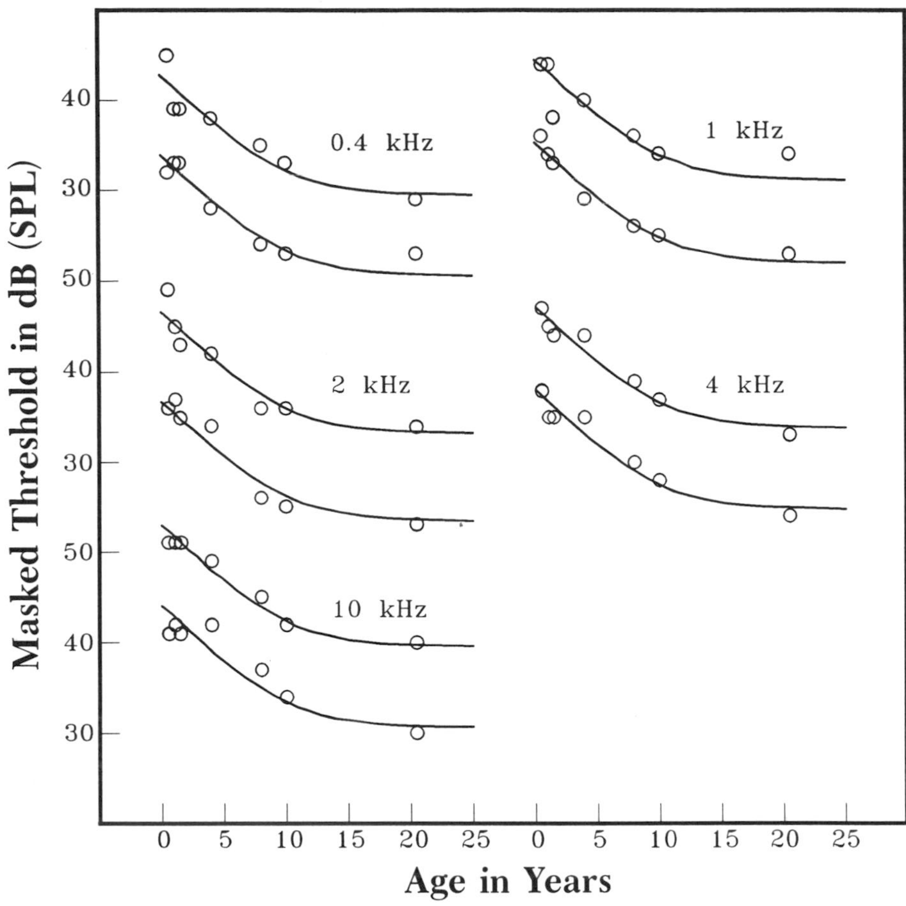

FIGURE 13 Masked thresholds as a function of age for five octave-band noises. Thresholds for two masker levels (0 and 10 dB/cycle) are shown. Exponential decay functions identical in the extent and rate of decline but differing in asymptote are fit to the data. From Schneider, Trehub, Morrongiello, and Thorpe (1989). Copyright 1989 by the Acoustical Society of America. Adapted by permission.

old listeners were elevated above adult thresholds by about 4 to 6 dB, which is very nearly the value found in our experiments. Allen et al. (1989), Hall and Grose (1991) and Veloso et al. (1990) have found elevated masked thresholds in preschool children. However, Hall and Grose (1991) and Veloso et al. (1990) found that the masked thresholds of 6-year-olds were equivalent to those of adults. The discrepancies in estimates of masked thresholds at 6 years of age may reflect the fact that it is difficult to get a good estimate of average performance in young children when the number of subjects tested is small, because of the large intersubject variability that is often observed (see chapter 4 in this volume). The evidence clearly shows that the signal-to-noise ratio required for detection declines with age, with this decline continuing until at least 6 years of age, and possibly longer in some listeners. Later, we will consider possible reasons for this decline.

Now that we know how masked thresholds change with age we can return to the question of absolute thresholds. If we incorporate age-related changes in signal to-noise ratio at threshold into our general equation, we obtain

$$\frac{\int_0^\infty F_{cf}(f) * M(f,a) * S(f)df}{\int_0^\infty F_{cf}(f) * M(f,a) * N_e(f)df + \int_0^\infty F_{cf}(f) * N_i(f,a)df} = C(cf) * (1 + 20.7 \exp[-a/3.2]). \quad (9)$$

Equation 9 identifies the remaining factors that may contribute to changes in sensitivity with age. Aside from changes in the criterion signal-to-noise ratio (which we have already estimated), they include age-related changes in mechanical advantage and in the distribution and amount of internal noise.

Throughout infancy, there will be progressive changes in ear-canal size that will affect the amount of resonance that occurs at particular frequencies. Changes in middle-ear impedance could also affect the amount of energy that is actually delivered to the inner ear. These mechanical factors could affect absolute threshold. It is also possible that the amount and distribution of internal noise changes with age. In the absolute threshold experiment, Equation 9 reduces to

$$\frac{\int_0^\infty F_{cf}(f) * M(f,a) * S(f)df}{\int_0^\infty F_{cf}(f) * N_i(f,a)df} = C(cf) * (1 + 20.7 \exp[-a/3.2]). \quad (10)$$

Equation 10 indicates that developmental changes in absolute threshold will depend on age-related changes in the criterion signal-to-noise ratio (a known factor), mechanical advantage (an unknown factor), and the amount and distribution of internal noise (also an unknown factor). Figure 14 shows how absolute thresholds change as a function of age (after Trehub et al., 1988). In contrast to age-related changes in masked thresholds, the rate and extent of the decline in absolute thresholds is frequency-dependent, with infant and adult thresholds being closer at 10 kHz than at lower frequencies. Indeed, at even higher frequencies (Trehub et al., 1989), infants and adults have comparable thresholds.

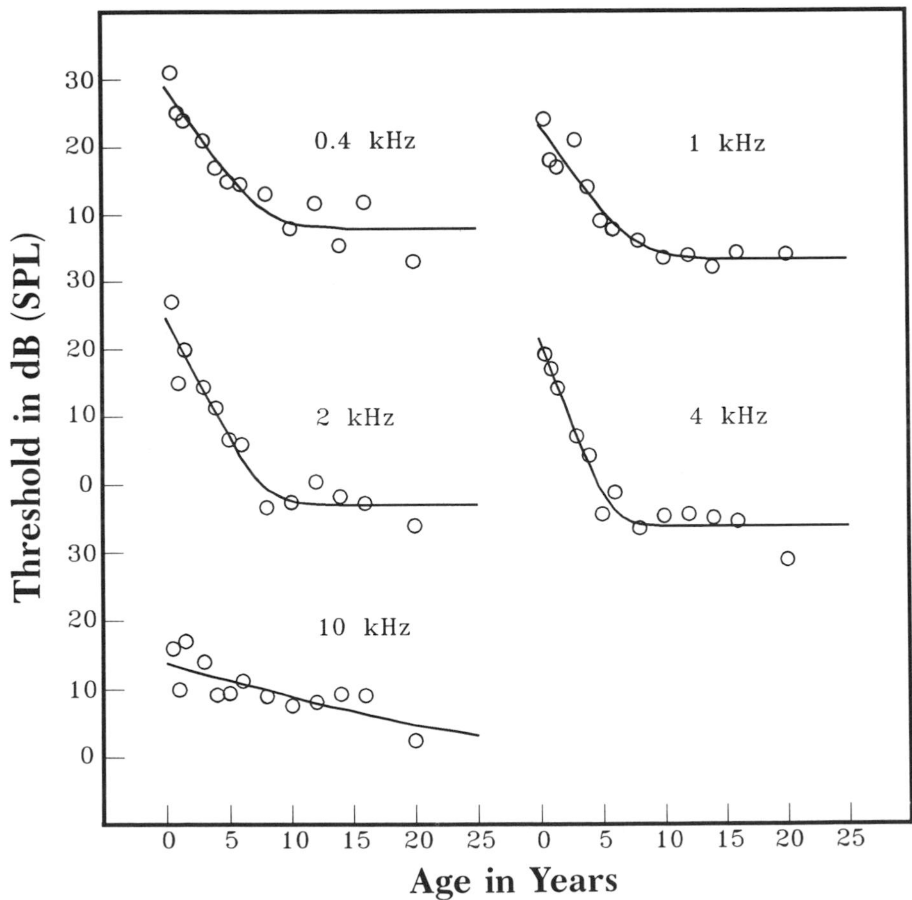

FIGURE 14 Absolute thresholds as a function of age for five octave-band noises. Individual exponential decay functions have been fit to the data at each frequency. From Trehub, Schneider, Morrongiello, and Thorpe (1988). Copyright 1988 by Academic Press. Adapted by permission.

As noted, a part of the observed decline is attributable to changes in the criterion signal-to-noise ratio. Because changes in the signal-to-noise ratio required for threshold are independent of frequency, the frequency-dependent effects in absolute threshold must be due to age-related changes in mechanical efficiency or in internal noise. If the mechanical advantage is approximately constant within a critical band, and if the spectrum level of the internal noise is also approximately constant within a critical band, then the joint effect of these two factors can be expressed as a single ratio of mechanical advantage to amount of internal noise. Under these conditions, Equation 10 becomes

$$\left[\frac{M(cf,a)}{\omega_{cf}N_{i}(cf,a)}\right]\int_{0}^{\infty}F_{cf}(f)*S(f)df = C(cf)*(1 + 20.7\exp[-a/3.2]), \qquad (11)$$

where $M(cf,a)$ is the mechanical efficiency at cf, ω_{cf} is the bandwidth of the filter at cf, and $N_{i}(cf,a)$ is the spectrum level of the internal noise at cf. Clearly, Equation 11 can be solved to determine how the ratio of mechanical advantage to internal noise changes with age. Figure 15 plots these functions for the five frequencies of octave-band noise. It can be seen that this ratio improves dramatically with age over the frequency range from 0.4 to 4 kHz up to about 5 years of age, beyond which there do not seem to be further changes. Note, however, that for the 10-kHz stimulus, there is no significant change in this factor with age. Unless mechanical advantage and internal noise are varying in a reciprocal fashion, Figure 15 indicates that 6-month-old infants already have adult-like sensitivities at the very high frequencies (for a discussion of the development of high-frequency sensitivity, see Trehub et al., 1989).

With respect to the low frequencies, what is unclear is the extent to which changes in threshold are due to mechanical factors or to internal noise. Kruger (1987) has found that the neonate's peak resonant frequency is about 6 to 7 kHz and that infants do not acquire the adult peak of about 2.7 kHz until about 24 months of age. If less resonance is developed in the infant ear than in the adult ear between 2 and 5 kHz, this would contribute substantially to observed adult–infant differences. Because the infant's outer ear canal reaches adult length by about 2 to 3 years of age (Kruger, 1987), the contribution of outer-ear resonance to adult–infant differences could be expected to disappear at about this age. It is

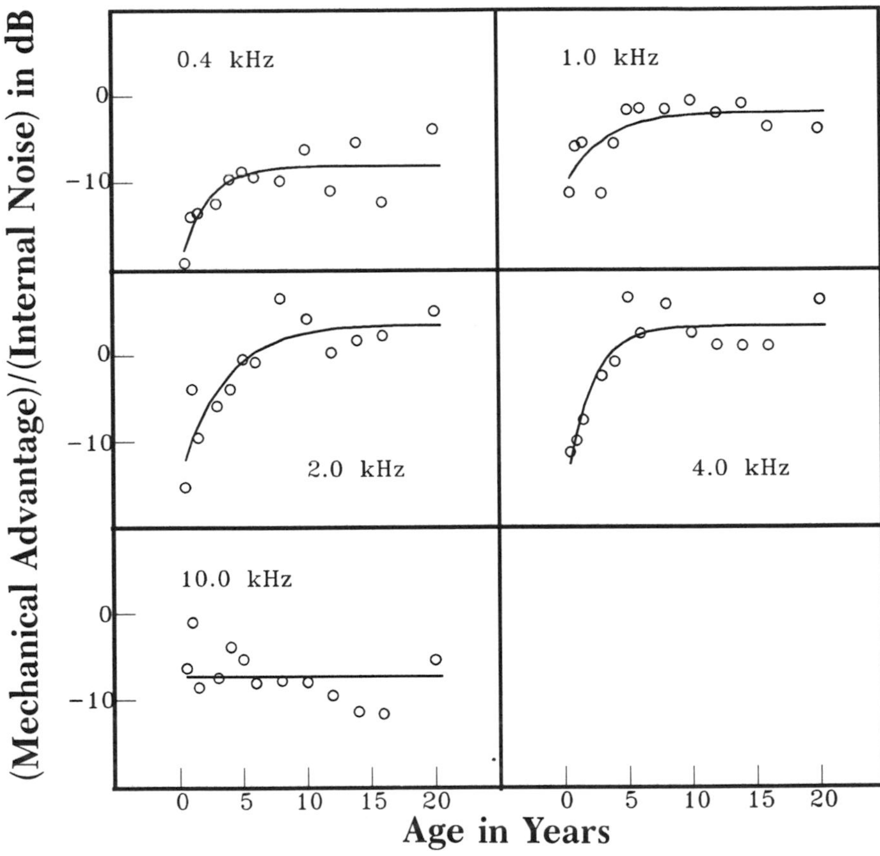

FIGURE 15 The ratio of mechanical advantage to level of internal noise as a function of age for five frequencies of an octave-band noise.

interesting to note that there are substantial changes in the ratio of mechanical advantage to internal noise in the 2-to-4-kHz range over the first 2 to 3 years of life. It is quite likely that much of this change is due to changes in outer-ear resonance. To evaluate how much of the change is attributable to this factor, it is necessary to determine the transfer function relating sound pressure in the sound field (the place occupied by the listener's head) to sound pressure developed at the eardrum over the entire age range. At present, this transfer function is known only for adults (Shaw, 1974). Once comparable information is available for infants, it will be possible to correct adult–infant differences for this factor, leaving us with an estimate of how the amount and distribution of internal noise changes with age.

It is of considerable interest to note that if we include only the data points from children over 3 years of age in Figure 15 (all but the four data points at the farthest left), we would be hard-pressed to argue for further developmental changes in the ratio of mechanical advantage to internal noise, because the remaining variation is within our error of measurement. This implies that beyond 3 years of age, adult–child threshold differences are independent of frequency (for frequencies $\leq$10 kHz) for both absolute and masked thresholds. Within our model, then, all changes beyond 3 years of age are attributable entirely to changes in the signal-to-noise ratio required for detection.

Motivational and Attentional Factors

As noted, changes in mechanical efficiency and in the level of internal noise can potentially affect thresholds in quiet but not in noise. Recall that Schneider et al. (1989) showed that adult–infant differences in masked thresholds were on the order of 12 to 13 dB at all frequencies tested. Within our model, then, these differences were interpreted as differences in the signal-to-noise ratio required for detection. It was assumed that such differences were also present in the absolute threshold data. To indicate how the ratio of mechanical advantage to internal noise varied with age, it was necessary to factor out the effect of changes in the signal-to-noise ratio required for threshold. Thus, in both absolute and masked threshold experiments (for frequencies $\leq$10 kHz), we have found adult–infant threshold differences that cannot be attributed to changes in mechanical efficiency or in the level of internal noise. The extent of these changes is indicated in Figure 16.

What is responsible for this 12-to-13-dB shift in threshold from 6 months of age to adulthood? One explanation that readily comes to mind is motivational and/or attentional. We have shown that one model of inattention can account for about 1 dB of this difference. In this model, it was assumed that the infant was inattentive on about 14% of the trials and that these inattentive trials were scattered randomly throughout the session. Even if we assume that inattention is increased to about 20–25% of the trials, it is easy to show that this has a relatively inconsequential effect on the group psychometric functions derived from a 2AFC-L experiment. Although Wightman and Allen (this volume) and Viemeister and Schlauch (this volume) have shown that inattention may have a somewhat

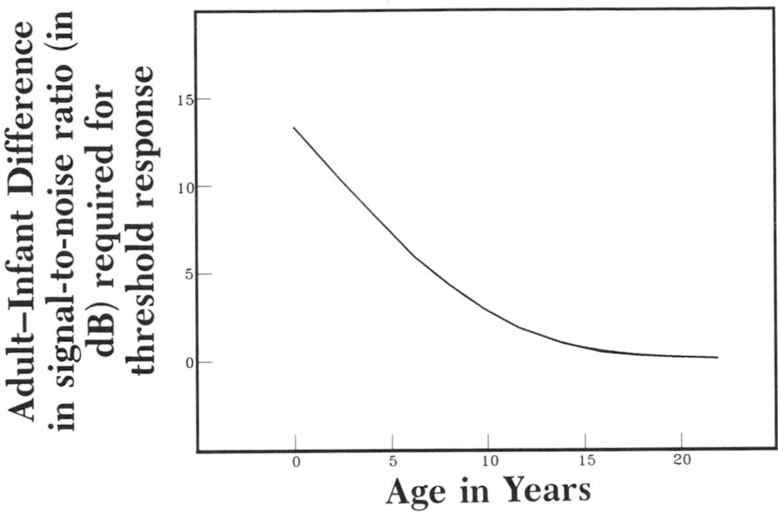

FIGURE 16 Adult–infant difference in signal-to-noise ratio (in dB) required for threshold as a function of age.

greater effect in adaptive G/NG-D tasks, the effect of randomly dispersed inattentive trials is too small to account for the full extent of adult–infant differences. In the 2AFC-L task, moreover, attentional models of this sort produce negligible effects.

There is, however, a model of inattention that could account for adult–infant threshold differences. Suppose that inattentive trials, instead of being randomly dispersed, were level-dependent. This seems unlikely in the 2AFC-L case, where the different intensity levels are randomly distributed throughout the session. It is more likely to be a point of difficulty for adaptive techniques where the intensity level declines over a session. Nevertheless, suppose that adult–infant differences are due to the correlation of attention with stimulus intensity. To implement this model, we constructed a group psychometric function for adults from the Schneider et al. (1989) masking study just as we had done for infants. If attention is all that distinguishes infant from adult listeners, we can determine how infant attention would have to vary as a function of signal-to-noise ratio in order to transform the adult psychometric function into the observed infant psychometric function. Figure 17 indicates that attention must quickly drop to zero as signal-to-noise ratio decreases in order to completely account for the adult–infant differences. Indeed, if adult–infant differences are to be based solely on

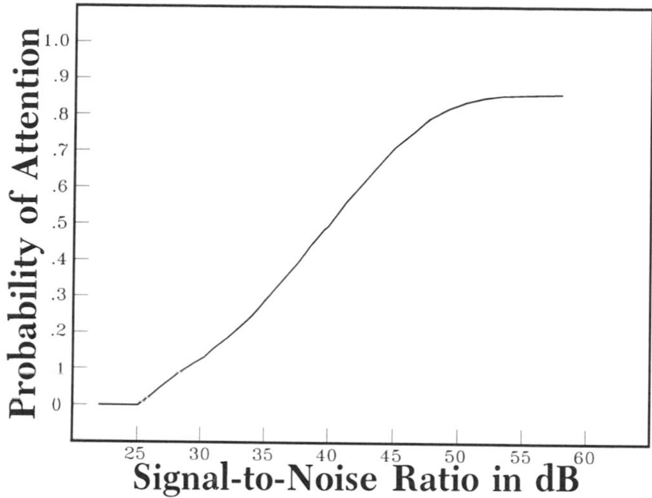

FIGURE 17 Hypothetical psychometric function for "attention" in the 6-month-old. This function specifies how the probability of attention would have to change with signal-to-noise ratio to convert the psychometric function of an adult into that of a 6-month-old infant (see text).

attentional factors, Figure 17 represents the "psychometric function for attention," specifying how the probability of attention varies as a function of stimulus intensity.

Is this a reasonable way of accounting for adult–infant differences? According to this model, stimulus intensity must be well above the "perceptual" threshold before the infant "attends" to it. If the adult psychometric function specifies how detection improves with signal-to-noise ratio in infants (i.e., no adult–infant differences in perceptual or sensory thresholds), then for infants to perform as poorly as they did, a stimulus that is theoretically detectable 99% of the time must be attended to only 15% of the time. Indeed, if infants and adults have the same sensory thresholds, then the psychometric functions shown in Figure 6 reflect "attention thresholds" rather than sensory thresholds. Such an attentional threshold model is unlikely to characterize infant performance for the reasons that follow.

One assumption of attentional models is that, if the experimenter were able to instruct and motivate the listener sufficiently, the "attentional" threshold would soon converge on the "sensory" threshold. We have argued elsewhere

(Schneider et al., 1991) that the 2AFC-L task places minimal cognitive demands on the infant insofar as it capitalizes on a natural component of the orienting response to sound. According to principles of learning, reinforcing a "natural" response to a stimulus should produce the quickest learning and the strongest conditioning. In this sense, the task is about as well-structured for the infant as possible, producing the lowest behavioral thresholds of any procedure. Moreover, we have ensured that all infants used for threshold determination are properly "instructed" by passing a training criterion before proceeding to the test phase. Beyond this, we have arranged for reinforcement conditions to be as rewarding and motivating as is ethically possible. In other words, we have maximized the likelihood of obtaining a sensory or perceptual threshold rather than an attentional threshold.

It is always possible, of course, that increased motivation on the part of infant listeners would lead to dramatic improvements in threshold. We believe this to be unlikely for several reasons. First, there is no evidence once subjects are appropriately instructed and familiarized with the situation that further manipulation of motivational variables has any appreciable effect on psychophysical thresholds. In the case of adults, masked thresholds are relatively stable across individuals (Green, 1976), showing negligible practice effects so long as listeners have some pre-exposure to the stimulus (Gundy, 1961; Swets & Sewall, 1963). Moreover, such thresholds cannot be shifted by more than 1 or 2 dB by substantial changes in reward structure (Green & Swets, 1966; Lukaszewski & Elliot, 1962). Because the infants in our test situation seem to be under good stimulus control, and because our reinforcement conditions are highly motivating, it seems unlikely that our thresholds could be moved appreciably by increasing infants' motivation to listen (assuming that it were possible to do so).

Although it is not clear how to increase motivation in 2AFC-L, it is certainly possible to decrease it. Trehub, Schneider, and Bull (1981) compared performance on 2AFC-L with and without reinforcement. The 2AFC-L procedure used in that experiment differed slightly from our usual procedure in that trial duration was limited to 5 seconds. Thus, if a head turn did not occur within 5 seconds of stimulus onset, the stimulus was terminated and no response was scored. Omitting reinforcement substantially reduced the number of head turns scored, indicating that reinforcement was having a clear motivational effect. For example, infants turned on 91% of the trials for a 4-kHz stimulus when reinforcement was present, but only on 69% of the trials when reinforcement was absent. However, when percentage correct was computed for only those trials on which a head turn occurred, there was very little difference between the psychometric functions for reinforced versus nonreinforced sessions. Clearly, reinforcing the response boosted attentive behavior, increasing the percentage of head turns by one third. However, increases in attention and/or motivation did not result in a lower threshold once the psychometric functions were corrected for attention. Thus, what little data we have for infant listeners suggests that, like adults, increases in motivation *do not* result in a substantial improvement in sensitivity. We conclude, therefore, that motivational factors do not play a significant role in the observed developmental changes in the criterion signal-to-noise ratio shown in Figure 16.

With respect to the relevance of these issues to young children, our experience has been that children 4 to 6 years of age are highly motivated and attentive. In fact, they sometimes become upset about their incorrect responses despite warnings that some signals would be too soft to hear. Nevertheless, thresholds in this age range are higher than those of adults independent of the psychophysical technique used to measure them (see also chapter 4 in this volume). These results also imply that observed changes in sensitivity cannot be attributed solely to age related motivational or attentional changes.

Peripheral and Central Processing Factors

If attentional or motivational factors cannot account for developmental changes in the signal-to-noise ratio required for detection, what is responsible for these changes? Whereas it may be difficult to identify the factors that are actually responsible for these developmental changes, it is possible to eliminate some potential candidates and identify some possibilities. If we examine the auditory information flow, we note that there are several stages at which information is converted from one medium to another, and several points at which noise or error can enter. Initially, the information is conveyed by sound waves. The eardrum translates the sound wave into mechanical motion, which in turn through the action of the ossicles produces a traveling wave on the basilar membrane. Because the mechanics of the outer and middle ear are thought to be essentially linear over a wide intensity range throughout life, age-related changes in the sensitivity of such a linear system could not produce changes in signal-to-noise ratio. As we have seen earlier, an increase in sensitivity increases signal and noise, leaving the ratio unchanged. Similarly, if the mechanics of the inner ear remain linear throughout life, simple changes in sensitivity will also leave the signal-to-noise ratio unaffected. Therefore, it is unlikely that developmental changes in the signal-to-noise ratio required for detection result from changes in mechanical efficiency.

The vibration of the basilar membrane, through the action of the hair cells, activates the neurons of the spiral ganglion. Starting with the point at which mechanical activity is transduced into neural activity, it is reasonable to assume that the system becomes nonlinear. It is possible that developmental changes in the nonlinear portion of the auditory system could affect the magnitude of the internal representation of signal and noise (see Schneider et al., 1989), effectively changing the discriminability of a signal in noise. To illustrate this point, consider the electrical circuit in Figure 18. In this circuit, the waveform, $g(t)$, after passing through an amplifier, is fed to a power meter, which computes the power in the amplified signal in successive x-ms periods. The power meter produces a DC voltage, V, that is directly proportional to power (suppose $V = W$, where W is power in watts), with a feedback loop from the output of the power meter to the amplifier. Assume that the amplification factor, k, the amount by which the signal is amplified, is a nonlinear function of the control voltage V. In particular, let us assume that $k = V^{-p}$, for $p < .5$. It is easy to show that the steady-state voltage output from the meter is $V = [W(g(t))]^{1/(1+2p)}$, and that

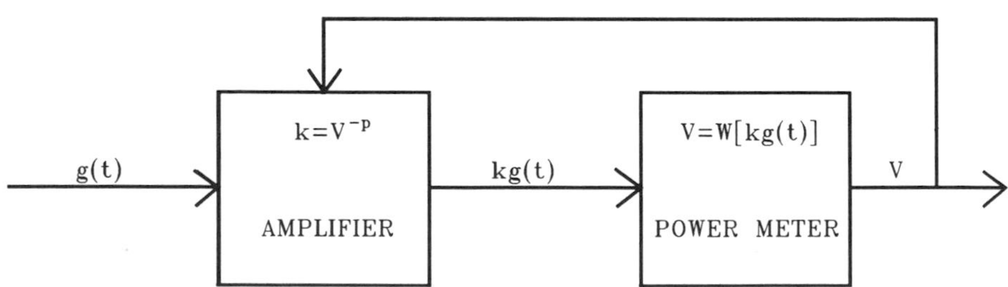

FIGURE 18 Circuit diagram for a hypothetical nonlinear auditory transducer. In this circuit, the power output of the amplifier is used to control the degree of amplification. Changes in the parameter p will produce changes in the function relating d' to signal-to-noise ratio (see text). V = voltage; W = power in watts; $g(t)$ = waveform as a function of time; k = amplification factor.

$k = [W(g(t))]^{-p/(1+2p)}$. Therefore, the voltage output from the meter after the initial period of oscillation will be a power function of signal intensity. Suppose $p = .25$ for infants and $p = 0$ for adults. Consider what happens when noise alone is presented to the circuit. If the power in the noise is 0.4 W, the steady-state power output from the circuit for the adult will be 0.4 W. According to signal-detection theory, the listener takes a sample of the noise. Values of the noise sample will vary from trial to trial, giving rise to a distribution of noise values with a mean of 0.4 and standard deviation σ, where σ depends on the bandwidth of the noise and the integration time of the power meter. If a pure tone of intensity 0.4 W is added to the background noise, the average power of the signal-plus-noise is 0.8 watts and the noise distribution is shifted 0.4 units along the abscissa (with a negligible change in variance) to become the signal-plus-noise distribution. Therefore d' for the adult is $0.4/\sigma$. For the infant, the mean value of the same noise is $0.4^{(2/3)} = 0.543$ W, and the average amplification factor, k, is $0.4^{(-1/6)} = 1.165$. Because the standard deviation of the noise distribution equals $k^2\sigma$, the standard deviation of the infant's noise distribution is therefore 1.357σ. If the signal is 0.4 W, the power going into the circuit is 0.8 W and the steady-state power for the signal-plus-noise at the output of the circuit is $0.8^{(3/3)} = 0.862$, and the amplification factor, k, is $0.8^{(-1/6)} = 1.038$. Therefore, the SN distribution for the infant will have a mean of 0.862 and a standard deviation of approximately 1.077σ, so that d' for the infant will be smaller than that of the adult. Note that, according to this model, the same signal-to-noise ratio produces a different d' value for infants and adults because of nonlinear changes in the transfer function mapping sound pressure onto neural activity. It should be apparent, then, that infants would require a greater external signal-to-noise ratio to produce a d' equivalent to that of the adults.

This example shows how a change in the nonlinear portion of the auditory pathway can affect the signal-to-noise ratio required for detection. A second possible source of adult–infant differences is that internal or neural noise can be added at any point in the nervous system. Indeed, some form of internal noise is needed to explain why human performance differs from that of the ideal observer. If the amount of neural noise added at various stages decreases with age, then the signal-to-noise ratio required for threshold would decrease with age.

A third possible reason relates to sampling strategy. If the human observer is an energy detector, then the variance of both the N and SN distributions will depend on the integration time of the detector, with longer integration times producing smaller variances in the N and SN distributions. Why is this the case? Assume, for example, that we are computing the power in a continuous noise. Measures based on independent and random 10-ms samples of noise will be more variable than those based on independent and random 20-ms samples of the same noise, that is, the shorter the time period, the more variable the measurements. If adult listeners used a longer sampling time, or if their observations were based on averages of many samples, then their N and SN distributions would have lower variances and, consequently, they would have lower thresholds than infants.

Obviously the available data do not permit the definitive selection of any of these alternative explanations. They are offered, rather, as heuristics for future investigations. If, as seems to be the case, motivational and attentional factors cannot account for developmental changes in auditory sensitivity, then other stages in auditory processing must be searched for the factors responsible for these changes. As noted, it is unlikely that the mechanics of the peripheral system will provide a full explanation. Once basilar membrane motion is converted to neural impulses, and nonlinearities enter into the processing stream, there are many possible levels of processing that may differ for infant, child, and adult listeners. We know, for example, that developmental changes in auditory neural pathways continue after birth (see Eggermont, 1985). Indeed, at least one such change has a time course equivalent to that shown in Figure 16. Fabiani, Sohmer, Tait, Gafni, and Kinarti (1979) measured differences in latency between wave I and the vertex-negative wave following wave V from 1 to 12 years of age. Eggermont (1985) fitted an exponential decay function to their data and arrived at a time constant of 3.15 years, which is close to that reported by Schneider et al. (1989). The relations between such electrophysiological changes and behavioral thresholds are difficult to establish, but changes of this nature nevertheless indicate that adultlike states of neural processing may not develop until late childhood. If this is the case, then developmental changes in absolute and masked thresholds, which also continue until late childhood, may arise from maturational changes in the auditory pathways.

Conclusions

Over the past 15 years, two different varieties of visual reinforcement audiometry (go/no-go detection, and two-alternative, forced-choice localization) have been used to measure auditory sensitivity in infants. A consideration of these two techniques from a signal-detection viewpoint indicates that both methods yield equivalent estimates of adult–infant threshold differences when the G/NG-D threshold estimates are corrected for adult–infant differences in false-alarm rate. Further analyses show (a) that inattention does not substantially affect the size of these adult–infant threshold differences, and (b) that the presence of undetected otitis media would have a negligible effect on the extent of such differences.

Masked threshold studies in infants, children, and adults indicate that (a) at all ages, detection occurs when the signal-to-noise ratio reaches a criterion value; (b) the size of the ratio required for detection declines with age; and (c) the size of the critical band or auditory filter does not change from infancy to adulthood. A comparison of absolute and masked thresholds from infancy to adulthood shows that, in the high-frequency region (≥10 kHz), there are no changes in either mechanical efficiency or in the amount of internal physiological noise. At lower frequencies, however, changes in mechanical efficiency (e.g., outer-ear resonance), and/or internal noise continue to occur until about 3 years of age. It is only after 3 years of age that all changes in sensitivity are considered due to changes in the signal-to-noise ratio required for detection.

A review of several studies indicates that motivational and/or attentional factors are unlikely to account for more than a small portion of the observed adult–infant difference in sensitivity that remains after thresholds are corrected for differences in either mechanical efficiency or internal noise. Because changes in the linear portion of the auditory pathway cannot affect signal-to-noise ratio, we are left with the conclusion that age-related changes in the nonlinear portions of the auditory pathways are responsible for the observed changes in auditory sensitivity. Possible ways in which this could occur include (a) age-related, nonlinear changes in the encoding of stimulus intensity; (b) age-related changes in the amount of internal noise in the nonlinear pathways, or (c) age-related changes in sampling strategy.

References

Allen, P., Wightman, F., Kistler, D., & Dolan, T. (1989). Frequency resolution in children. *Journal of Speech and Hearing Research*, *32*, 317–322.

Banks, M. S., & Bennett, P. J. (1988). Optical and photoreceptor immaturities limit the spatial and chromatic vision of human neonates. *Journal of the Optical Society of America*, *5*, 2059–2079.

Berg, K. M., & Smith, M. (1983). Behavioral thresholds for tones during infancy. *Journal of Experimental Child Psychology, 35*, 409–425.

Bull, D., Schneider, B. A., & Trehub, S. E. (1981). The masking of octave-band noise by broad-spectrum noise: A comparison of infant and adult thresholds. *Perception & Psychophysics, 30*, 101–106.

Chun, R. W. M., Pawsat, R., & Forster, F. M. (1960). Sound localization in infancy. *Journal of Nervous & Mental Disease, 130*, 472–476.

Egan, J. P., & Benson, W. (1966). Lateralization of a weak signal presented with correlated and with uncorrelated noise. *Journal of the Acoustical Society of America, 40*, 20–26.

Eggermont, J. J. (1985). Physiology of the developing auditory system. In S. E. Trehub & B. A. Schneider (Eds.), *Auditory development in infancy* (pp. 21–46). New York: Plenum.

Fabiani, M., Sohmer, H., Tait, C., Gafni, M., & Kinarti, R. (1979). A functional measure of brain activity: Brain stem transmission time. *Electroencephalography and Clinical Neurophysiology, 47*, 483–491.

Green, D. M. (1976). *An introduction to hearing*. Hillsdale, NJ: Erlbaum.

Green, D. M., & Swets, J. A. (1966). *Signal detection theory and psychophysics*. New York: Wiley.

Gundy, K. F. (1961). Auditory detection of an unspecified signal. *Journal of the Acoustical Society of America, 33*, 1008–1012.

Hall, J. W., III, & Grose, J. H. (1991). Notched-noise measures of frequency selectivity in adults and children using fixed-masker-level and fixed-signal-level presentation. *Journal of Speech and Hearing Research, 34*, 651–660.

Irwin, R. J., Stillman, J. A., & Schade, A. (1986). The width of the auditory filter in children. *Journal of Experimental Child Psychology, 41*, 429–442.

Jeffress, L. A. (1967). Stimulus-oriented approach to detection re-examined. *Journal of the Acoustical Society of America, 41*, 480–488.

Klein, J. O. (1986). Risk factors for otitis media in children. In J. F. Kavanaugh (Ed.), *Otitis media and child development*. Parkton, MD: York Press.

Kruger, B. (1987). Hearing aids and aural rehabilitation: An update on the external ear resonance in infants and young children. *Ear and Hearing, 8*, 333–336.

Lukaszewski, J. S., & Elliot, D. N. (1962). Auditory threshold as a function of forced choice techniques, feedback, and motivation. *Journal of the Acoustical Society of America, 34*, 223–228.

Marchant, C. D., Shurin, P. A., Turczyk, V. A., Wasikowski, D. E., Tutihasi, M. A., & Kinney, S. E. (1984). Course and outcome of otitis media in early infancy: A prospective study. *Journal of Pediatrics, 104*, 826–831.

Moore, J. M., Thompson, G., & Thompson, M. (1975). Auditory localization of infants as a function of reinforcement conditions. *Journal of Speech and Hearing Disorders, 40*, 29–34.

Nozza, R. J., & Wilson, W. R. (1984). Masked and unmasked pure-tone thresholds of infants and adults: Development of auditory frequency selectivity and sensitivity. *Journal of Speech and Hearing Research, 27*, 613–622.

Olsho, L. W. (1985). Infant auditory perception: Tonal masking. *Infant Behavior and Development, 8*, 371–384.

Olsho, L. W., Koch, E. G., Carter, E. A., Halpin, C. F., & Spetner, N. B. (1988). Pure-tone sensitivity of human infants. *Journal of the Acoustical Society of America*, *84*, 1316–1324.

Schneider, B. A., Morrongiello, B. A., & Trehub, S. E. (1990). The size of the critical band in infants, children, and adults. *Journal of Experimental Psychology: Human Perception and Performance*, *16*, 642–652.

Schneider, B. A., & Trehub, S. E. (1985). Infant auditory psychophysics: An overview. In G. Gottlieb & N. A. Krasnegor (Eds.), *Measurement of audition and vision during the first year of life: A methodological overview* (pp. 113–126). Norwood, NJ: Ablex.

Schneider, B. A., Trehub, S. E., & Bull, D. (1979). The development of basic auditory processes in infants. *Canadian Journal of Psychology*, *33*, 306–319.

Schneider, B. A., Trehub, S. E., & Bull, D. (1980). High-frequency sensitivity in infants. *Science*, *207*, 1003–1004.

Schneider, B. A., Trehub, S. E., Morrongiello, B. A., & Thorpe, L. A. (1986). Auditory sensitivity in preschool children. *Journal of the Acoustical Society of America*, *79*, 447–452.

Schneider, B. A., Trehub, S. E., Morrongiello, B. A., & Thorpe, L. A. (1989). Developmental changes in masked thresholds. *Journal of the Acoustical Society of America*, *86*, 1733–1742.

Schneider, B. A., Trehub, S. E., & Thorpe, L. A. (1991). Developmental perspectives on the localization and detection of auditory signals. *Perception & Psychophysics*, *49*, 10–20.

Shaw, E. A. G. (1974). Transformation of sound pressure level from the free field to the eardrum in the horizontal plane. *Journal of the Acoustical Society of America*, *56*, 1848–1861.

Sinnott, J. M., Pisoni, D., & Aslin, R. (1983). A comparison of pure tone auditory thresholds in human infants and adults. *Infant Behavior and Development*, *6*, 3–18.

Sokolov, E. N. (1963). *Perception and the conditioned reflex*. New York: Macmillan.

Suzuki, T., & Ogiba, Y. (1961). Conditioned orientation reflex audiometry. *Archives of Otolaryngology*, *74*, 192–198.

Swets, J. A., & Sewall, S. T. (1963). Invariance of signal detectability over stages of practice and levels of motivation. *Journal of Experimental Psychology*, *66*, 120–126.

Teele, D. W., Klein, J. O., & Rosner, B. A. (1980). Epidemiology of otitis media in children. *Annals of Otology, Rhinology, and Laryngology*, *89*, 5–6.

Trehub, S. E., Bull, D., & Schneider, B. A. (1981). Infants' detection of speech in noise. *Journal of Speech and Hearing Research*, *24*, 202–206.

Trehub, S. E., Schneider, B. A., & Bull, D. (1981). Effect of reinforcement on infants' performance in an auditory detection task. *Developmental Psychology*, *17*, 872–877.

Trehub, S. E., Schneider, B. A., & Endman, M. (1980). Developmental changes in infants' sensitivity to octave-band noises. *Journal of Experimental Child Psychology*, *29*, 282–293.

Trehub, S. E., Schneider, B. A., Morrongiello, B. A., & Thorpe, L. A. (1988). Auditory sensitivity in school-age children. *Journal of Experimental Child Psychology*, *46*, 273–285.

Trehub, S. E., Schneider, B. A., Morrongiello, B. A., & Thorpe, L. A. (1989). Developmental changes in high-frequency sensitivity. *Audiology*, *28*, 241–249.

Trehub, S. E., Schneider, B. A., Thorpe, L. A., & Judge, P. (1991). Observational measures of auditory sensitivity in early infancy. *Developmental Psychology*, *27*, 40–49.

Veloso, K., Hall, J. W., III, & Grose, J. H. (1990). Frequency selectivity and comodulation masking release in adults and in 6-year-old children. *Journal of Speech and Hearing Research*, *33*, 96–102.

Zwislocki, J. J. (1978). Masking: Experimental and theoretical aspects of forward, backward, and central masking. In E. C. Carterette & M. P. Friedman (Eds.), *Handbook of perception: Vol. IV. Hearing* (pp. 283–336). New York: Academic Press.

CHAPTER 2

Interpreting Developmental Psychoacoustics

Lynne A. Werner

Psychophysics is one of the few techniques that can be applied to both human and nonhuman organisms and can thus bridge the gap between the fields of sensory anatomy and physiology and human sensory behavior. Most of what researchers know of the functional characteristics of human sensory systems is in the form of psychophysical data. Psychophysical data represent what sénsory anatomists and physiologists must explain: How is the nervous system organized in such a way as to accomplish the performance measured psychophysically? What aspect of the visual system accounts for differential sensitivity to different wavelengths of light? How does the auditory nervous system allow a listener to make fine discriminations between different frequencies of sound?

If one were interested in the development of a sensory system, it would seem reasonable to use the psychophysical approach. With few exceptions (e.g.,

The preparation of this chapter was supported by National Institutes of Health Grants DC00396 and DC00520.

I thank Lincoln Gray, Jill Bargones, and Cam Marean for insightful reviews of the chapter, and Jo Ann Chavira-Bash and Janelle Constantino for assistance in the preparation of the manuscript.

Hoversten & Moncur, 1969), however, psychophysical techniques have only recently been used to study sensory development during infancy. The pioneering work of Davida Teller and her colleagues (e.g., Teller, 1979; Teller, Morse, Borton, & Regal, 1974; Teller, Peeples, & Sekel, 1978) in visual development and, subsequently, the work of Sandra Trehub, Bruce Schneider, and their co-workers (e.g., Schneider, Trehub, & Bull, 1979; Schneider, Trehub, & Bull, 1980; Trehub, Schneider, & Endman, 1980) on auditory sensitivity established that the psychophysical approach could be applied to the study of sensory function in human infants. These investigators were able to demonstrate that infant performance varies in a predictable fashion with stimulus parameters and that thresholds, the traditional measure of psychophysics, could be reliably estimated in infants.

Despite the apparent success with which psychophysical methods have been applied to the study of development, there is no consensus on what the resulting data mean. A small, but vocal, minority of psychophysicists holds that psychophysical data from infant subjects are essentially uninterpretable. At the other extreme are those who argue that developmental data should be interpreted in the same way as any other psychophysical data. Most investigators appear to believe that developmental psychophysical data require special interpretive strategies. Consideration of the goals and approaches of the two parent disciplines, developmental psychology and psychophysics, may clarify the source of this controversy.

The developmentalist is faced with explaining age-related behavioral change: Given the multitude of processes that mature, which actually contribute to the behavioral change in question? In the context of psychophysical development, one is generally interested in age-related change in the sensory system. There are, however, age-related changes that occur concurrently in nonsensory processes, such as the motor system and cognition. Is it development of the sensory system or development of some nonsensory system that is responsible for changes in psychophysical performance with age? The developmentalist comes armed with an array of research strategies to address such questions. Chief among these strategies are designing experiments that lead to interactions between experimental condition and age and using correlational techniques that take advantage of the variability among individuals that characterizes development (e.g., Gottlieb, 1983). To a developmental psychologist, psychophysical data are just one more type of developmental data that can be addressed with such strategies.

From the earliest days of psychophysics it has been recognized that processes other than sensory function influence an observer's performance in a psychophysical experiment (Fechner, 1860); however, the psychophysicist controls such factors by reducing or eliminating the contributions of nonsensory factors to performance. Unfortunately, the tools that psychophysicists use to control these nonsensory factors—including extensive practice and statistically well-characterized, efficient psychophysical methods—are typically not applicable to the study of infants. Even if one were able to use these techniques with infants, it is likely that immature nonsensory processes would limit performance in ways that mature processes would not. Finally, because individuals develop at different rates, there would be variability in performance at any given age that is not due to "error" in the usual sense but rather to an inherent property of developing organisms. No amount of rigor in measurement can eliminate that variability. To a psychophysicist used to dealing with mature human observers, then, the facts that developmental psychophysical methods do not include many of the controls applied to adults and that the performance of infants is relatively poor and variable cast doubt on whether psychophysical data can reveal anything about sensory development.

Developmental psychophysics is, then, faced with a dilemma: How does the field take advantage of the methods and substance of psychophysics given, first, that developmental psychophysics must adapt conventional methods and, second, that infant performance will rarely be as stable or as good as that of adults? The purpose of this chapter is to address both aspects of that dilemma. The first part of the chapter examines the effects of procedural variations on infant performance in psychophysical tasks. If deviations from conventional psychophysical methods are important, then one would predict that measures of infant sensitivity would be strongly dependent on procedural variables. Substantial variability in outcome that can be accounted for by procedural factors would support the position that it is difficult to interpret developmental psychophysical data in a meaningful way. The second part of the chapter addresses the problem of interpreting differences in psychophysical performance between infants and adults. Examples from two areas of research, detection in noise and frequency discrimination, are used to illustrate possible developmental research strategies. The chapter focuses on studies of developmental psychoacoustics in infant listeners, but the same general issues and approaches are important to any subfield of developmental psychophysics.

Effects of Procedural Variations on the Outcome of Developmental Psychoacoustics Experiments

Only a few researchers have directly assessed the effects of procedural variables on infant psychophysical performance. However, because different investigators tend to use different procedures to assess infant hearing, between-study comparisons can provide some idea of what these effects might be. Olsho, Koch, Carter, Halpin, and Spetner (1988) made such comparisons in examining infants' detection of sounds in quiet, the most studied infant auditory capacity. Their summary provides the basis of the discussion that follows.

Olsho, Koch, Carter, Halpin, and Spetner (1988) identified seven studies of detection by 6-to-8-month-olds in which investigators tested both infants and adults. They calculated the difference between the infant thresholds and the adult thresholds reported in each study; this difference will be referred to as the *infant relative threshold*. The range of infant relative thresholds, plotted in Figure 1, was rather large.

The studies varied in the stimulus used, the mode of stimulus presentation, the response measured, whether the infant's response was reinforced, the number of response alternatives, the psychophysical method, and whether individual thresholds were estimated. The degree to which each of these variables could have contributed to the differences between the studies is addressed in the remainder of this section. Any available data that directly assess the effects of a variable will also be considered. Surprisingly, this review leads to the conclusion that many procedural variations, in fact, have little impact on infant performance.

Stimulus

Absolute sensitivity is typically assessed in both clinic and laboratory using pure tones of different frequencies. Some studies of infants have used noise bands as stimuli (Trehub et al., 1980) or warbled (FM) tones (Moore & Wilson, 1978). Adults' detection thresholds, of course, vary with the frequency and bandwidth of the stimulus, but the question is whether infant thresholds change, relative to

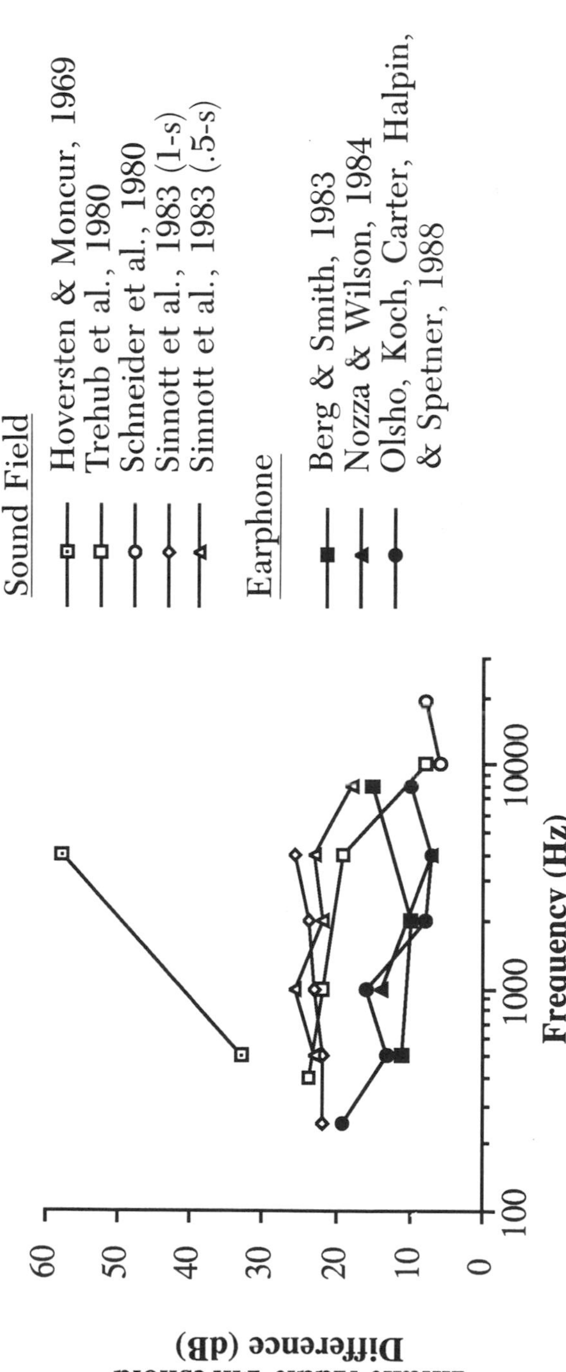

FIGURE 1 A comparison among seven studies in absolute detection thresholds of 6-to-8-month-old infants, relative to adults tested in the same study, as a function of frequency. From Olsho, Koch, Carter, Halpin, and Spetner (1988). Copyright 1988 by the Acoustical Society of America. Reprinted by permission.

adult thresholds, in a stimulus-dependent way. There is, in fact, little evidence in Figure 1 that they do. For example, Trehub et al. (1980) presented infants with octave bands of noise, whereas Sinnott, Pisoni, and Aslin (1983) used pure tones as stimuli. The results of these two studies are quite similar. Moreover, Sinnott et al. (1983) measured infant thresholds for tones of two durations, 0.5 s and 1 s, and found that duration did not have a significant effect on infant relative threshold. Finally, Werner and Bargones (in press) also compared infant relative thresholds in three studies using stimuli differing in duration and presentation rate. Neither of these variables appeared to have a significant effect on infant relative threshold. In general, then, stimulus appears to have little effect on infant relative threshold.

Mode of stimulus presentation

Some investigators present sounds over loudspeakers (e.g., Berg & Smith, 1983; Trehub et al., 1980), whereas others use earphones (e.g., Nozza & Wilson, 1984; Olsho, Koch, Carter, Halpin, & Spetner, 1988). There are two reasons that one would predict different infant thresholds for these modes of stimulus presentation. First, as one might expect, it is not always easy to get an infant to wear earphones, although the investigators who use them have devised various means for keeping the earphones in place. To the extent that infants find the earphones bothersome, their performance might be expected to be affected. The second and more important issue is that of "calibration": How does the investigator know the amplitude of sound being delivered to the infant's ear? When sounds are presented over loudspeakers, or in sound field, the amplitude of sound delivered to the ear will vary with the position of the head. Thus, the fact that infants are typically mobile during a test session could introduce variability in infant performance. Schneider, Trehub, and colleagues (e.g., Schneider, Trehub, & Thorpe, 1991) have dealt with this problem by using as stimuli octave bands of noise rather than pure tones because the problem of amplitude variations is reduced for the former (Dillon & Walker, 1982). However, octave bands of noise are less frequency specific than are pure tones so that variations in performance as a function of frequency may be obscured when octave bands of noise are used. Because earphones move with the infant, this sort of amplitude variation would not occur as long as the position of the earphones is stable. Changes in earphone position, however, can cause leakage, which would reduce the amplitude of the sound delivered. This effect would be more pronounced at low frequencies (e.g., Arlinger, 1991).

Sound amplitude is also measured differently for loudspeaker and earphone presentations. When sound-field presentation is used, amplitude is usually measured at the position of the listener's head. Thus, the amplitude arriving at the head is estimated. Earphones are calibrated using a microphone that is held in a cavity, the volume and resonance of which are approximately those of the external ear. In this case, the amplitude in the ear canal is estimated. As a result of resonance, the difference between the amplitude at the head and the amplitude in the ear canal will vary with sound frequency. Furthermore, because the volume and resonant properties of the infant external ear are likely to be different from those of the adult external ear (Keefe, Burns, Bulen, & Campbell, 1991; Kruger, 1987; Kruger & Ruben, 1987), the amplitude estimated in a cavity approximating an adult ear is not a good estimate of the amplitude in the infant ear. Specifically, because the infant's ear-canal volume is smaller, delivering the same stimulus to infants and adults would result in a higher amplitude being delivered to infants, and the size of the difference would depend on stimulus frequency.

The infant relative thresholds shown in Figure 1 tended to be lower for earphone presentation than for sound-field presentation. Excluding for the moment the Hovcrsten and Moncur (1969) data, the maximum size of the effect was approximately 10 dB. A large part of this effect can probably be accounted for by the calibration factors described above: Earphone studies will tend to underestimate sound pressure level (SPL) for infants when the earphones are calibrated in an adult-size coupler. The differences between sound-field and earphone studies appear to be smaller at the highest frequencies (>8000 Hz) and possibly at the lowest frequencies (200–250 Hz) than they are in the midfrequency range. The low-frequency earphone thresholds may be overestimated as a result of leakage from under the earphones. It is not clear why the high-frequency sound-field and earphone relative thresholds converge; possible contributors to this are the difficulties in sound-field calibration at high frequencies and the differences between the resonant characteristics of infant and adult ears at high frequencies.

Only one study has directly compared infant thresholds under earphones with those measured under sound-field conditions. Berg and Smith (1983) compared pure-tone thresholds of 10-month-olds under earphones with those obtained in sound field. Infant relative thresholds were about 5 dB lower under earphones than in sound field at 2000 Hz and about 2 dB lower at 8000 Hz. This is the same pattern that is evident in the between-study comparison. However, Berg and Smith also found that infant relative thresholds were 8–9 dB higher under earphones at 500 Hz. Because they noted difficulty keeping earphones in place on older infants, this effect probably resulted from earphone leakage.

To conclude, both between-study and direct comparisons suggest that infant relative thresholds are lower when sounds are presented under earphones and that the sound field–earphone difference tends to be greatest in the midfrequency range. In addition, low-frequency infant thresholds may be difficult to estimate under earphones because of leakage. Thus, mode of stimulus presentation is an important methodological variable in studies of infants' detection of sound in quiet. However, the effects of this variable are readily understood in terms of the acoustical properties of the infant's external ear. Once accurate measures of these properties are in hand, it is expected that sound-field and earphone results will be found to be in substantial agreement.

Response

The procedure that is used in the vast majority of laboratories is some modification of a discrimination learning paradigm, visual reinforcement audiometry (VRA), first described by J. M. Moore, Thompson, and Thompson (1975). In this procedure, the infant is trained to make a head turn in response to a sound. Another audiometric procedure for assessing infant hearing is behavioral observation audiometry (BOA; Northern & Downs, 1991). In BOA, any response that occurs in temporal proximity to the presentation of a sound is taken as evidence of hearing. A somewhat different approach, observer-based procedures (OBP), accepts any response that reliably distinguishes between sound and no-sound or between two different sounds (Olsho, Koch, Halpin, & Carter, 1987; Trehub, Schneider, Thorpe, & Judge, 1991). Thus, OBP and BOA are similar in that they both use a variety of infant responses, whereas VRA requires a specific response, the head turn.

Of the studies summarized in Figure 1, five used the head-turn response (Berg & Smith, 1983; Nozza & Wilson, 1984; Schneider et al., 1980; Sinnott et al., 1983; Trehub et al., 1980), one used BOA (Hoversten & Moncur, 1969), and one used OBP (Olsho, Koch, Carter, Halpin, & Spetner, 1988). Notice that although the BOA relative thresholds were much higher than were all the others, the OBP relative thresholds fall in the lower cluster. Thus, it appears unlikely that response is an important variable here. In fact, Olsho, Koch, Halpin, and Carter (1987) found no difference between head-turn thresholds and OBP thresholds in 6-month-olds.

Reinforcement

Responses are not reinforced in BOA, are sometimes reinforced in OBP, and always reinforced in VRA and other head-turn procedures. The typical reinforcer used is an interesting visual event (e.g., the activation of a mechanical toy). Notice that the Hoversten and Moncur (1969) thresholds in Figure 1 are considerably higher than are any of the others shown; this is the only study in the group that did not use reinforcement. This suggests that reinforcement has substantial effects on infant relative threshold.

The effects of reinforcement have been addressed directly in several studies. Moore et al. (1975) compared the number of head turns that 12- to 18-month-olds made in response to a noise in the following four reinforcement conditions: no reinforcer, blinking light reinforcer, social reinforcer, and mechanical toy reinforcer. All reinforcers increased the number of responses relative to no reinforcer; of the three reinforcers, the mechanical toy was most effective in increasing the number of head turns. Moore, Wilson, and Thompson (1977) showed that visual reinforcement substantially increased the number of head turns by 5- to 11-month-olds in response to a noise stimulus. Although neither of these studies examined the effect of reinforcement on threshold, one could argue that thresholds would have been high if infants had rapidly habituated to the sounds. Trehub, Schneider, and Bull (1981), however, showed that detection thresholds of 12-month-olds were lower when a mechanical toy reinforcer was used, and Werner and Feeney (1990) found that thresholds of 2- to 4-week-old infants were lower when an audiorecording of women reading from children's books was used as a reinforcer in an OBP. Clearly, reinforcement is an important procedural variable.

A final note on the effects of reinforcement on auditory behavior: Although Moore et al. (1977) reported that a mechanical toy reinforcer had no effect on the number of head turns that 4-month-olds made in response to a noise, the same mechanical toy was used to estimate thresholds in infants of this age in other experiments (e.g., Olsho, Koch, Carter, Halpin, & Spetner, 1988). The most likely explanation for this apparent discrepancy is that 4-month-olds do not make directional head turns toward sounds (Clifton, Morrongiello, Kulig, & Dowd, 1981). Thus, the apparent ineffectiveness of reinforcement in this age group probably results from the fact that these infants make few head turns under any condition. However, the same reinforcer may be effective in increasing the probability of other responses. Werner and Feeney's (1990) findings with 2- to 4-week-olds also support the contention that reinforcement is an effective way to increase responsiveness of young infants when a response within the infant's existing repertoire is used. Whether other yet untried reinforcers would be more effective remains to be explored.

Psychophysical Method

Two different procedures have been used to estimate infant thresholds. The most commonly used method is an adaptive, or staircase, method (Levitt, 1971). In this method, the stimulus is varied over the course of the session depending on the listener's performance. For example, in a detection experiment, the amplitude of the stimulus would be reduced if the listener correctly detected the stimulus, but the amplitude would be increased if the listener did not detect the stimulus. Depending on the rules used to decide when to change the stimulus amplitude, after a number of trials the amplitude of the stimulus can be shown to oscillate around a given level of performance (e.g., the amplitude at which the listener detects the stimulus 70% of the time). Although adaptive methods tend to be more efficient than do other methods, they can be difficult to use with infants because they may track the infant's level of attentiveness or boredom rather than auditory sensitivity. Adaptive methods have also been criticized on the basis that in the single-alternative procedures in which they are typically used, the threshold on which the "staircase" will converge has not been established (Trehub et al., 1991).

The other class of methods used to estimate infant thresholds has been the method of constant stimuli. In this case, several stimuli are presented over a range of values around the expected threshold. The same stimuli are presented to all subjects. Performance is evaluated for each stimulus; threshold is defined as the stimulus value that would have led to an arbitrary level of performance (e.g., 70% correct). In the adult literature, all the trials for a given stimulus are typically presented in a block of trials in which only that stimulus is presented. Although this procedure has sometimes been used with infants (Trehub et al.,

1991; Werner & Marean, 1991a, 1992), it is more typical for stimuli to be presented in random order in a single block. Although changes in infant attentiveness, for example, would not be expected to affect thresholds estimated in the method of constant stimuli as much as adaptive thresholds, the method of constant stimuli is inefficient in that it does not concentrate trials in the vicinity of threshold. In addition, one must know at the outset the approximate threshold level. This is a particular problem if there is substantial between-subject variability because the stimuli chosen may be ill-placed relative to threshold for many subjects.

Of the studies included in Figure 1, all of the earphone studies used adaptive procedures. However, among the sound-field studies, Trehub et al. (1980) and Schneider et al. (1980) used the method of constant stimuli, whereas Sinnott et al. (1983) used an adaptive procedure. The similarity between the Trehub et al. and Sinnott et al. relative thresholds implies that this procedural difference had little effect.

There are two studies that have compared adaptive procedures and procedures using the method of constant stimuli for measuring thresholds in infants. Trehub, Bull, Schneider, and Morrongiello (1986) developed an adaptive procedure specifically for infant testing. Average individual adaptive thresholds estimated for 6-month-olds using this procedure were about the same as those estimated by Trehub et al. (1980) with procedures using the method of constant stimuli to detect a 4000-Hz, octave-band noise. Werner and Marean (1991b) also compared adaptive and method-of-constant-stimuli thresholds of 3- and 6-month-old infants. The stimulus was a 16-ms, 1000-Hz tone burst. Because infants may be less responsive to short-duration stimuli (e.g., Gray, 1990) and because adaptive procedures are believed to be vulnerable to inattentiveness, this stimulus would be expected to give the worst-case scenario. Two different adaptive procedures were used to estimate thresholds: a modification of the hybrid adaptive procedure described by Hall (1981; Spetner & Olsho, 1990) and a one-up, two-down method (Levitt, 1971; Yost, 1978). Psychometric functions for individual infants were also constructed on the basis of proportion of "signal" responses made at four stimulus levels presented in random order. Thresholds were estimated as the 70% "signal" point on these functions. The results of this comparison are shown in Figure 2. Too few hybrid thresholds were obtained from 3-month-olds to make meaningful comparisons. When thresholds were obtained, there was no dif-

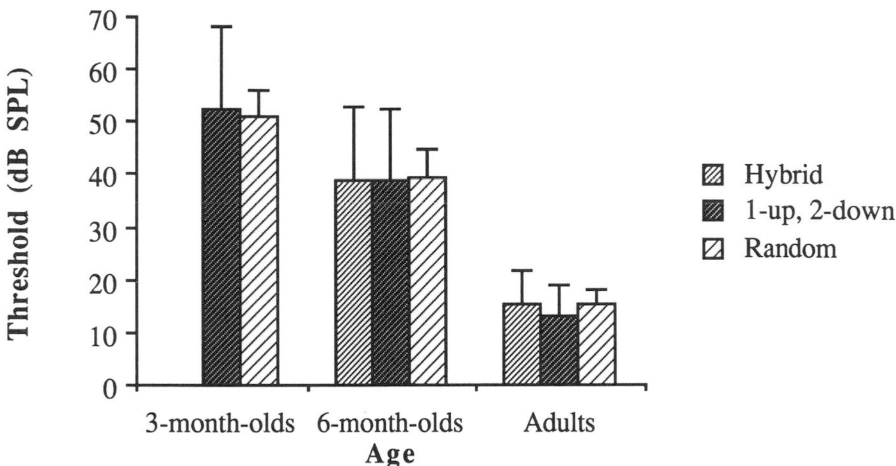

FIGURE 2 Thresholds of infants and adults tested using three different psychophysical procedures (see text). SPL = sound pressure level. Error bars indicate ±1 standard deviation. From Werner and Marean (1991b). Copyright 1991 by the Acoustical Society of America. Reprinted by permission.

ference between the average thresholds obtained using an adaptive method and those obtained using the method of constant stimuli at any given age. This result suggests factors such as inattentiveness make no greater contribution to adaptive thresholds than they do to method of constant-stimuli thresholds. Variability was lower, however, for method of constant-stimuli thresholds—an important factor in many experiments. Both between-study and direct comparisons, then, suggest that adaptive methods and the method of constant stimuli give similar results with respect to infant detection thresholds.

Number of Response Alternatives

In most cases, the infant is trained to respond if a sound is heard and to withhold a response if no sound is heard (Berg & Smith, 1983; Nozza & Wilson, 1984; Olsho, Koch, Carter, Halpin, & Spetner, 1988; Sinnott et al., 1983). This single-alternative paradigm is also known as a *go/no-go procedure*. Schneider, Trehub, and colleagues (e.g., Schneider et al., 1979) developed a method in which the infant turns to the left if the sound comes from a speaker to the left but to the right if the sound comes from a speaker to the right. This is a two-alternative, forced-choice paradigm. A criticism of the single-alternative procedure has been that thresholds may be influenced by response bias. The number of times the infant responds when a sound is heard is actually influenced by two factors: the infant's sensitivity to sound and the infant's tendency to respond, or response bias. For example, if the infant responded on every no-sound trial, the fact that he or she also responded on every sound trial says little about the infant's sensitivity to the sound. Laboratories that use the single-alternative paradigm generally control response bias by only accepting an infant's data if the rate of response when no sound is presented, the false-alarm rate, is below some criterion rate, say .25 or .30 of no-sound trials. However, as Schneider et al. (1991) pointed out, because infants who are unbiased but insensitive may also have high false-alarm rates, this practice may have the effect of making infants seem more sensitive as a group than they actually are. The two-alternative, forced-choice procedure controls for response bias in that the same tendency to respond should apply to both left and right responses; thus, response bias "cancels out." However, the two-alternative procedure developed by Trehub, Schneider, and their colleagues has been criticized on the grounds that it requires that the listener both detect and localize the sound.

A comparison between the relative thresholds (Figure 1) reported by Sinnott et al. (1983), Trehub et al. (1980), and Schneider et al. (1980) suggests that there is little difference between single-alternative and two-alternative methods. Furthermore, Schneider et al. (1991) recently presented data showing that infant thresholds estimated by two-alternative and single-alternative methods are not substantially different when a bias-free measure of sensitivity is used.

The effects of bias on infant threshold in a single-alternative paradigm have been examined in two studies. Trehub et al. (1991) looked at the relation between false-alarm rate and sensitivity in 1.5- to 3.5-month-olds in the detection of 4000-Hz, octave bands of noise in an OBP. Average d', a bias-free estimate of sensitivity, was lower for infants with false-alarm rates greater than 25% than it was for infants with false-alarm rates less than 25%. Thus, eliminating these infants from a sample as is the usual practice would overestimate the sensitivity of infants as a group. It is difficult to precisely estimate the effects that this would have on threshold estimates, but it appears that the threshold estimates would change by only a few decibels. Werner and Marean (1991a) addressed the same question in several different ways. First, they examined the correlation between false-alarm rate and detection threshold in 3- and 6-month-olds. The correlations were significant for the 6-month-olds tested using a hybrid adaptive procedure (Hall, 1981) but were not in the one-up, two-down adaptive procedure or in the method of constant stimuli. Second, they calculated average thresholds when infants with false-alarm rates greater than 25% were included in the sample and compared these with the averages that excluded these infants. For the method of constant stimuli, average threshold changed by less than 1 dB. For the hybrid adaptive procedure, the difference was greater, on the order of 8 dB. Thus, average thresholds are affected by the methods that are used to control response bias in single-alternative paradigms; however, with few exceptions, the size of the effect is quite small.

Finally, there has been some controversy in this field about the use of adaptive procedures to estimate thresholds in a single-alternative paradigm. Different adaptive rules estimate different points on the psychometric function (Levitt, 1971); the point estimated is termed the *convergence point*. Trehub et al. (1991), for example, argued that the statistical properties of these procedures were established for the two-alternative, forced-choice case and that the convergence point is unknown in the single-alternative case. In addition, as false-alarm rates are typically controlled in single-alternative infant experiments, variation in false-alarm rates could affect the properties of the staircase in unknown ways. Differences between infants and adults in false-alarm rates, for example, could result in estimating different points on the psychometric function for the two groups, which would thus provide misleading information about sensitivity differences.

One can approach the importance of this methodological variable using computer simulations. An example of the results of computer simulations of the behavior of the one-up, two-down adaptive rule in the single-alternative paradigm is shown in Figure 3. For the simulation, a psychometric function was assumed that had a slope and intercept typical of infant detection. This psychometric function was used to decide on each trial whether the infant made a response. The starting level of the adaptive run in each session, the step size, and the stopping rule were the same as those reported by Werner and Marean (1991a); 1,000 sessions were completed for each simulation. Two parameters were varied in the simulations: β, a measure of bias, and an "attentiveness factor," which determined the hypothetical maximum performance achieved by the infant. Only

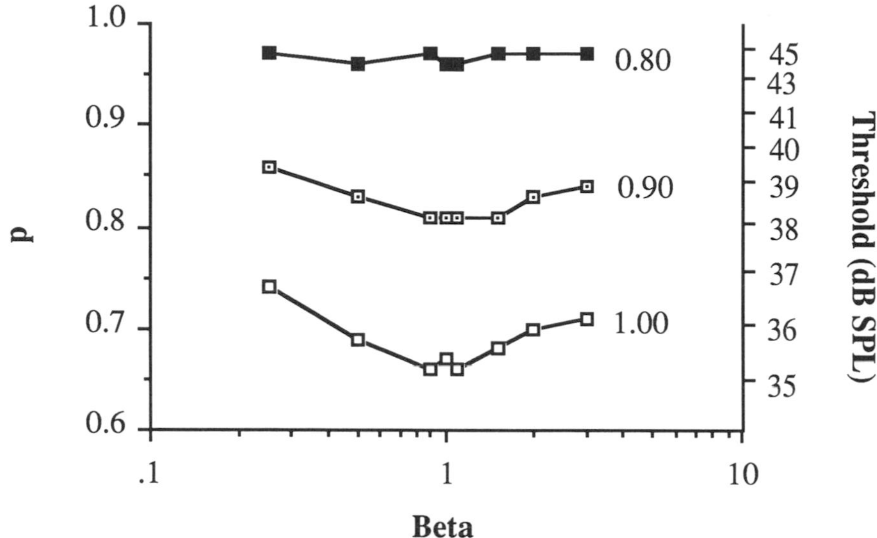

FIGURE 3 Results of simulation of one-up, two-down adaptive procedure as a function of beta. SPL = sound pressure level. Parameter is an "inattentiveness" factor that determines the maximum level of performance achieved by the listener. Right axis shows results in terms of expected threshold; left axis shows results in terms of *p*, the point on the underlying psychometric function on which the adaptive algorithm would converge.

sessions that met the criteria for inclusion in the Werner and Marean study were used to calculate the average threshold and the convergence point.

As Figure 3 shows, for a given maximum performance, changes in β result in shifts of the convergence point, *p*. For example, assume that both infants and adults achieve maximum performance of 1.0 correct. Werner and Marean (1991a) found that infants tended to be unbiased, on average, in the one-up, two-down procedure but that adults tended to be rather conservative. The simulations indicate that if the observer were unbiased (β = 1.0), the algorithm would estimate the .66 correct point; if the observer were very conservative in responding "yes" (β = 3.0), the algorithm would estimate the .71 correct point. The predicted difference between infants and adults in adaptive convergence points would lead to an underestimate of the actual difference in thresholds. Note, however, that the predicted change in threshold, even for a large shift in β, on an infant's shallow psychometric function is on the order of 1 or 2 dB (Figure 3). Given that the standard deviation in infant adaptive thresholds is on the order of 15 dB, this effect is quite small. It is clear that for this adaptive rule, at least, age differences in bias probably contribute little to age differences in threshold or to variability among infants in thresholds.

The effect of maximum performance achieved by the listener, on the other hand, is more dramatic (Figure 3). If the listener never achieves better than .90 correct, the convergence point is .15 higher and threshold increases by about 3 dB. If the listener never achieves better than .80 correct, the convergence point increases by .30 and threshold increases by 8 dB. These observations suggest that differences between infants and adults in maximum performance could make a substantial contribution to age differences in adaptive threshold. Variability among infants in this parameter could contribute substantial variability to adaptive thresholds.

Werner and Marean's (1991a) report of no differences between one-up, two-down adaptive procedures and procedures using the method of constant stimuli to measure thresholds in infants argues that poor infant maximum performance does not differentially affect adaptive thresholds. However, to address this question directly, it is necessary to establish the shape of the psychometric function for individual infants. It has been suggested that 60–100 trials are needed to have any idea what a psychometric function looks like (McKee, Klein, & Teller, 1985), and few laboratories routinely collect that many trials from infants (but see chapter 8, this volume). Recently, however, Werner and Marean (1991b) were able to collect 120 trials from 10 6-month-olds detecting the 16-ms, 1000-Hz tone burst used in the other studies described earlier. Four levels of the tone were chosen to surround the average threshold estimated by Werner and Marean (1991a), about 40 dB SPL. At each level, 30 test trials were presented in a block at a fixed intensity. The results for two infants are shown in Figure 4. The performance of the subject whose data are shown in Figure 4A tended to level off quickly, reaching an asymptote near .80 correct. These data could be reasonably described by the solid curve drawn with the data points. The performance of the other subject, however, did not appear to level off within the range of levels tested. These data could be reasonably described by a function with an upper asymptote of 1.00 correct, as shown. But because the latter subject never actually

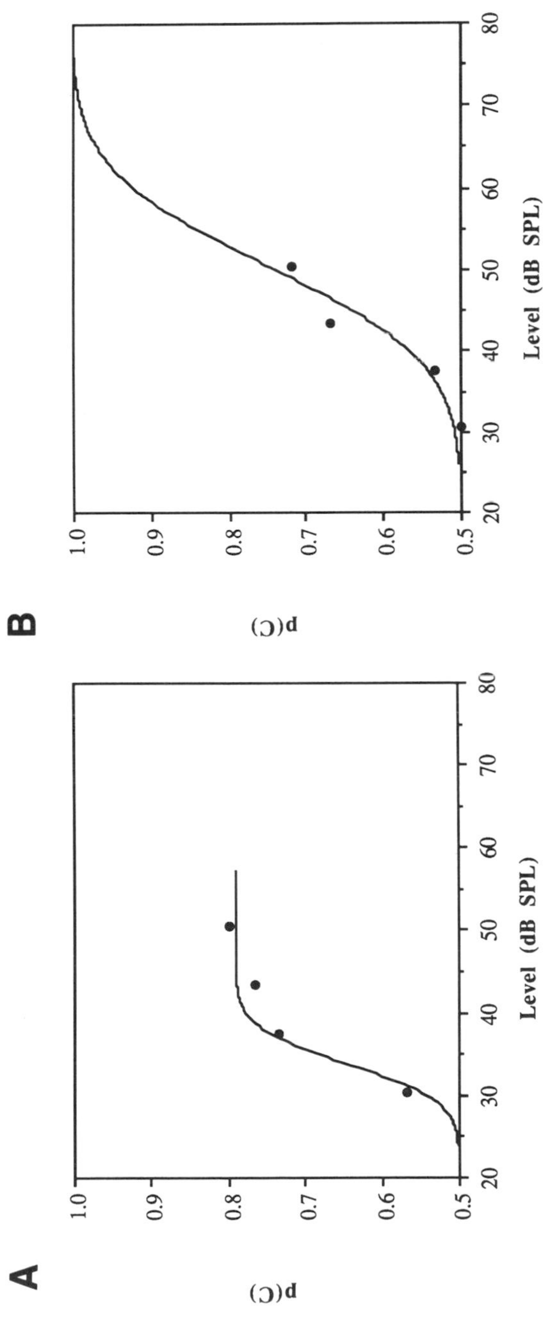

FIGURE 4 Examples of performance of two individual infants as a function of stimulus level in the detection of a 16-ms, 1000-Hz tone burst presented at near-threshold levels. SPL = sound pressure level. Curves are best fitting psychometric functions fit by probit analysis. (*A*) shows performance of subject S55008 and (*B*) shows performance of subject S55006.

did better than .70 or .75 correct, it is difficult to know where the upper asymptote of the function actually falls.

In a second study, Werner and Marean (1992) tested 6-month-olds' detection of the 16-ms, 1000-Hz tone burst at levels predicted from the first study (Werner & Marean, 1991b) to yield asymptotic performance. On average, infants achieved about .85 correct detections at these levels. This result is consistent with that of the initial psychometric function study (Werner & Marean, 1991b). Thus, one can be fairly confident that the upper asymptote of the 6-month-olds' psychometric function in detection of a 16-ms, 1000-Hz tone burst is .85 correct.

To return to the original question, how will this difference in maximum performance be reflected in adaptive thresholds? Computer simulations with maximum performance of .85 correct show that an adaptive threshold would be about 5 dB higher than it would be if the level of maximum performance was 1.0 correct. Keep in mind, however, that the stimulus in these experiments was chosen to maximize infant inattentiveness. Thus, one would expect that the extent to which adaptive thresholds for other stimuli are affected by the level of maximum performance would be smaller.

To summarize, then, single-alternative and two-alternative methods yield similar results in terms of infant detection threshold. Both between-study and direct comparisons of these methods support that conclusion. Furthermore, using adaptive procedures in a single-alternative paradigm should not substantially influence threshold estimates.

Individual Versus Group Thresholds

In traditional psychophysics, thresholds based on hundreds of trials are estimated for each observer, typically in numerous conditions. Because it is unlikely that one will get hundreds of trials from an infant listener, investigators typically take one of two approaches. One approach is to estimate thresholds from each infant but to base the threshold estimate on a relatively small number of trials (e.g., Berg & Smith, 1983; Olsho, Koch, Carter, Halpin, & Spetner, 1988; Sinnott et al., 1983). These are referred to here as *individual thresholds*. The other approach is to present each infant with only a few trials at several stimulus values, then to combine the data of all infants, defining average threshold as that stimulus value where the infants as a group achieve some level of performance, say .65 correct (Schneider et al., 1980; Schneider, Trehub, Morrongiello, & Thorpe, 1989; Trehub et al., 1980). These are referred to here as *group thresholds*. The arguments in favor of the group threshold approach have been that it is an effort to get even the minimum number of trials that one would want to estimate an individual threshold from an infant and that such threshold estimates are likely to include many trials at which the infant has lost interest or patience with the task. If one uses the group threshold approach, one need only get a few trials from each of many infants so that it is more certain that the infant is in an attentive state. There are two arguments against the group threshold approach. One is that when the variability among subjects is high, the group threshold may not correspond to the average individual threshold; the other is that the group threshold gives no indication of the variability among infants (Werner & Gillenwater, 1990).

Of the studies summarized in Figure 1, only Trehub et al. (1980) and Schneider et al. (1980) estimated group thresholds. Their results, as noted before, are quite similar to those of Sinnott et al. (1983), who estimated individual thresholds. This suggests that the two approaches yield the same results. Trehub et al. (1986) also reported that average individual thresholds were similar to the group thresholds reported by Trehub et al. (1980). One limitation in these comparisons, however, is that the group thresholds were estimated using the method of constant stimuli, whereas the individual thresholds were estimated using adaptive methods.

Werner and Marean's (1991b) psychometric function data for 6-month-olds in detecting a short duration tone burst provide the opportunity to compare group and individual thresholds obtained using the method of constant stimuli. Recall that in that study 30 trials were collected at each of four intensities from 10 infants. A threshold can be calculated for each infant from the individual psychometric function. In addition, one can construct a group psychometric function from these data and estimate a group threshold. The group curve is shown in Figure 5, along with the average individual threshold. The average individual threshold falls on the group psychometric function. A threshold estimated by simple linear interpolation from the group psychometric function at .70 correct would be about 40 dB SPL. This is the same value obtained by Werner and Marean (1991b) by averaging individual thresholds. Thus, 6-month-olds detecting the 16-ms, 1000-Hz tone burst produced the same threshold by both methods of estimation.

Werner and Gillenwater (1990), however, found substantial differences between group thresholds and average individual thresholds in 2- to 5-week-old in-

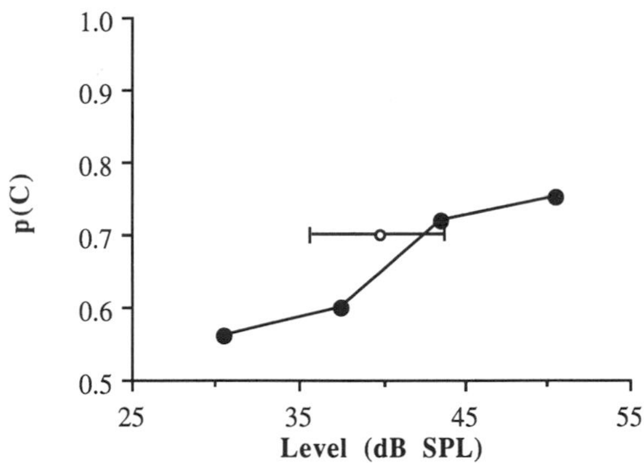

FIGURE 5 Average performance of 10 infants as a function of stimulus level in the detection of a 16-ms, 1000-Hz tone burst (filled symbols) and average individual threshold (open symbol), ±1 standard deviation. SPL = sound pressure level.

fants, both estimated by the method of constant stimuli. Moreover, the difference between group and average individual thresholds was greater at 4000 Hz than it was at 500 Hz. The difference between the young infants in the Werner and Gillenwater study and the 6-month-olds in the Werner and Marean (1991b) and Trehub et al. (1986) studies seems to be in the between-subject variability. Younger infants were more variable in performance, particularly at higher frequencies (Werner & Gillenwater, 1990). As a result, the group psychometric function is very shallow, and the group threshold estimate tends to be high. Thus, one might tentatively conclude that as long as the group psychometric function is reasonably steep, there will be little difference between thresholds estimated from group psychometric functions and average individual threshold. It remains, however, for the relationship between psychometric function slope and average individual threshold to be systematically explored.

Conclusions

The goal of this section was to ask whether procedural factors can account for variability in the outcome of developmental psychoacoustics studies. Of the seven methodological variables considered, only two appear to have consistent and substantial effects on infant detection thresholds: method of stimulus presentation and reinforcement. Whether thresholds are estimated for individuals or for the group also matters, but apparently only under extreme conditions.

These conclusions should not be taken to mean that blind application of any method is justified. For example, some of Werner and Marean's (1992) results illustrate the importance of choosing stimulus levels carefully. Recall that stimulus levels were chosen in that experiment so that asymptotic levels of performance were expected. In fact, most subjects did not vary in performance across levels. However, a few subjects produced data like that shown in Figure 6, where performance ($p[C]$) increased monotonically with level. If one were to fit the data of this infant with a psychometric function like that shown and calculate a threshold, the threshold would be 30 dB higher than that estimated when lower levels were presented to infants at the same age (e.g., Werner & Marean, 1991a, 1991b). Similarly, it is likely that if an adaptive run were begun at, say 80 dB SPL, the threshold estimate would be high because the infant would miss more trials at 65 dB SPL. I do not believe that infants like the one whose data are shown in Figure 6 are actually 30 dB less sensitive than are their peers. Rather, it seems that infants sometimes do not respond as well to moderately high sound levels as one would predict from near-threshold responses. I have seen infants who get .70 or .80 correct at low levels but consistently miss higher

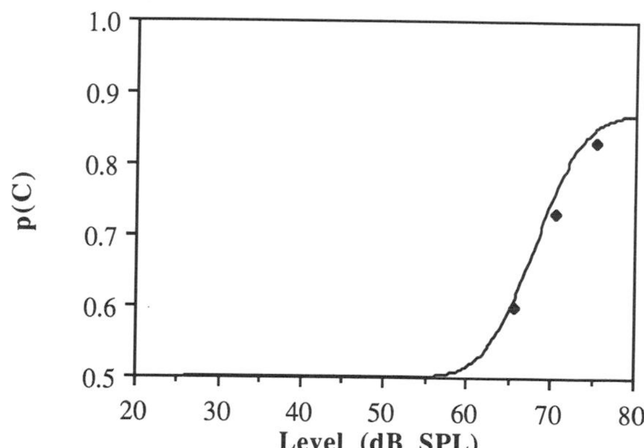

FIGURE 6 Examples of performance of one infant as a function of stimulus level in the detection of a 16-ms, 1000-Hz tone burst presented at moderately high levels. SPL = sound pressure level. Curve is best fitting psychometric function fit by probit analysis.

level "probe" trials in the same test run (Werner & Marean, 1988). This finding implies that it is very important to choose stimulus levels carefully when estimating infant thresholds. Such range effects may also make it difficult to determine what the infant's psychometric function looks like; it appears to be critical that a broad range of stimulus values be sampled.

Given reasonable precautions, however, this review supports the applicability of the psychophysical approach to the study of auditory development. Despite the facts that infants are not well-trained listeners and that threshold estimates are based on few trials from each subject, the thresholds obtained are stable across studies and methods. Although stability of results does not guarantee that the thresholds measured only reflect auditory sensitivity, it does offer promise that the sources of age-related change in threshold can be identified. These results also suggest that an investigator who uses reasonable care in choosing stimulus values and designing a test procedure need not be overly concerned with the details of the psychophysical method. As a field, developmental psychoacoustics is now in a position to move away from an exclusive concern with method to a concern for generating testable hypotheses about the differences found in performance between infants and adults.

Accounting for Differences Between Infants and Adults in Psychoacoustical Performance

The dilemma of developmental psychoacoustics outlined at the beginning of this chapter has two parts. The first part is the problem that the methodological adjustments made to accommodate infant subjects may make it impossible to measure anything meaningful about infant hearing. The analyses presented in the previous section, as well as the simple fact that infant psychoacoustical performance varies with stimulus parameters in a reasonable way, suggest that this problem is not as serious as some have argued. The second problem stems from the fact that infants do not perform as well as adults do. Getting consistent, stimulus-driven performance from infants does not necessarily imply that age-related change in performance results from age-related change in the auditory system. The purpose of this section is to consider how psychoacoustical measurements of infant auditory capacity can be used to develop hypotheses about the mechanisms that underlie infant–adult performance differences.

As one might gather from the discussion to this point, detection of sounds in quiet has been the most frequently examined infant psychoacoustical capacity. As previously noted, infants have higher detection thresholds than do adults. Peripheral immaturity (Keefe et al., 1991; Kruger, 1987; Kruger & Ruben, 1987), sensory neural immaturity (Schneider et al., 1989), and immaturity of attention and motivation (Olsho, Koch, Carter, Halpin, & Spetner, 1988) have been offered as possible explanations for this result. Direct measurements of the characteristics of the external and middle ear during development (e.g., Keefe et al., 1991) and comparisons between evoked potential and behavioral measures of detection (e.g., Werner, Rickard, & Folsom, 1990) promise to establish the contributions of these factors to age-related improvements in behavioral absolute thresholds.

Other measures, however, will be more important in understanding how infants perceive the complex sounds that they hear every day. Organisms rarely process sounds in quiet; the world is a noisy place. Furthermore, most auditory processing involves not detection but discrimination and identification of suprathreshold sounds. The remainder of this chapter, then, uses two potentially important measures that have been examined in infants, detection in noise and frequency discrimination, to illustrate the application of developmental research strategies to the interpretation of age-related change in psychophysical performance.

Detection of Sounds in Noise

In the laboratory, the effects of noise or other competing sounds on detection are referred to as *masking*. Infants have consistently been shown to have higher masked thresholds than adults do. For example, Figure 7 shows data published by Nozza and Wilson in 1984 representing detection thresholds for 1000- and 4000-Hz pure tones in broadband noise at 26-dB spectrum level for 6- and 12-month-olds and for adults. The infants' masked thresholds were about 8 dB higher than were the adults' at both frequencies. Figure 8 shows data by Schneider et al. (1989) of 6-month-olds', 12-month-olds', and adults' masked thresholds in 10-dB spectrum level noise for octave bands of noise at several frequencies. The infants' masked thresholds were 10–15 dB higher than were those of the adults. Finally, Figure 9 shows psychophysical tuning curves in simultaneous masking (Olsho, 1985). The maskers in this study were pure tones. The figure shows the average masker level at threshold as a function of masker frequency for the detection of 25-dB sensation level (SL) tones at 500, 1000, 2000, and 4000 Hz. Notice that the

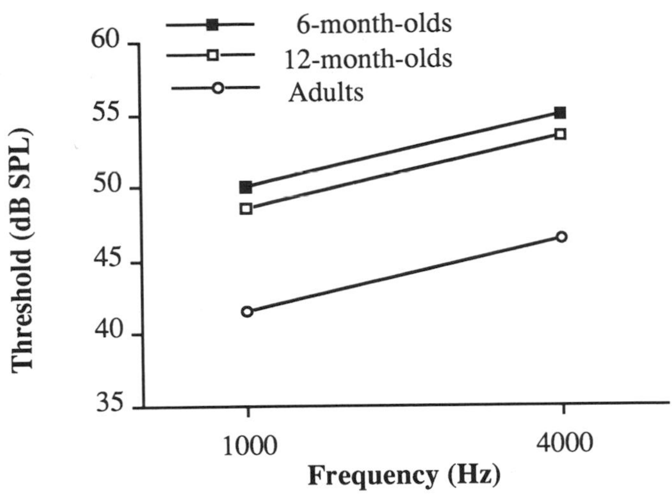

FIGURE 7 Average thresholds for detection of a tone in broadband noise, as a function of tone frequency for 6-month-olds, 12-month-olds, and adults. SPL = sound pressure level. From Nozza and Wilson (1984). Copyright 1984 by the American Speech-Language-Hearing Association. Reprinted by permission.

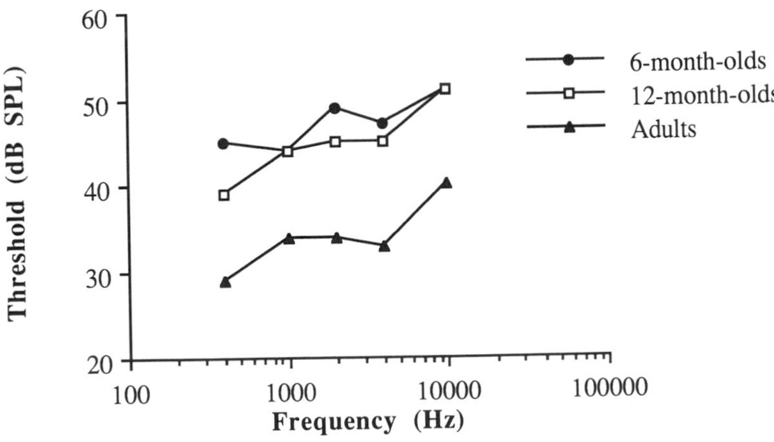

FIGURE 8 Average thresholds for detection of an octave-band noise in 10 dB spectrum level broadband noise as a function of frequency for 6-month-olds, 12-month-olds, and adults. SPL = sound pressure level. From Schneider, Trehub, Morrongiello, and Thorpe (1989). Copyright 1989 by the Acoustical Society of America. Reprinted by permission.

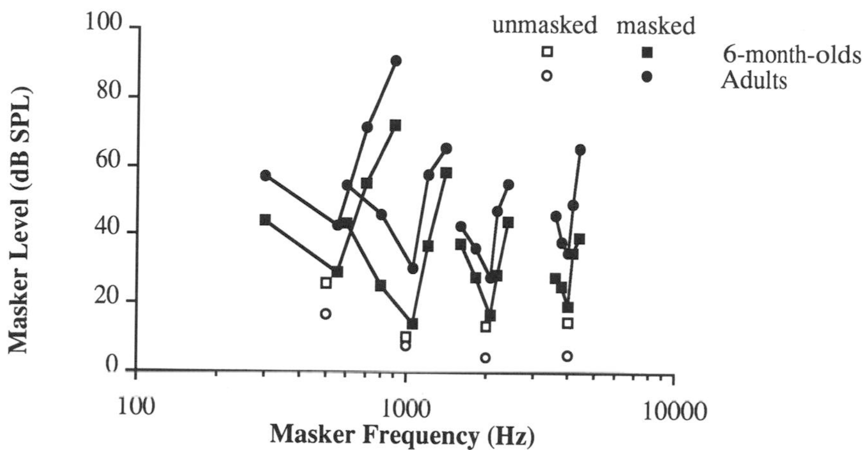

FIGURE 9 Psychophysical tuning curves for 6-month-olds and adults. Each curve shows masker level at threshold for the detection of a tone at the frequency plotted at the open symbols below it. SPL = sound pressure level. From Olsho (1985). Copyright 1985 by Ablex. Reprinted by permission.

infants exhibited masking when the masker level was 10–15 dB lower than when adults did so; that is, the infants needed a 10–15 dB higher signal-to-masker ratio to detect the probe.

Current models of masked threshold posit two underlying mechanisms, auditory filter width, reflecting the frequency-resolving power of the auditory system, and efficiency, reflecting the signal-to-noise ratio required for detection (Patterson, Nimmo-Smith, Weber, & Milroy, 1982). Several studies have shown that auditory frequency resolution is adultlike by 6 months of age in humans (Olsho, 1985; Schneider, Morrongiello, & Trehub, 1990; Spetner & Olsho, 1990), eliminating filter width as an explanation for infants' elevated masked thresholds. Unfortunately, labeling the problem *efficiency* does not explain anything: Either sensory immaturity, nonsensory immaturity, or both could make the infant inefficient at detecting sounds in noise.

One frequently mentioned nonsensory contributor is inattentiveness. Casual observation suggests that infants can hardly be characterized as vigilant subjects. Schneider et al. (1989) argued that inattentiveness cannot substantially contribute to the age difference in masked thresholds on the basis that the slope of the group psychometric function for detection in noise does not appear to change with age, although they admitted that 6-month-olds are a possible exception. Until there are data that accurately assess the slope of the psychometric function for infant detection of sound in noise, it will be difficult to evaluate this hypothesis.

Werner and Bargones (1991) took a somewhat different approach to the question of how attention affects infant psychophysical performance by asking not whether the infant is directing his or her attention to the task at hand but rather whether the infant is able to direct his or her attention selectively to the signal when there is also energy in other regions of the spectrum, as is the case in most masking situations. Adults are generally able to listen through a single auditory filter to optimize detection of a tone (e.g., Dai, Scharf, & Buus, 1991; Greenberg & Larkin, 1968; Schlauch & Hafter, 1991). Werner and Bargones's question was whether infants would have difficulty listening in this optimal way in the case in which the spectrum of the masker was known but was at some distance in frequency from the signal to be detected.

In the experiment, 6-month-old infants were trained to respond when they heard a repeated tone burst presented simultaneously with a noise band but not to respond when they heard the noise band alone. However, the tone and noise band did not overlap spectrally: The tone was 1000 Hz in frequency, the noise band had cutoffs of 4000 and 10000 Hz, and the filter slopes were 90 dB/octave. One would not expect this noise band to cause any peripheral interference with detection of the tone because it is spectrally distant from the tone and because high-frequency sounds tend to be ineffective maskers of lower frequency sounds. Such a noise band is referred to as a *distraction masker*. Thresholds for the tone with and without the noise band were estimated using an adaptive procedure. The distraction masker was turned on at the beginning of each trial. In one condition, the masker level was 40 dB SPL; in another, the masker level was 50 dB SPL. Figure 10 plots average threshold as a function of distraction masking condition for 6-month-olds and for adults. Notice first that the adults showed essentially no effect of the distraction masker. On the other hand, the infants showed significantly higher thresholds in the distraction masking conditions than they did in quiet. The difference between the 40-dB and 50-dB conditions was not significant. This is another argument against the idea that any kind of sensory masking effect is operating here: Adults showed a 10-dB increase in threshold for every

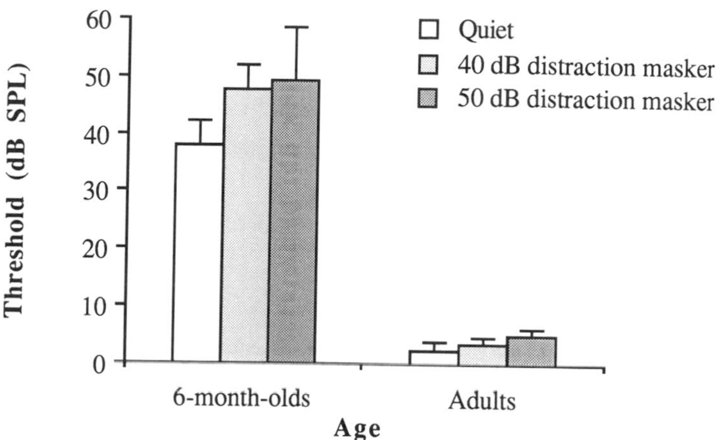

FIGURE 10 Thresholds for detection of a 1000-Hz tone in quiet and in two distraction-masking conditions for 6-month-olds and adults. SPL = sound pressure level. Error bars indicate ±1 standard error. From Werner and Bargones (1991). Copyright 1991 by the Psychonomic Society. Reprinted by permission.

10-dB increase in the level of a broadband masker (Hawkins & Stevens, 1950); Schneider et al. (1989) demonstrated that the same was true for 6-month-olds. In a second experiment, Werner and Bargones (1991) kept the distraction masker on continuously and reported the same effect: Infant thresholds were significantly higher in the presence of the distraction masker than in quiet. Finally, note that the size of the distraction masking effect is on the order of 5–10 dB and thus could account for a large portion of the typically reported 10–15 dB difference between infants and adults in masked thresholds.

The conclusion, then, is that attentional effects, as defined by Werner and Bargones (1991), are likely to be important in the development of masked thresholds. This is not to deny that other factors, such as neural variability or rate of response growth (Schneider et al., 1989), do not contribute to age-related change in masked threshold. In order to assess the contributions of the latter factors, however, additional data are needed. To begin with, psychometric functions for the detection of tones in noise from infant subjects would establish whether some of these hypotheses should be considered more directly.

In terms of developmental research strategies, the Werner and Bargones (1991) study illustrates two points. First, both sensory and nonsensory processes must be taken as serious explanations for infant psychophysical performance. As long as one treats nonsensory processes as nuisance factors that can be eliminated by choosing the correct procedure, one will neither eliminate nor understand them. Immature nonsensory processes are as much a characteristic of infants as are immature sensory processes. Moreover, the distraction masking experiment suggests that immature nonsensory processes can substantially affect what the infant perceives. Second, the Werner and Bargones (1991) study shows that infant performance cannot always be accounted for by models that have been developed to account for adult performance. Adult detection of a tone in noise is only affected by noise that falls within the same auditory filter as the tone; infant detection is clearly affected by noise falling outside that filter. Specific models of the detection process that include both sensory and nonsensory mechanisms are needed. As far as attention is concerned, the recent work of Schlauch and Hafter (1991), Dai et al. (1991), and Neff and Callaghan (1988) may provide some direction to this effort.

Frequency Discrimination

In the case of detection in noise, the psychophysical approach has been used to measure nonsensory contributions to masked thresholds. In the case of frequency discrimination, psychophysical studies of several infant sensory processes have been used to try to understand the way in which infants discriminate between different frequencies of sound. Olsho, Koch, and Halpin's (1987) study of frequency discrimination in infants is the most comprehensive study in the literature. In the experiment, infants learned to respond when a repeated tone burst changed in frequency and not to respond when the tone burst did not change in frequency. The size of the frequency change, Δf, ranged from 0.3% to 12.8% of the standard frequency, which was either 500, 1000, or 4000 Hz. Frequency difference thresholds were estimated from individual psychometric functions on the basis of 10 trials at each of six values of Δf. Thresholds were defined as the value of Δf responded to 70% of the time and were expressed as a proportion of the standard frequency. The tones were presented at two levels, 40 and 80 dB SL. The average frequency difference thresholds obtained are shown in Figure 11. Although infants as a group do not do as well as adults in this task, they can generally detect a frequency change on the order of 2–3%. Similar results have been reported in two other studies (Olsho, 1984; Olsho, Schoon, Sakai, Turpin, & Sperduto, 1982; Sinnott & Aslin, 1985). The most interesting aspect of infant fre-

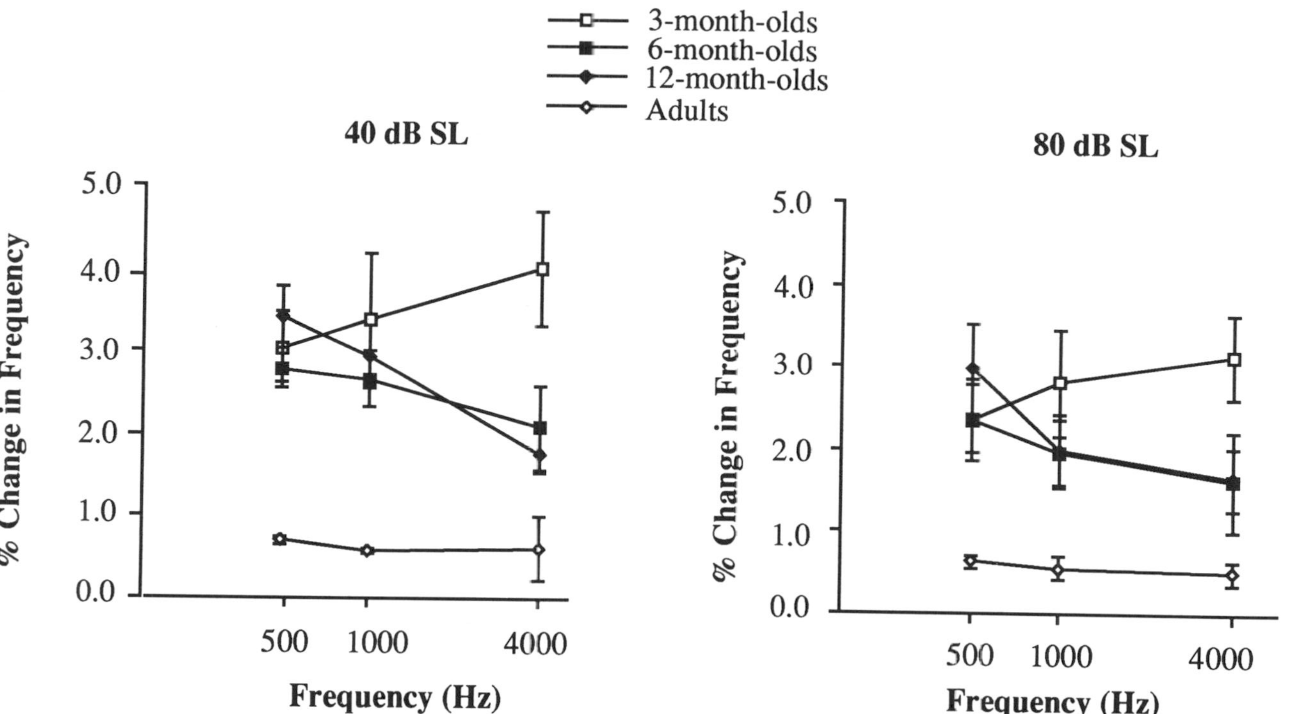

FIGURE 11 Frequency difference limens expressed as a percentage of standard frequency, as a function of standard frequency for infants and adults. Error bars indicate ±1 standard error. SL = sensation level. From Olsho, Koch, and Halpin (1987). Copyright 1987 by Acoustical Society of America. Reprinted by permission.

quency discrimination is that the effect of standard frequency on the difference threshold depends on the infant's age: Three-month-old infants get relatively worse at frequency discrimination as the standard frequency is increased, but 6- and 12-month-old infants get relatively better. All infants are poorer than are adults at 500 and 1000 Hz, but 6- and 12-month-olds approach adult performance at 4000 Hz. These results indicate that frequency discrimination follows a different developmental time course at high and low frequencies.

There are indications in adults that the mechanisms underlying frequency discrimination at high frequencies are different from those underlying frequency discrimination at low frequencies. For example, Dye and Hafter (1980) found that when tones were presented in noise, frequency discrimination improved with increasing level at high frequencies but grew worse with increasing level at low frequencies. B. C. J. Moore (1973) showed that the effects of tone duration on frequency discrimination were different at low and high frequencies. Both Dye and Hafter (1980) and Moore (1973) found a transition point in frequency discrimination around 2000–3000 Hz. It has been suggested that human listeners use temporal information to make frequency discriminations at low frequencies, whereas place or excitation pattern provide information at high frequencies.

These observations suggest an explanation for infant frequency discrimination performance. Infant frequency discrimination at a high frequency improves between 3 and 6 months of age. If frequency discrimination in this frequency range is limited by the excitation pattern, maturation of frequency resolution, the basis of the excitation pattern, during this period could account for this result. Similarly, if frequency discrimination in the low-frequency range is limited by temporal resolution, then immaturity of temporal resolution, persisting to 12 months, could account for infants' relatively poor low-frequency discrimination.

The existing data on frequency resolution in infants are consistent with these predictions. Spetner and Olsho (1990) examined frequency resolution in 3- and 6-month-olds in the psychophysical tuning curve paradigm using pulsation threshold masking. In this experiment, the subject hears two tones, designated *probe* and *masker*. If the masker and probe are alternated in close temporal proximity, the subject will hear two alternating tones when the masker level is low but will hear an intermittent masker against a continuous probe when the masker level is high. The masker level at which the perception of the probe changes from intermittent to continuous is the pulsation threshold. When the masker and probe are close in frequency, the pulsation threshold is low; the pulsation threshold increases as the masker and probe frequencies diverge. The degree to which the pulsation threshold changes with the masker frequency at a fixed probe frequency provides a measure of frequency resolution. Spetner and Olsho taught infants to respond when masker and probe were intermittent and alternating and to not respond when the masker was continuous. The probe frequency was either 500, 1000, or 4000 Hz, and the pulsation threshold was estimated for each subject at three different masker frequencies, one equal in frequency to the probe, one higher in frequency than the probe, and one lower in frequency than the probe. The thresholds were used to calculate a measure of frequency resolution, Q_{10}. Higher values of Q_{10} indicate better frequency resolution. The average Q_{10} obtained in this experiment are shown in Figure 12. There was no difference between 6-month-olds and adults at any of the probe frequencies examined. Other studies have also found that 6-month-olds have adultlike frequency resolution (Olsho, 1985; Schneider et al., 1990). Three-month-olds, on the other hand, were similar to older listeners at 500 and 1000 Hz but were sig-

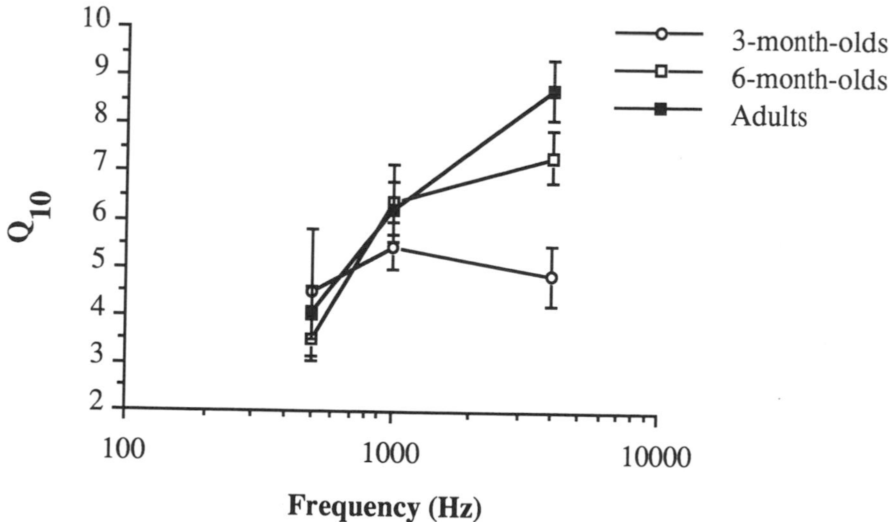

FIGURE 12 Q_{10} as a function of probe frequency in pulsation threshold procedure for 3- and 6-month-old infants and adults. Error bars indicate ± 1 standard error. From Spetner and Olsho (1990). Copyright 1990 by the Society for Research in Child Development. Reprinted by permission.

nificantly poorer than 6-month-olds and adults at 4000 Hz. This result is entirely consistent with the frequency discrimination data in that frequency resolution is improving between 3 and 6 months, the same age range in which improvement occurs in discrimination at high frequencies.

Because frequency resolution is adultlike at both 3 and 6 months at lower frequencies, Spetner and Olsho's (1990) findings are also consistent with the dual-mechanism account of frequency discrimination: Something other than frequency resolution must account for the infants' poor frequency discrimination at low frequencies. One suggestion has been that learning to use low-frequency information to make discriminations takes longer than does learning to use high-frequency information to do the same. This suggestion is based on the observation that adult listeners with little training tend to be relatively worse at low-frequency discrimination than at high-frequency discrimination compared with well-trained adult listeners (e.g., Harris, 1952; Wier, Jesteadt, & Green, 1977). However, although Olsho, Koch, and Carter (1988) found a greater effect of training on adult frequency discrimination at lower frequencies, this effect did not appear to completely account for the reported differences in low-frequency discrimination between infants and adults.

The data on infant temporal resolution at this point are not conclusive. For example, Morrongiello and Trehub (1987) reported a progressive increase in duration discrimination between infancy and adulthood. Werner, Marean, Halpin, Spetner, and Gillenwater (1992) also examined temporal resolution in 3-, 6-, and 12-month-old infants using the gap detection paradigm. Subjects were presented with a continuous broadband noise. Infants learned to respond when they heard brief interruptions or gaps in this noise but not to respond when the noise was continuous. The duration of the gap was varied adaptively to estimate the gap-detection threshold. In order to examine the effects of frequency on gap detection, in some conditions a continuous high-pass masker was introduced that would allow the listener to use only those frequencies below the pass band of the masker to detect gaps. The masker cutoff frequencies were 500, 2000, and 8000 Hz in different conditions. Average gap-detection thresholds are shown in Figure 13. Notice that the adults improved in gap detection as the masker cutoff frequency was increased and that with an 8000-Hz masker cutoff, adults performed as well as they did when the interrupted noise was not masked. The infants' performance was quite poor relative to adults', but there was no evidence that infant

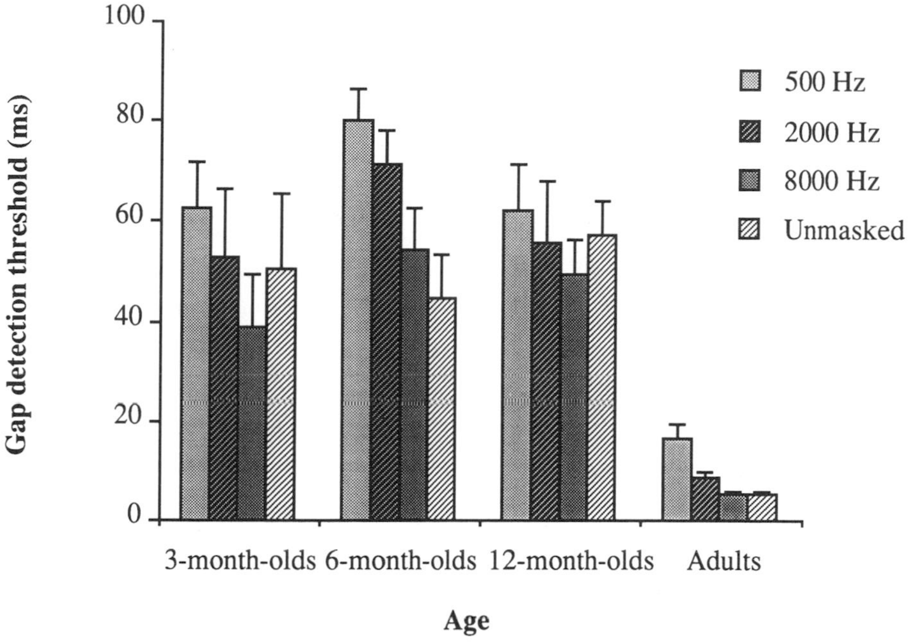

FIGURE 13 Gap detection threshold in broadband noise as a function of masking condition for 3-, 6-, and 12-month-old infants and for adults. Error bars indicate +1 standard error. From Werner, Marean, Halpin, Spetner, and Gillenwater (1992). Copyright 1992 by the Society for Research in Child Development. Reprinted by permission.

performance was affected by the masker condition any differently than was that of the adults.

Both the Morrongiello and Trehub (1987) and the Werner et al. (1992) results are difficult to interpret: On the one hand, one might take the fact that all the infants did poorly in this task to mean that they had poor temporal resolution. On the other hand, infant temporal resolution varied across frequency in the same way as did adult temporal resolution. Infants performed qualitatively like adults, and there are many reasons besides poor temporal resolution that could account for the main effect of age.

There are only preliminary data at this time to suggest that temporal resolution is immature during infancy. Marean and Werner (1991) examined forward masking, another measure of the temporal resolving power of the auditory system, in 3-month-olds. The subject was trained to detect a 1000-Hz tone, here called the *probe*, when it was preceded by a broadband noise masker at 65 dB SPL. The amount of forward masking depends on the temporal separation of the masker and probe, Δt. In this experiment, probe detection thresholds were estimated for values of Δt of 5, 10, and 25 ms. In another condition, the detection threshold was estimated for a Δt of 200 ms. This Δt is so long that one would not expect any forward masking to occur, but if just having a masker of any kind has a detrimental effect on infant performance, this condition would provide a control. Figure 14 shows amount of masking (i.e., the difference between masked and unmasked thresholds) as a function of Δt for 3-month-olds and adults (Elliott, 1962; Marean & Werner, 1991). First, notice that when Δt was 200 ms, there was no difference between infants and adults in amount of masking. This suggests that there is little in the way of a nonsensory contribution to the infant masked threshold. Second, notice that for values of Δt where masking would be expected, the infants exhibited much more masking than did adults. This suggests that they have poorer temporal resolution than do adults.

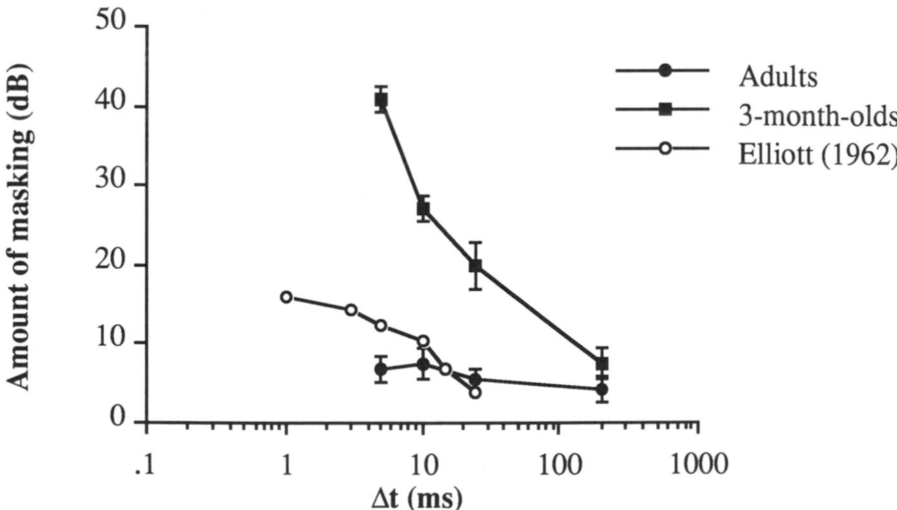

FIGURE 14 Amount of forward masking of a 1000-Hz probe masked by a 65 dB sound pressure level (SPL) broadband noise as a function of masker-probe interval, Δt, for 3-month-old infants and for adults. Error bars indicate ±1 standard error. From Elliott (1962). Copyright 1962 by the Acoustical Society of America. Reprinted by permission.

These data suggest that 3-month-olds have poor temporal resolution, at least at 1000 Hz, and there is reason to believe that this is not due to some general performance deficit. In order to make any statements about the relation between the development of temporal resolution and that of frequency discrimination, additional forward masking data from older infants is required. One would predict little development of forward masking during the first 12 months of life.

The data on infant frequency discrimination, frequency resolution, and temporal resolution represent, at least to a first approximation, an internally consistent set of observations about the way that the infant auditory system works, based on psychophysical measures. This is very encouraging in terms of what the psychophysical approach to the study of auditory development can accomplish. It appears that one can actually use developmental psychoacoustical data to help figure out the way that the mature system works. If the data show that temporal resolution matures along with low-frequency discrimination, whereas frequency resolution matures along with high-frequency discrimination, this would lend support to a general model of frequency discrimination. This is not a new approach, even in the study of the auditory system (e.g., Pujol, Carlier, & Lenoir, 1980), but it is the first time that such an approach has been possible with respect to auditory behavior in human infants. Thus, developmental psychoacoustical data can not only lead to testable hypotheses about infant hearing, but they can contribute to a general understanding of auditory function.

Conclusions

This chapter set out to solve a dilemma: How can researchers use the psychophysical approach to study the development of the auditory system in human infants? The application of psychophysical methods to the study of development has been questioned on two major grounds. First, it can be argued that methodological adjustments necessary to do psychophysics with infants violate so many of the assumptions underlying psychophysical methods that the results are essentially meaningless. Second, it can be argued that when infant performance is so poor relative to that of adults, it is unlikely that the operation of the sensory system is being reflected in that performance to any significant degree. I have attempted to address each of these arguments.

The analysis of procedural effects on measures of infant sensitivity led to the conclusion that many of the factors that have concerned researchers—bias, number of response alternatives, stimulus, psychophysical method, whether thresholds are calculated for the group or individual—in fact have little effect on infant thresholds. That different investigators have obtained similar answers about infant performance, despite variation in the methods used, argues strongly that these thresholds are meaningful.

It is understandable and appropriate that developmental psychoacoustics, as a fairly new field, has concentrated on developing accurate and sensitive methods. Methodological issues cannot, moreover, be completely ignored even now. As the analysis of reinforcement effects indicates, thresholds can be strongly influenced by whether or not the infant's response to sound is reinforced; although researchers have apparently found quite effective reinforcers for older infants, that may not be the case for the 0- to 5-month-old group. Thus, some effort at developing reinforcers for this group is probably in order. At the same time, although the introduction of reinforcement reduced thresholds by as much as 30 dB, one can expect that improving the effectiveness of reinforcers will have much smaller effects, on the order of 5 or 10 dB. Thresholds were also shown to be dependent on mode of stimulus presentation, with thresholds under earphones being lower than thresholds measured in sound field. The issue here is not whether one method is superior to the other; rather, the fact that thresholds measured in these two ways differ suggests that the acoustical properties of the infant ear are an important contributor to differences between infant and adult detection thresholds. Understanding this effect, then, depends on additional data with respect to the development of the external ear. Finally, as work on infant psychometric functions shows, infant performance is sometimes unpredictable. As a consequence, there will be no substitute for careful pilot work, particularly when a stimulus or psychophysical paradigm is being used for the first time.

Perhaps a more important implication of the procedural analysis is that much of the effort and energy that has been expended on methodological issues can now be turned to explaining why infants' thresholds consistently come out the way they do. As far as absolute sensitivity is concerned, it is clear that there are reliable differences between infants and adults. It is time to generate hypotheses about the nature of the differences and to test those hypotheses. Although other auditory capacities have not been as extensively described in infants, there is enough information about frequency discrimination, masked thresholds, frequency resolution, and binaural processing to warrant attention to possible explanations.

How one goes about testing hypotheses about age differences, of course, lies at the heart of the second part of the original dilemma. If solving the first part of the dilemma required an exclusive concern with psychophysics, solving this part will require that researchers place themselves squarely within the realm of developmental psychology. In a sense, the critics are correct when they argue that the age differences in performance reported are uninterpretable: Simply finding that infants do not perform as well as adults do does not necessarily mean that infants' primary auditory systems are immature. What the critics fail to recognize is that interpreting age differences is the business of developmental psychologists.

Developmental research strategies, for example, have as their aim not only to document but to explain age-related change. Banks and Dannemiller (1987) provide an elegant summary of such approaches in the context of developmental psychophysics, and their application is illustrated in the treatment of the infant frequency discrimination earlier. By looking for interactions and comparing performance on different measures, for example, one can not only make a case that maturation of the sensory system contributes to age-related improvement in psychophysical performance, but one can eliminate certain nonsensory variables as potential contributors.

Developmentalists have also long recognized that models of adult behavior are often inadequate to account for behavior during development. This idea is a common theme in the areas of cognitive development (e.g., Flavell, 1985; Piaget, 1954) and language development (e.g., Brown, 1973; Peters, 1986). In the area of perceptual development, Gottlieb's (1985) work on the effects of experience on ducklings' preference for maternal calls illustrates this point nicely. Work on distraction masking indicates that the development of appropriate models of infants' detection of sounds will be necessary to account for age-related change in this capacity. Models of adult psychophysical performance often ignore processes such as attention and memory because psychophysical procedures make the effects of these processes on performance negligible. Such factors are probably not negligible in infant performance, first, because the procedures used to test infants cannot eliminate their contributions, and, second, because immaturity of processes like attention and memory make their effects difficult to eliminate. Thus, although attention and other higher level perceptual processes are included, but essentially ignored, in models of adult performance, they cannot be ignored in models of infant performance. It seems unlikely that the primary auditory system mechanisms that underlie detection operate in a qualitatively different way during development. However, given that the "task" of the developing organism is different from that of the mature organism, it seems likely that the way that behavior is organized around auditory input does change during development. Because behavior provides the basis for psychophysical measures, then, it is critical that researchers take such differences into account in trying to understand age-related change in psychophysical performance. This observation suggests that successful models of infant psychophysical performance will depend as much on an understanding of general theories of development as they do on an understanding of the mature perceptual process.

Finally, it is hoped that this review broadens the role of developmental psychoacoustics as a scientific endeavor. Certainly researchers are interested in learning "what a baby hears"—the most direct product of research efforts. However, the implications of the findings go beyond that. The models of infant auditory processing developed in the course of this work are obviously relevant to the general field of perceptual development. Moreover, the developmental approach offers the opportunity to test models of mature auditory processing in a unique way. It is the potential for such interactions between the field and its parent disciplines that makes developmental psychoacoustics interesting and important.

References

Arlinger, S. D. (1991). Normal hearing threshold levels in the low-frequency range determined by an insert earphone. *Journal of the Acoustical Society of America*, *90*, 2411–2414.

Banks, M. S., & Dannemiller, J. L. (1987). Infant visual psychophysics. In P. Salapatek & L. Cohen (Eds.), *Handbook of infant perception: From sensation to perception* (pp. 115–184). San Diego, CA: Academic Press.

Berg, K. M., & Smith, M. C. (1983). Behavioral thresholds for tones during infancy. *Journal of Experimental Child Psychology*, *35*, 409–425.

Brown, R. (1973). *A first language: The early stages*. Cambridge, MA: Allen & Unwin.

Clifton, R., Morrongiello, B. A., Kulig, J. W., & Dowd, J. M. (1981). Developmental changes in auditory localization in infancy. In R. N. Aslin, J. R. Alberts, & M. R. Petersen (Eds.), *Development of perception* (Vol. 1, pp. 141–160). San Diego, CA: Academic Press.

Dai, H., Scharf, B., & Buus, S. (1991). Effective attenuation of signals in noise under focused attention. *Journal of the Acoustical Society of America*, *89*, 2837–2842.

Dillon, H., & Walker, G. (1982). Comparison of stimuli used in sound field audiometric testing. *Journal of the Acoustical Society of America*, *71*, 161–172.

Dye, R. H., & Hafter, E. R. (1980). Just-noticeable differences of frequency for masked tones. *Journal of the Acoustical Society of America*, *67*, 1746–1753.

Elliott, L. L. (1962). Backward and forward masking of probe tones of different frequencies. *Journal of the Acoustical Society of America*, *34*, 1116–1117.

Fechner, G. T. (1860). *Element der psychophysik*. Leipzig: Breitkopf & Harterl.

Flavell, J. H. (1985). *Cognitive development* (2nd ed.). Englewood Cliffs, NJ: Prentice-Hall.

Gottlieb, G. (1983). The psychobiological approach to developmental issues. In M. M. Haith & J. J. Campos (Eds.), *Handbook of child psychology* (Vol. 2, 4th ed., pp. 1–26). New York: Wiley.

Gottlieb, G. (1985). On discovering significant acoustic dimensions of auditory stimulation for infants. In G. Gottlieb & N. A. Krasnegor (Eds.), *Measurement of audition and vision in the first year of life: A methodological overview* (pp. 3–29). Norwood, NJ: Ablex.

Gray, L. (1990). Development of temporal integration in newborn chickens. *Hearing Research*, *45*, 169–178.

Greenberg, G. Z., & Larkin, W. D. (1968). The frequency response characteristic of auditory observers detecting signals of a single frequency in noise: The probe-signal method. *Journal of the Acoustical Society of America*, *44*, 1513–1523.

Hall, J. L. (1981). Hybrid adaptive procedure for estimation of psychometric functions. *Journal of the Acoustical Society of America*, *69*, 1763–1769.

Harris, J. D. (1952). Pitch discrimination. *Journal of the Acoustical Society of America*, *24*, 750–755.

Hawkins, J. E., & Stevens, S. S. (1950). The masking of pure tones and of speech by white noise. *Journal of the Acoustical Society of America*, *22*, 6–13.

Hoversten, G. H., & Moncur, J. P. (1969). Stimuli and intensity factors in testing infants. *Journal of Speech and Hearing Research*, *12*, 677–686.

Keefe, D. H., Burns, E. M., Bulen, J. C., & Campbell, S. L. (1991, April). *Pressure transfer function from the diffuse field to the human infant ear canal*. Paper presented at the 121st Meeting of the Acoustical Society of America, Baltimore.

Kruger, B. (1987). An update on the external ear resonance in infants and young children. *Ear and Hearing*, *8*, 333–336.

Kruger, B., & Ruben, R. J. (1987). The acoustic properties of the infant ear: A preliminary report. *Acta Otolaryngologica*, *103*, 578–585.

Levitt, H. (1971). Transformed up–down methods in psychoacoustics. *Journal of the Acoustical Society of America*, *49*, 467–477.

Marean, G. C., & Werner, L. A. (1991, April). *Forward masking functions of 3-month-old infants*. Paper presented at the 121st Meeting of the Acoustical Society of America, Baltimore.

McKee, S. P., Klein, S. A., & Teller, D. Y. (1985). Statistical properties of forced-choice psychometric functions: Implications of probit analysis. *Perception & Psychophysics*, *37*, 286–298.

Moore, B. C. J. (1973). Frequency difference limens for short-duration tones. *Journal of the Acoustical Society of America*, *54*, 610–619.

Moore, J. M., Thompson, G., & Thompson, M. (1975). Auditory localization of infants as a function of reinforcement conditions. *Journal of Speech and Hearing Disorders*, *40*, 29–34.

Moore, J. M., & Wilson, W. (1978). Visual Reinforcement Audiometry (VRA) with infants. In S. E. Gerber & G. T. Mencher (Eds.), *Early diagnosis of hearing loss* (pp. 177–213). New York: Grune & Stratton.

Moore, J. M., Wilson, W. R., & Thompson, G. (1977). Visual reinforcement of head-turn responses in infants under 12 months of age. *Journal of Speech and Hearing Disorders*, *42*, 328–334.

Morrongiello, B. A., & Trehub, S. E. (1987). Age-related changes in auditory temporal perception. *Journal of Experimental Child Psychology*, *44*, 413–426.

Neff, D. L., & Callaghan, B. P. (1988). Effective properties of multicomponent simultaneous maskers under conditions of uncertainty. *Journal of the Acoustical Society of America*, *83*, 1833–1838.

Northern, J. L., & Downs, M. P. (1991). *Hearing in children* (4th ed.). Baltimore: Williams & Wilkins.

Nozza, R. J., & Wilson, W. R. (1984). Masked and unmasked pure-tone thresholds of infants and adults: Development of auditory frequency selectivity and sensitivity. *Journal of Speech and Hearing Research*, *27*, 613–622.

Olsho, L. W. (1984). Infant frequency discrimination. *Infant Behavior and Development*, *7*, 27–35.

Olsho, L. W. (1985). Infant auditory perception: Tonal masking. *Infant Behavior and Development*, *8*, 371–384.

Olsho, L. W., Koch, E. G., & Carter, E. A. (1988). Nonsensory factors in infant frequency discrimination. *Infant Behavior and Development*, *11*, 205–222.

Olsho, L. W., Koch, E. G., Carter, E. A., Halpin, C. F., & Spetner, N. B. (1988). Pure-tone sensitivity of human infants. *Journal of the Acoustical Society of America*, *84*, 1316–1324.

Olsho, L. W., Koch, E. G., & Halpin, C. F. (1987). Level and age effects in infant frequency discrimination. *Journal of the Acoustical Society of America*, *82*, 454–464.

Olsho, L. W., Koch, E. G., Halpin, C. F., & Carter, E. A. (1987). An observer-based psychoacoustic procedure for use with young infants. *Developmental Psychology*, *23*, 627–640.

Olsho, L. W., Schoon, C., Sakai, R., Turpin, R., & Sperduto, V. (1982). Auditory frequency discrimination in infancy. *Developmental Psychology*, *18*, 721–726.

Patterson, R. D., Nimmo-Smith, I., Weber, D. L., & Milroy, R. (1982). The deterioration of hearing with age: Frequency selectivity, the critical ratio, the audiogram, and speech threshold. *Journal of the Acoustical Society of America*, *72*, 1788–1803.

Peters, A. M. (1986). Early syntax. In P. Fletcher & M. Garman (Eds.), *Language acquisition* (2nd ed., pp. 307–325). New York: Cambridge University Press.

Piaget, J. (1954). *The construction of reality in the child*. New York: Basic Books.

Pujol, R., Carlier, E., & Lenoir, M. (1980). Ontogenetic approach to inner and outer hair cell function. *Hearing Research*, *2*, 423–430.

Schlauch, R. S., & Hafter, E. R. (1991). Listening bandwidths and frequency uncertainty in pure-tone signal detection. *Journal of the Acoustical Society of America*, *90*, 1332–1339.

Schneider, B. A., Morrongiello, B. A., & Trehub, S. E. (1990). The size of the critical band in infants, children, and adults. *Journal of Experimental Psychology: Human Perception and Performance*, *16*, 642–652.

Schneider, B. A., Trehub, S. E., & Bull, D. (1979). The development of basic auditory processes in infants. *Canadian Journal of Psychology*, *33*, 306–319.

Schneider, B. A., Trehub, S. E., & Bull, D. (1980). High-frequency sensitivity in infants. *Science*, *207*, 1003–1004.

Schneider, B. A., Trehub, S. E., Morrongiello, B. A., & Thorpe, L. A. (1989). Developmental changes in masked thresholds. *Journal of the Acoustical Society of America*, *86*, 1733–1742.

Schneider, B. A., Trehub, S. E., & Thorpe, L. (1991). Developmental perspectives on the localization and detection of auditory signals. *Perception & Psychophysics*, *49*, 10–20.

Sinnott, J. M., & Aslin, R. N. (1985). Frequency and intensity discrimination in human infants and adults. *Journal of the Acoustical Society of America*, *78*, 1986–1992.

Sinnott, J. M., Pisoni, D. B., & Aslin, R. N. (1983). A comparison of pure tone auditory thresholds in human infants and adults. *Infant Behavior and Development*, *6*, 3–17.

Spetner, N. B., & Olsho, L. W. (1990). Auditory frequency resolution in human infancy. *Child Development*, *61*, 632–652.

Teller, D. Y. (1979). The forced-choice preferential looking procedure: A psychophysical technique for use with human infants. *Infant Behavior and Development*, *2*, 135–153.

Teller, D. Y., Morse, R., Borton, R., & Regal, D. (1974). Visual acuity for vertical and diagonal gratings in human infants. *Vision Research*, *14*, 1433–1439.

Teller, D. Y., Peeples, D. R., & Sekel, M. (1978). Discrimination of chromatic from white light by two-month-old infants. *Vision Research*, *18*, 41–48.

Trehub, S. E., Bull, D., Schneider, B. A., & Morrongiello, B. A. (1986). PESTI: A procedure for estimating individual thresholds for infant listeners. *Infant Behavior and Development*, *9*, 107–118.

Trehub, S. E., Schneider, B. A., & Bull, D. (1981). Effect of reinforcement on infants' performance in an auditory detection task. *Developmental Psychology*, *17*, 872–877.

Trehub, S. E., Schneider, B. A., & Endman, M. (1980). Developmental changes in infants' sensitivity to octave-band noises. *Journal of Experimental Child Psychology*, *29*, 282–293.

Trehub, S. E., Schneider, B. A., Thorpe, L. A., & Judge, P. (1991). Observational measures of auditory sensitivity in early infancy. *Developmental Psychology*, *27*, 40–49.

Werner, L. A., & Bargones, J. Y. (1991). Sources of auditory masking in infants: Distraction effects. *Perception & Psychophysics*, *50*, 405–412.

Werner, L. A., & Bargones, J. Y. (in press). Psychoacoustic development of human infants. In C. Rovee-Collier & L. Lipsitt (Eds.), *Advances in infancy research* (Vol. 7). Norwood, NJ: Ablex.

Werner, L. A., & Feeney, M. P. (1990). *Pure-tone sensitivity of 2- to 4-week-old infants assessed with auditory reinforcement*. Paper presented at the International Conference for Infant Studies, Montreal, Quebec, Canada.

Werner, L. A., & Gillenwater, J. M. (1990). Pure-tone sensitivity of 2- to 5-week-old infants. *Infant Behavior and Development*, *13*, 355–375.

Werner, L. A., & Marean, G. C. (1988). [Performance of infants on "probe" trials]. Unpublished raw data.

Werner, L. A., & Marean, G. C. (1991a). Methods for estimating infant thresholds. *Journal of the Acoustical Society of America*, *90*, 1867–1875.

Werner, L. A., & Marean, G. C. (1991b). *Psychometric functions of human infants for short duration tone bursts*. Paper presented at the Midwinter Research Meeting of the Association for Research in Otolaryngology, St. Petersburg Beach, FL.

Werner, L. A., & Marean, G. C. (1992). *The upper asymptote of the infant psychometric function in detection of short duration tone bursts*. Paper presented at the Midwinter Research Meeting of the Association for Research in Otolaryngology, St. Petersburg Beach, FL.

Werner, L. A., Marean, G. C., Halpin, C. F., Spetner, N. B., & Gillenwater, J. M. (1992). Infant auditory temporal acuity: Gap detection. *Child Development*.

Werner, L. A., Rickard, L. K., & Folsom, R. C. (1990). *Correlation between frequency-specific ABR and behavioral thresholds in 3-month-old infants*. Paper presented at the 120th Meeting of the Acoustical Society of America, San Diego, CA, *63*, 260–272.

Wier, C. C., Jesteadt, W., & Green, D. M. (1977). Frequency discrimination as a function of frequency and sensation level. *Journal of the Acoustical Society of America*, *61*, 178–184.

Yost, W. A. (1978). A forced-choice adaptive procedure for measuring auditory thresholds in children. *Behavioral Research Methods & Instrumentation*, *10*, 671–677.

CHAPTER 3

Interactions Between Sensory and Nonsensory Factors in the Responses of Newborn Birds to Sound

Lincoln Gray

This chapter reviews a decade of research on the hearing of newborn chickens and focuses on how both sensory and nonsensory factors affect the responsiveness of neonates. Discussions of nonsensory effects would be relatively uninteresting without some evidence that such experiments tap sensory processes. Accordingly, an introductory section reviews evidence that valid psychoacoustical measurements can be made from newborn chickens. The remainder of the chapter describes nonsensory factors that influence these results. Given that neonatal subjects do not maintain the constant vigil that characterizes the performance of mature human observers, the bulk of this chapter reviews the consequences of neonates' inattention. The chapter concludes with some suggestions for future experiments.

Caroline Petrin helped prepare the manuscript and the figures. Constantine Trahiotis ably served as a consultant throughout this research program. Bernie Mathes and Kathleen Philbin reviewed the manuscript. Work on the effects of habituation was done in collaboration with Kathleen Philbin and Diane Ballweg.

This research has been supported by the National Institutes of Health grants NS17520 to L. Gray and E. W Rubel, NS20474 and DC243 to L. Gray, and HD28261 to L. Gray and M. Kathleen Philbin.

The two major sections of this chapter constitute a dichotomy; they are separate discussions of sensory and nonsensory effects. This separation is unfortunate, however, because it is probably not productive to ask whether a particular response is due solely to either a sensory or nonsensory effect. A similar problem emerged from an attempt to determine if behaviors are due solely to either genetic or environmental influences. The resolution of this nature/nurture controversy came from experiments that investigated interactions between the formative factors (Lippe, 1976). Similarly, sensory and nonsensory factors interact to determine neonates' responsiveness to sound. Thus, this chapter shows how nonsensory effects change with age, species, and experience and lead to various nonparallel changes in auditory responsiveness as a function of state, distraction, duration, and habituation. Such nonparallel trends are indicative of important interactions.

In conclusion, the goal of this review is to facilitate an appreciation for the fascinating mix of sensory and nonsensory factors in developmental psychoacoustics. Some general trends in perceptual development are suggested by the similarity in results from human and avian neonates. There are three "take-home" messages. The most important of these is that neonatal psychophysics must include an analysis of interactions between sensory and nonsensory factors. Second, stimuli may need to be presented at relatively low levels to minimize the effect of inattention. Finally, nonsensory factors are not just nuisance variables; they are interesting dependent variables in their own right, and important experiments can be designed to further investigate their influence on sensory information processing by developing organisms.

Sensory Effects

Consistent and interpretable psychoacoustical measurements can be made from newborn chickens. These subjects have an unconditioned response that is useful for such studies. They peep nearly incessantly but momentarily delay their ongoing vocalizations when they detect a sound (Kerr, Ostapoff, & Rubel, 1979). An unbiased measure of performance, the area under a receiver operating characteristic (ROC), can be derived from the pooled responses of many chicks (Gray, 1987, 1990a, 1992b). A two-alternative, forced-choice testing procedure can also be devised when stimulus and control trials are presented in pairs, and a "correct" response is inferred whenever the delay on a stimulus trial is greater than that on a control trial (Gray, 1990b; Gray & Rubel, 1985).

The following brief review of a series of experiments strongly suggests that this unconditioned response can tap sensory processes. First, ROCs from these subjects closely resemble those from mature human and animal observers. Second, psychometric functions from chicks are well described by a cumulative normal distribution, as in mature humans. Third, low-frequency thresholds are mature at birth. Fourth, masked pure-tone thresholds are proportional to the level of a broadband masker. Fifth, there is a strong effect of duration on threshold. Finally, thresholds of a pure tone are elevated by the presence of a second tone of a similar frequency in the same pattern in newborn chickens and mature humans. The first three results (ROCs, psychometric function, and audiogram) show that the techniques used were sensitive. Because responses under some conditions are as sensitive as those obtained from mature subjects, one can comfortably surmise that the procedures were appropriate. The last three results (growth of masking, temporal integration, and tuning curves) generally follow the laws of physical acoustics and contribute to confidence in a sensory effect. Of course, inferences about the perceptions of nonverbal neonates will always be somewhat speculative. A failure to respond may be due to an inability to detect the stimulus, to an inappropriate procedure, or to a nonsensory factor such as lapsing attention. Despite this uncertainty, an accumulation of consistent observations leads to some confidence that these results reflect an underlying sensory process.

General Methods

Subjects are white leghorn chicks, incubated and hatched in the university laboratory and tested at 0 days and again at 4 days of age (Gray, in press). Subjects are individually tested in a small (2-L) Plexiglas chamber suspended below a microphone and above a speaker built to produce a relatively uniform sound field. The microphone provides the input to a specially built "peep detector" that signals a computer with 99% accuracy at the end of the loud regular peeps of the subjects (Severns, Gray, & Rubel, 1985). Subjects are acclimated to the chamber for about 2 min, after which they begin to peep at a regular rate. Various stimulus and control trials are then presented for up to 15–20 min for each subject. A sensitive dependent variable, termed *delay,* is the elapsed time between the start of a trial and the end of the second poststimulus peep (Gray, 1987). Discarding data from a small number of somnolent subjects (defined a priori as those that fail to peep for 2 min at any time during the test) ensures that delays are elicited by acoustic stimuli. Different rules for when to start the trials have been used. A simple criterion used in initial experiments of at least two peeps in 2 s ensured that trials were started when the birds were peeping. Recently, more precisely defined intervals between a peep and the start of a trial have been shown to enhance responsiveness (Gray, 1990a).

Receiver Operating Characteristics, a Psychometric Function, and an Audiogram

An acoustic stimulus can cause a delay in the otherwise regular peeping of newborn chickens. The response is variable, however, and it is not easy to determine if the subjects heard a stimulus on the basis of a small number of delays. ROCs provide a sensitive analysis of this response because they combine a large number of delays in a way that can be thought of as including all possible definitions of how much delay is considered to be a "yes" response. ROCs are constructed from comparisons of delays accumulated over many stimulus and control trials (Gray, 1987, 1990a, 1992). Briefly, these delays are treated as if they were sensitive rating scales. The duration of the delay is taken to indicate the chick's confidence that a stimulus was presented, and traditional methods are used to construct ROCs (Watson & Nichols, 1976; Watson, Rilling, & Bourbon, 1964). A detailed discussion of these methods is beyond the scope of this chapter. The methods are computationally demanding but conceptually straightforward. A computer pools delays on control trials, plots the area under this histogram, and compares it with the area under a similar histogram from stimulus trials given all possible definitions of how much delay is considered to indicate that the subject heard the sound. For example, if any delay greater than some low value (e.g., 0.3 s) were taken as an indication that the subject heard a sound, then there would be many "hits" but also many false alarms from a collection of stimulus and control trials. Increasing this criterion should decrease the rate of false alarms on control trials faster than it should the rate of hits on stimulus trials; the form of this function is a careful quantification of responsiveness.

The ROCs from chicks and mature humans are similar (see Figure 1). ROCs from these different forms of ratings—delays from chickens and latencies and confidence scales from humans—suggest that the unconditioned response in chicks is a reasonable representation of signal detection.

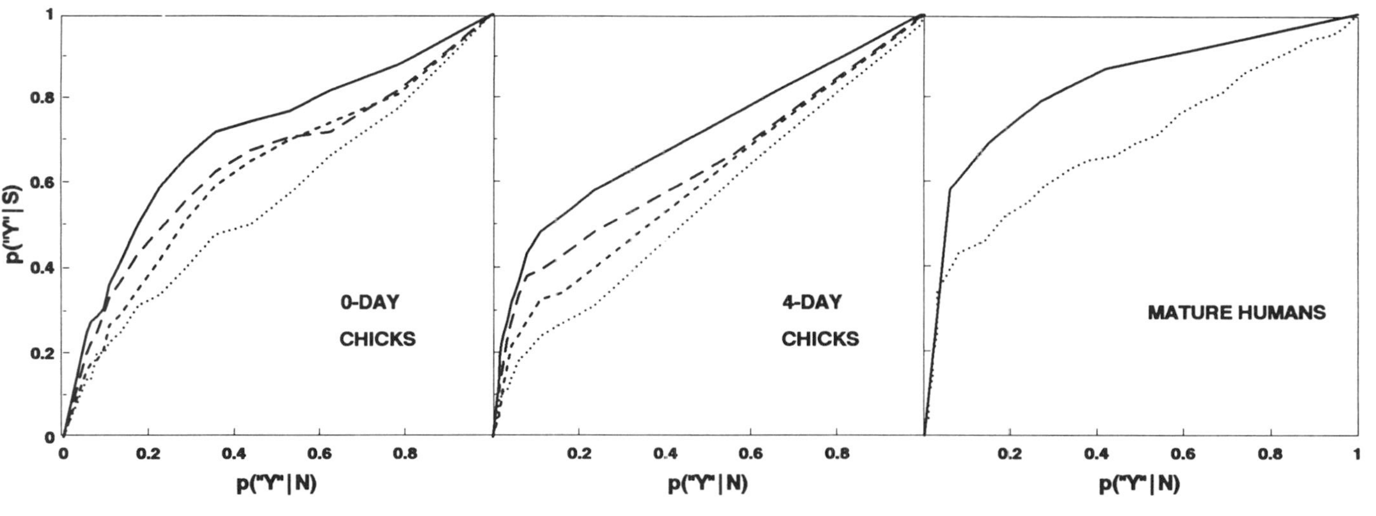

FIGURE 1 Examples of receiver operating characteristics. Chick data are delays resulting from 3-dB increases in intensity, shown by dotted to dashed to solid lines. (From Gray, 1992a. Copyright 1992 by the Acoustical Society of America.) Human data are from response latencies (dotted line, Emmerich, Gray, Watson, & Tanis, 1972. Copyright 1972 by the Psychonomic Society) and a 6-point rating procedure (solid line, Green & Swets, 1974. Copyright 1973 by D. M. Green and J. A. Swets). All material reprinted by permission.

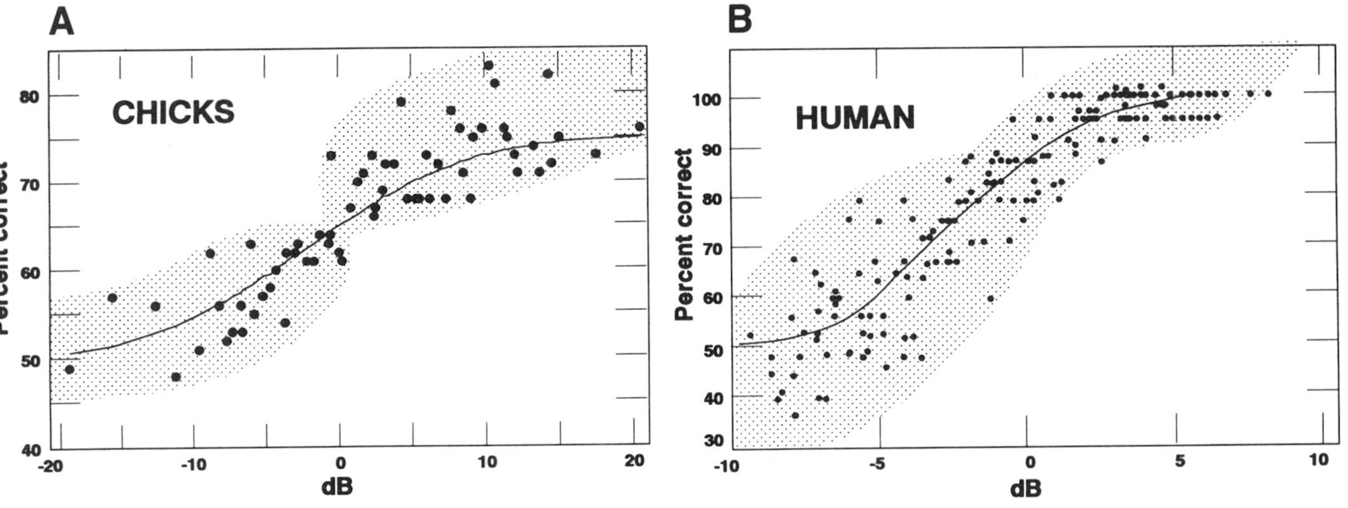

FIGURE 2 Examples of psychometric functions. Chick data are areas under ROCs. (From 1992a Gray, Copyright 1992 by the Acoustical Society of America.) Human data are from the forced-choice performance of a single subject. (From Green & Swets, 1974. Copyright 1973 by D. M. Green and J. A. Swets.) Shading has been added to represent expected variability. Decibels are relative to the approximate "sweet point," a desirable estimate of threshold with minimum variability as discussed in the text. All material reprinted by permission.

Psychometric functions can be derived from areas under these ROCs. The responsiveness of both chicks and mature humans, for example, can be described by the S-shaped ogive of the cumulative normal distribution (see Figure 2).

Absolute thresholds can be estimated for various frequencies at various ages (see Figure 3). Note that low-frequency thresholds are similar for chicks at ages 0 days and 4 days and are similar to data from other species of mature birds collected with time-consuming operant-conditioning techniques that would not have been possible in a developmental analysis. These similarities, both within

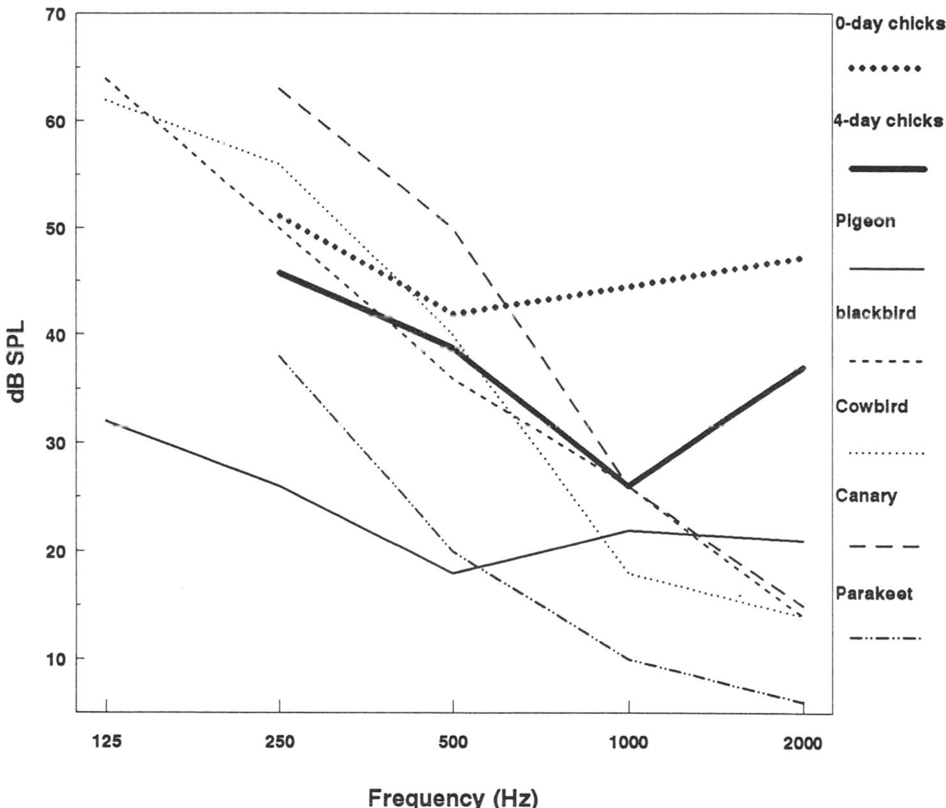

FIGURE 3 Avian audiograms. Absolute thresholds for various species of birds are shown. Chick data are estimates of the psychometric function at 65% correct. The other data are from mature birds (reviewed in Fay, 1988). From Gray (1992a). Copyright 1992 by the Acoustical Society of America. Reprinted by permission. SPL = sound pressure level.

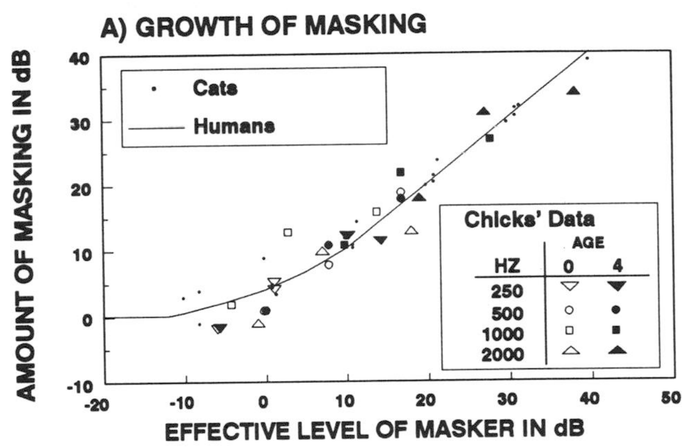
A) GROWTH OF MASKING
Cats
Humans
Chicks' Data
AGE
HZ 0 4
250
500
1000
2000
AMOUNT OF MASKING IN dB
EFFECTIVE LEVEL OF MASKER IN dB
40
30
20
10
0
-10
-20
-10
0
10
20
30
40
50

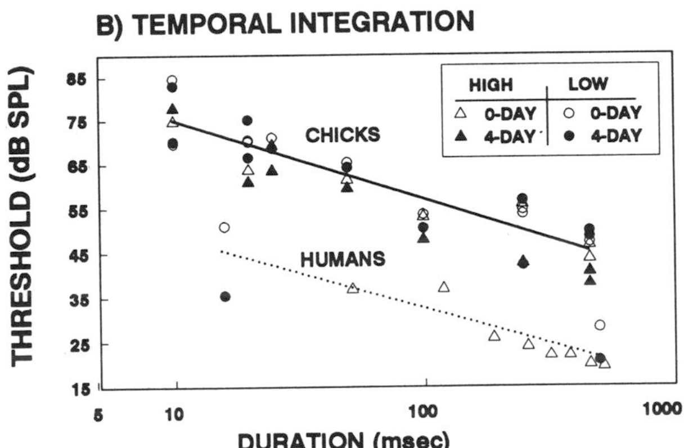
B) TEMPORAL INTEGRATION
HIGH
LOW
0-DAY
4-DAY
0-DAY
4-DAY
CHICKS
HUMANS
THRESHOLD (dB SPL)
DURATION (msec)
85
75
65
55
45
35
25
15
5
10
100
1000

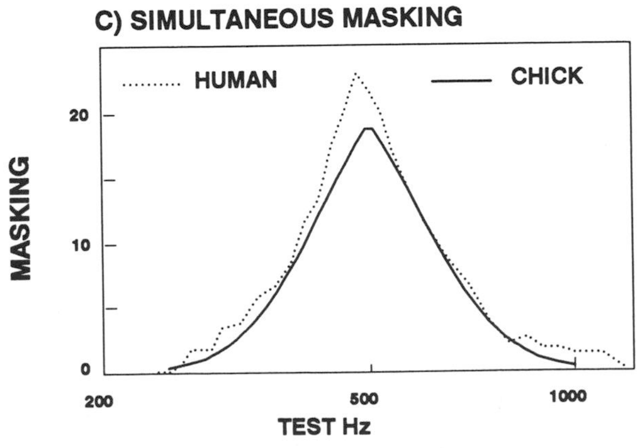
C) SIMULTANEOUS MASKING
HUMAN
CHICK
MASKING
TEST Hz
20
10
0
200
500
1000

and between species, indicate that the procedure used in this experiment was appropriate for these newborn subjects. It is, in other words, unlikely that a different procedure would result in much lower estimates of sensory sensitivity. Rapidly changing thresholds at high frequencies are thus likely to reflect a sensory process. Fortunately, this trend has been replicated in other behavioral studies of chickens (Gray, 1990b; Gray & Rubel, 1981, 1985), and consensus on a similar trend in young humans seems to be emerging (Werner & Bargones, in press).

Frequency and Temporal Effects

Figure 4A shows the way in which the thresholds of pure tones change in the presence of a broadband masker (Gray, in press). Thresholds increase 1 dB for every decibel of increase in the spectrum level of the masker in chicks as they do in mature humans and other animals. This shows that the chicks follow a fundamental principle of acoustics (linear integration of energy), strongly suggesting that these estimates are related to a sensory process.

Further evidence for a sensory process comes from the effect of duration on thresholds. As seen in Figure 4B, thresholds in both chicks and humans fall as durations increase (Gray, 1990b). This suggests that both species of neonates respond to accumulated acoustic energy.

The final evidence for a sensory process that will be presented in this chapter is simultaneous masking. The presence of a pure tone interferes with the ability to detect the presence of another tone of similar frequency. The pattern of this interference, termed a *masking function,* is similar in chicks and humans (see Figure 4C; Ehmer, 1959; Gray, 1992b).

FIGURE 4 Sensory effects. (*A*) shows a consistent growth of masked thresholds with the level of a broadband masker. (From Gray, in press, Copyright John Wiley & Sons; with data from Hawkins & Stevens, 1950, and Watson, 1963. Also from Fay, 1988. Copyright 1988 by Hill-Fay Associates.) (*B*) shows temporal integration functions in newborn chicks and humans. (From Gray, 1990b. Copyright 1990 by Elsevier; with human data from Olsho & Marean, 1988, Thorpe & Schneider, 1987.) (*C*) shows simultaneous masking, the amount that the threshold of a 500-Hz tone is increased by constant pure tones of various frequencies. Chick data are from Gray (1992b). Human data are from Ehmer (1959, Copyright 1959 by the Acoustical Society of America). In humans, the maskers were approximately 40 dB above threshold and in chicks were about 25 dB above threshold. All material reprinted by permission.

Summary of Sensory Effects

These six examples (ROCs, psychometric function, the audiogram, growth of masking, temporal integration, and simultaneous masking) show remarkable similarity in the responses of newborn chicks and humans. It is unlikely that changes in the testing procedures would dramatically improve the sensitivity of these estimates. The data show that delays vary with physical properties of acoustic stimuli.

The remainder of this review will highlight possible consequences of inattention to these stimuli. Throughout this discussion, however, remember the overall evidence that the response taps sensory processes. The nonsensory effects to be described are interesting perturbations on predominately sensory effects.

Nonsensory Effects

Nonsensory factors are variables that affect responsiveness but are not related to the physical characteristics of the stimulus. Inattention is probably the most important nonsensory factor in neonates. Accordingly, the core of this chapter will review several ramifications of inattention. These include suboptimal performance, state-dependent changes, distraction, changing patterns of temporal integration, reactions to natural and unnatural sounds, and habituation. In each example, a nonsensory effect causes an interaction between auditory responsiveness and age, species, or experience, causing nonparallel trends across different groups.

Suboptimal Responsiveness

The most detailed assessment of inattention in these newborn listeners comes from the signal detection analyses. The psychometric function in Figure 2 shows that responsiveness rises to a maximum of only about 75% (Gray, 1992b). This less-than-perfect upper asymptote has an important implication for neonatal psychoacoustics.

Green (1990) determined, by theory and observation, that the "sweet point" (the level that leads to minimum variability) in human adaptive procedures occurs at about 90% correct. Finding the point of minimum variability at such high levels is not expected because the "steep point" (the point of maximum slope in the psychometric function) is at 75%, halfway between chance and perfection. Consequently, it has been popular to use the two-down, one-up rule, which is both simple and tracks a level eliciting 71% correct responses, very close to the steep point but not sweet point. Nevertheless, variability in threshold estimates is reduced at higher levels.

The sweet point is, however, lowered by inattention. As momentary lapses of attention become more frequent, the point of minimum variability decreases because misses have less effect when a lower proportion of correct responses is used to estimate threshold (Green, 1990). Chicks attain maximum responsiveness of about 75% (Gray, in press), equivalent to human observers who have lapses of attention half the time. If g is the probability of inattention, maximum responsiveness is $1 - g/2$ because an inattentive listener will be "correct" half the time by pure chance.

Green (personal communication) extended his calculations for levels of inattention as high as 50%, the level necessary to explain the maximum responsiveness of 75% observed in these chicks (Gray, in press). For 50% attention the sweet point is 67.6% (an extension of Green, 1990, Figure 7, for $g = .5$). Examination of the psychometric function in Figure 2 shows this to coincide closely with the data from Gray (in press). A shaded area, representing expected variability, has been drawn over the data to emphasize this congruence. A similarly shaded area has been drawn over mature human data to show a higher point of minimum variability.

In conclusion, chicks reach a maximum responsiveness of about 75% (Gray, in press). Human infants also show similar results, reaching maximum responsiveness at levels below perfection (Berg & Smith, 1983; Trehub, Schneider, & Endman, 1980; Werner & Gillenwater, 1990). This means that neonates are, for whatever reason, inattentive on a large percentage of trials. Fortunately, once this inattention is acknowledged and included in models of desirable procedures, variability in the responsiveness of chicks and humans appears to follow similar patterns. Chicks have the unique advantage that their sweet point and steep point are approximately the same. A take-home message is thus to track a level of about 65%.

Use of ROCs to estimate the level required to elicit 65% correct responses is an appropriate way to evaluate neonates' responsiveness, but it requires data from many subjects. Such a method of constant stimuli can be inefficient without some previous knowledge of thresholds. Some appropriate adaptive procedure would thus be helpful, if only for an initial estimate of sensitivity. The common

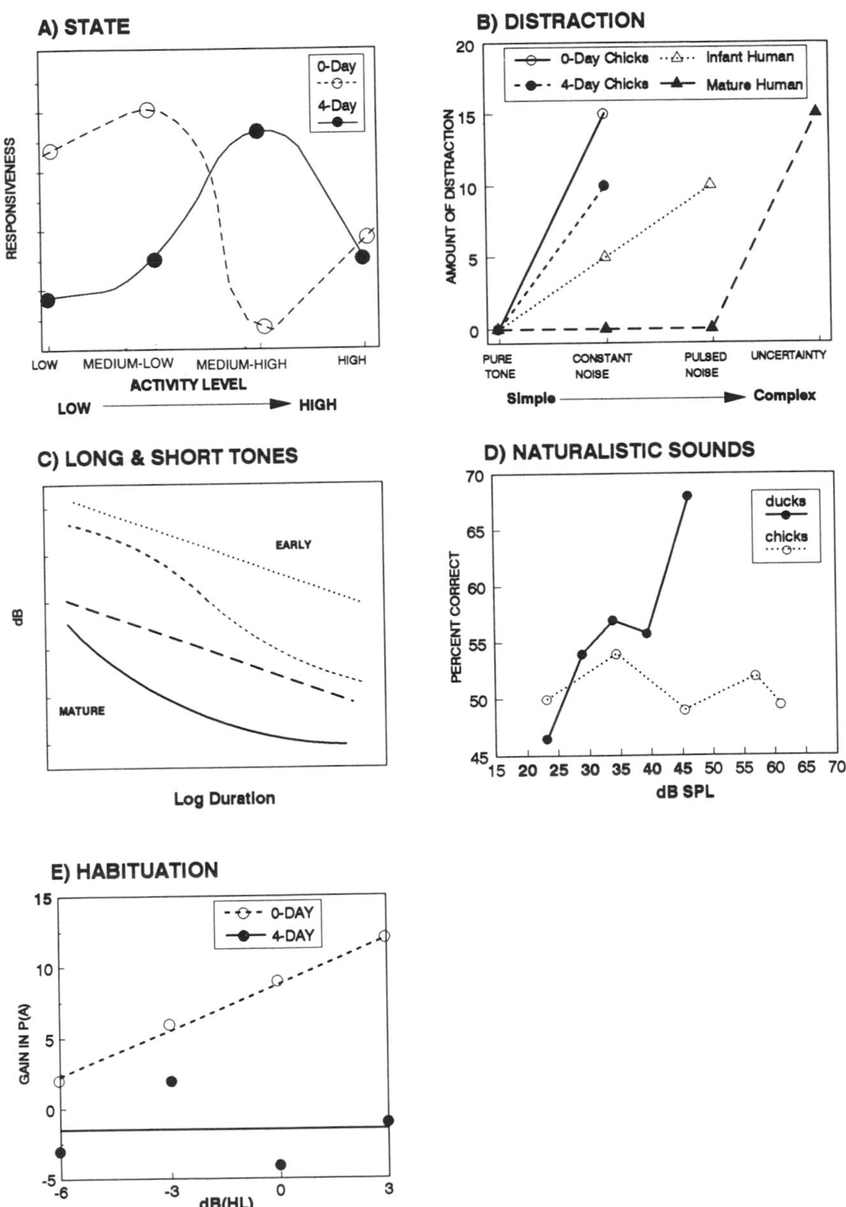

FIGURE 5 Nonsensory effects. Shown are six ways that nonsensory factors interact with age, species, and early experience to produce nonparallel trends. (*A*) shows relative responsiveness at different levels of prestimulus activity. (Adapted from Gray, 1990a. Copyright 1991 by John Wiley & Sons.) (*B*) is a speculative model of the amount of masking, termed *distraction*, that

two-down, one-up staircase procedure seems doomed to failure because it tracks a level (71%) above the steep point and sweet point and almost at the asymptote. A method of maximum likelihood could be devised to estimate the 65% point on the psychometric function and could also possibly include a correction for expected habituation.

State-Dependent Changes

Young chickens, like young humans, rapidly change their attentional status, oscillating between periods of somnolent and frenetic activity. One might hypothesize that maximum responsiveness should be observed at an intermediate state because this has been observed in humans (Wilson & Thompson, 1984). Human infants should be in a quiet alert state, not sleeping and not fussing, for maximum responsiveness. In chicks, a measure of prestimulus activity can be easily obtained from the rate of peeping immediately before the stimulus. A signal detection analysis of how prestimulus peeping affects poststimulus delays provides a detailed quantitative description of how responsiveness varies with the level of activity (Gray, 1990a). This function is bell shaped, as predicted, rising to a maximum at moderate levels of prestimulus activity (see Figure 5A). Interestingly, the curves are skewed differently at the two ages: Newborn chicks are maximally responsive when there is a slightly longer pause between their peeps and the onset of a stimulus, compared with the 4-day-old chicks. In other words, as animals mature, they are maximally responsive at increasing levels of activity. This view, that younger subjects need to be less active, is consistent with the theory

---

cannot be explained by peripheral or sensory effects. (From Werner & Bargones, 1991. Copyright 1991 by the Psychonomic Society.) Chick data are from Gray (1992a. Copyright 1992 by the Acoustical Society of America); infant data are from Werner and Bargones (1991); and the mature human data are averages based on Neff and Callaghan (1988). (*C*) is a model of developing temporal integration. (From Gray, 1990b. Copyright 1990 by Elsevier.) It suggests that mature responses are observed to long durations before short. (*D*) shows psychometric functions to a duck-like sound from ducklings and chicks. (From Gray & Jahrsdoerfer, 1986. Copyright 1986 by the American Psychological Association.) (*E*) shows the increase in areas under ROCs when chicks are exposed to multiple versus a single frequency. (From Gray, 1992a. Copyright 1992 by the Acoustical Society of America.) All material adapted by permission.

that immature auditory systems react more slowly (Morgan & Zimmerman, 1987; Olsho & Halpin, 1987).

In conclusion, there is an interaction of this nonsensory effect with age. The state in which these neonates are optimally responsive to the acoustic stimulus changes with age.

Distraction

Although the growth of masking (the increase in pure-tone thresholds caused by a white-noise background) is proportional to the spectrum level of the masker, (see Figure 4A), the amount of masking is too great to be caused by the masker alone. Such masking provides an unreasonable measure of frequency resolution. The extent that the auditory system can separate one frequency from others can be derived by subtracting the level of the background noise from the masked threshold to get a "critical ratio" (Scharf, 1970). It is like calculating the width of a rectangle by dividing its area by height. One can assume that the energy in a tone at threshold equals the energy in some band of frequencies surrounding the tone. If all frequencies contribute equally to the masking, then the number of frequencies that contribute to the masking multiplied by the noise level at each frequency would equal the amount of masking. This formula works well for mature subjects but not for neonates. The calculations suggest that frequencies that contribute to the masking of a pure tone extend beyond the range of frequencies that the animal can hear, which is absurd (Gray, in press). Sounds that are clearly different from the signal must somehow decrease the subject's attention.

Such a nonsensory factor, called *attentional* or *distraction masking* (Werner & Bargones, 1991), has also been shown to elevate thresholds in human infants. That is, background noise somehow distracts newborn chicks and humans, but once this distraction is subtracted, the results are completely consistent with those from acoustic theory and data from mature subjects. There are 15 dB of such distraction masking in 0-day-old chicks, 10 dB in 4-day-old chicks, and 5–10 dB in human infants depending on whether the noise is continuous (Gray, in press; Werner & Bargones, 1991).

This distraction does not occur with all maskers. Figure 4C shows simultaneous masking functions, the effect of a pure tone on the threshold of a second pure tone of similar frequency. The amount of masking reaches zero when the two tones are about an octave apart. *Zero masking* means that the presence of one tone has no effect on the threshold of another. Obviously, something is different between white noise and pure tones that leads to different amounts of distraction.

A speculative hypothesis (see Figure 5B) is that there might be an interaction between age and nonsensory masking. The hypothesis is that as subjects mature, the complexity of a masker has to be increased in order to get a given amount of distraction. The interaction is easiest to see at the extremes, where neonates appear to be distracted by all but the simplest maskers and where adults are only distracted by very complex maskers. Figure 5B shows the distraction caused by simple to complex maskers in two ages of chicks and humans. The simplest maskers are pure tones, which cause no distraction. The next most complex masker is continuous noise, which causes 15 dB of distraction in 0-day-old chicks, 10 dB in 4-day-old chicks, and 5 dB in human infants. The next most complex masker is pulsed noise, which causes 10 dB of distraction in human infants. The most complex masker is one that changes on every interval. This uncertainty causes between 0 and 30 dB of masking in mature humans (graphed as a group average like the other data) even though no component of the masker is close enough in frequency to the test tone to cause any peripheral sensory interference (Neff & Callaghan, 1988).

In conclusion, there appears to be an interaction between complexity and age in distraction. Youngsters are more easily distracted than are adults. It could be instructive to measure distraction by complex maskers at young ages to determine how this nonsensory effect changes with age.

Temporal Integration

The relation between threshold and duration is the same in both chickens and humans (see Figure 4B), but in both species thresholds decline more rapidly than normal as duration is increased. Thresholds decrease by almost 6 dB per doubling of duration, roughly twice the slope of 3 dB per doubling that describes the behavior of a perfect integrator of acoustic energy. The overall steeper slope in neonates can be explained by the effect of multiple looks (Viemeister & Wakefield, 1991), given a psychometric function that is twice as steep in adults as in neonates (see Figure 2). In other words, sensitivity should increase with stimulus duration because there is more opportunity for the external signal to be greater than the supposedly fluctuating internal noise. This effect of duration will be greater on a response that rises slowly with intensity. Detailed examination of the chick data, however, shows that as high-frequency thresholds improve, they do so at long durations before they do so at short ones (Gray, 1990b). A speculative model of shifting attention was used to explain these data. The model combines an attentional disadvantage that occurs at increasingly shorter intervals as subjects mature, alternating with general increases in sensitivity. This model of maturing sensitivity at long before short durations fits well with data from both human and avian neonates (see Figure 5C; Gray, 1990b). The data support a theory that the speed of auditory processing appears to increase with age, as do the state-dependent changes described above.

In conclusion, thresholds at short durations are likely explained by a nonsensory effect that limits the abilities of neonates to attend to brief stimuli. This is another example of a nonsensory factor interacting with age to produce a nonparallel trend in different ages (Figure 5C).

Species-Appropriate and Species-Inappropriate Stimulation

Neonatal animals appear to show enhanced sensitivity to species-typical acoustic stimulation. Chicks' responsiveness to changes in frequency, for example, is greatest at frequencies found in the maternal call (Gray & Rubel, 1981). Human infants are most responsive to their mothers' voices (DeCasper & Fifer, 1980). The responsiveness of ducklings drops off as the acoustic cues of the signal begin to differ from those of normal maternal calls (Miller, 1983).

A nonparallel, nonsensory effect is most clearly seen in a comparison of different species. Newborn birds are most responsive to changes that resemble important cues in the maternal call of their own species (Gray & Jahrsdoerfer, 1986). Ducklings' and chicks' psychometric functions to a ducklike sound are not parallel (see Figure 5D). Ducklings show a sensitive response, whereas chicks show no response above chance. The function is steep when the signal is appropriate (i.e., when ducklings respond to a ducklike sound) and flat when inappropriate (i.e., chicks responding to the duck call). This cannot be a sensory effect because the result is the opposite of that predicted by physiological recordings; peripheral evoked potentials are approximately 12 dB more sensitive in chicks than in ducklings in this frequency range (Saunders, Gates, & Coles, 1974). Increased attention to species-typical sounds thus provides another example of an interaction involving a nonsensory effect, in this instance between different species.

Inappropriate testing conditions also affect neonatal psychoacoustics. The responsiveness of newborn ducklings to their maternal call is enhanced if the testing conditions are similar to rearing conditions (Blaich, Miller, & Hicinbothom, 1989). Specifically, ducklings reared in groups but tested individually, and vice versa, do not show normal sensitivity. This is another example of an interaction between sensory and nonsensory effects.

Habituation

Rapid habituation appears to be a normal consequence of psychoacoustical testing in newborn chicks. That is, although mature humans may be as sensitive at the end of a session as at the beginning, newborn chicks require ever increasing levels of stimulation to maintain the same level of responsiveness. This decreasing responsiveness has been observed as steadily increasing staircases and as flattening psychometric functions. Each peak in an adaptive procedure, the level required for two successive correct responses, is approximately 5 dB above the previous peak in newborn chicks (Gray & Rubel, 1985, Figure 4). Psychometric functions (see Figure 2) may be as steep as about 2% per decibel on the first few trials, but they flatten to less than 0.5% per decibel after 5–10 trials and disappear (no reliable increase in responsiveness over intensity) after 15–20 trials (Gray, 1992b).

Habituation is also a normal consequence of psychoacoustical testing in humans and is used as a test of normal behavioral development in human infants (Brazelton, 1984). This assessment involves flashing a light or ringing a bell and observing the amount of movement by the infant. Healthy infants show decreasing responsiveness after several presentations. Thus, rapid habituation is interpreted as an indication of an intact and well-organized neurobehavioral system. This desirable response can be observed in healthy infants who sleep through repetitive distractions.

Attempts to prevent habituation in chicks have only been partially successful. Different procedural changes have different effects on different ages. That is, Age × Procedure interactions affect habituation. For example, responsiveness of 0-day-old but not 4-day-old chicks improves when they are presented with a variety of different frequencies during a test session. The amount of this improvement increases as stimuli get louder (Gray, 1992b; see Figure 5E). This figure shows the increased areas under ROCs when animals are presented with four versus one frequency at four different intensities. All levels in Figure 5E have been corrected for any age-related changes in sensitivity (Gray, 1992b). The interaction is likely due to rapidly decreasing attention to repeated presentations of loud tones at a single frequency in 0-day-old but not in 4-day-old chicks. This is a fifth nonsensory effect that is not parallel across ages.

Habituation in neonates is normal and may be unavoidable in prolonged testing of a single subject. Habituation should be expected and measured to assure that neonates are behaving normally. It should be viewed as an important part of neonatal psychoacoustics, not an unfortunate departure from the assumption of traditional psychoacoustical testing.

Habituation is usually thought of as a sensory effect because afferents stop responding to steady stimulation. Subjects cease to notice constant stimulation such as odors, the shadows of vessels on the retina, otoacoustic emissions, and pressure on the body in part because of decreasing sensory responsiveness. But habituation may also have a nonsensory component. If neonates were to tire of vigilance, then increasing inattention would combine with sensory habituation. The problem is how to separate different causes of similar behavioral changes. The Age × Procedure interaction provides a clue about the portion of the decreasing responsiveness that is due to nonsensory factors.

Effects of Experience on Habituation

If decreasing responsiveness were due to a nonsensory factor, and if a manipulation could be found that affected nonsensory but not sensory aspects of the response, then it might be possible to experimentally separate these components of a response. Studies of how early experience affects habituation provide such a way to quantify a nonsensory contribution. For example, a recent study showed that exposure to noise affects chicks' habituation (Philbin, Ballweg, & Gray, 1992). Chicks were exposed continuously to noises recorded in a neonatal intensive care unit (NICU) from before hatching until testing at 4 days of age. The birds exposed to noise showed no reliable habituation (Ballweg, 1991). It seems unlikely that this can be due to a sensory effect because exposure to noise made the subjects more responsive than normal at the end of the test. Noise is generally hypothesized to decrease responsiveness through a sensory effect of desensitization or receptor damage. But noise in this experiment caused the opposite result, suggesting that habituation may have an important nonsensory component. Habituation was measured as an important dependent variable, not just avoided as a nuisance. Interesting experiments can thus be designed to explore the effects of various manipulations (e.g., early experiences) on nonsensory processes (e.g., habituation).

Summary of Nonsensory Factors

Several nonsensory factors that affect the responsiveness of neonatal chicks to acoustic stimuli have been reviewed. Fortunately, there is ample evidence that current procedures successfully tap sensory processes in these newborn chicks. An understanding of the interactions between sensory and nonsensory factors provides the challenge of neonatal psychoacoustics.

Inattention is the primary nonsensory factor that decreases responsiveness in these subjects. Inattention appears in many forms: maximum responsiveness at moderate levels of prestimulus activity, distractions, changing temporal integration, and habituation beyond what is expected from sensory adaptation. Inattention also contributes to psychometric functions that form an asymptote at less than perfect performance and to the variability that seems to be inherent in the responses of neonates. An understanding of such nonsensory factors can be used to devise stimuli and testing conditions that maximize performance. For example, neonates are most responsive at middle levels of activity and are inattentive when sleepy or agitated; they are distracted by background noise. Habituation in newborn chicks is reduced when each subject hears multiple frequencies, possibly by maintaining their attention to novel stimuli. Atypical early experiences affect attention (through decreased habituation) and may contribute to later abnormal perceptual development.

Such nonsensory conditions are not unique to neonatal psychoacoustics. Attention in adult monkeys, for example, can affect cortical potentials (Spitzer, Desimone, & Moran, 1988). Nonsensory factors can also influence mature human observers. For example, subjects respond differently depending on whether they are told to expect speech or nonspeech stimuli (Bentin & Mann, 1990; Tomiak, Mullennix, & Sawusch, 1987). Relative responsiveness, that is, rates of hits and false alarms, can be altered by criterion shifts in the classic model of detection theory (Green & Swets, 1974). It is difficult to explain the masking caused by uncertain signals in terms of a peripheral sensory effect (Neff & Callaghan, 1988). In all of these examples, responsiveness depends on how the subject chooses to listen to the signal.

Conclusions

Nonsensory effects change with age, species, and experience. These nonsensory effects diminish, but may not always disappear, with maturity. Nonsensory factors need to be investigated, not avoided, for a full understanding of perceptual development.

What Is a Nonsensory Effect?

It is difficult to unambiguously define a nonsensory effect. Such usually unspecified variables include a combination of factors that influence responsiveness and are not directly related to physical characteristics of the manipulated stimulus. These might include attention, memory, motivation, state, motor coordination, tendency to be distracted, and others. No sensory effect can be observed without some nonsensory effect: No animal perceives without some attention or memory, no psychophysical response occurs without some motor activity, and all subjects are in some "state." Thus, sensory and nonsensory effects cannot be unambiguously separated. The challenge of neonatal psychophysics is to pursue the importance of their interaction.

Future Studies

Future studies to evaluate nonsensory effects on neonates' responsiveness might include (a) tests of how complexity affects distraction at different ages, (b) more comparisons of naturalistic and atypical stimuli and testing conditions, and (c) more experiments on the roles of early experience on nonsensory factors.

First, the compelling demonstration of distraction masking in human infants (pure-tone thresholds elevated by a band of noise that could not encroach on the critical band; Werner & Bargones, 1991) needs to be repeated in chicks. Then changing acoustic characteristics of these maskers could be used to evaluate Age × Complexity interactions in distractions. The distraction produced by a narrow band of flanking noise should decrease with age.

Developmental changes in the distractions caused by complex maskers are unknown. Uncertain maskers, even if all the acoustic energy is outside the critical band, still affect sensitivity of mature subjects, demonstrating that nonsensory effects may not disappear with age (Neff & Callaghan, 1988). The effect of these uncertain maskers on neonates could be used to determine an upper asymptote of distraction, which may or may not change with age.

Second, there have been few psychoacoustical experiments with naturalistic stimuli. Psychometric functions, for example, could be created to maternal sounds, and these might be steeper or less variable than functions elicited by pure tones. Difference limens to acoustic cues that vary along species-relevant dimensions could also be measured. Responsiveness in the controlled conditions of traditional psychoacoustics needs to be compared with that in naturalistic conditions.

Finally, attention should be given to the roles of early experience in nonsensory factors. An abnormal nonsensory process, such as habituation, could cascade to affect other nonsensory processes, such as distraction, and lead to a variety of attentional and perceptual disorders.

Summary

Hearing in newborn chicks can be measured by an unconditioned delay in their usually regular peeps. This responsiveness of neonates to sound is determined by an interaction between sensory and nonsensory factors. This interaction causes nonparallel changes in auditory responsiveness among developmentally different groups (due to age, species, or experience). Sensory factors are shown by ROCs, psychometric functions, thresholds, temporal integration, and masking to affect newborn chicks and humans in the same ways. Nonsensory factors cause less than perfect performance and cause responsiveness to vary with the subject's behavioral state, duration of the sound, and whether the sound was naturalistic. Nonsensory factors also cause distractions by background maskers and rapid habituation. These nonsensory factors are affected by age, species, and early experience. Suggestions from this review are to estimate neonates' thresholds at relatively low rates of responsiveness and to design more experiments that measure and manipulate the contribution of nonsensory factors.

References

Ballweg, D. (1991). *The effect of neonatal intensive care unit noise on the habituation of neonatal chicks*. Unpublished master's thesis, University of Texas Health Science Center at Houston, School of Nursing.

Bentin, S., & Mann, V. (1990). Masking and stimulus intensity effects on duplex perception: A confirmation of the dissociation between speech and nonspeech modes. *Journal of the Acoustical Society of America*, *88*, 64–74.

Berg, K. M., & Smith, M. C. (1983). Behavioral thresholds for tones during infancy. *Journal of Experimental Child Psychology*, *35*, 409–425.

Blaich, C., Miller, D., & Hicinbothom, G. (1989). Alarm call responsivity of mallard ducklings: VII. Interaction between developmental history and behavioral context. *Developmental Psychobiology*, *22*, 203–210.

Brazelton, T. (1984). *Neonatal behavioral assessment scale. Clinics in developmental medicine* (No. 88, 2nd ed.). Philadelphia: Lippincott.

DeCasper, A. J., & Fifer, W. P. (1980). Of human bonding: Newborns prefer their mothers' voices. *Science*, *208*, 1174–1176.

Ehmer, R. H. (1959). Masking patterns of tones. *Journal of the Acoustical Society of America*, *31*, 1115–1120.

Emmerich, D. S., Gray, J. A., Watson, C. S., & Tanis, D. C. (1972). Response latency, confidence, and ROCs in auditory signal detection. *Perception & Psychophysics*, *2*, 65–72.

Fay, R. R. (1988). *Hearing in vertebrates: A psychophysics data book*. Winnetka, IL: Hill-Fay.

Gray, L. (1987). Signal detection analyses of delays in neonates' vocalizations. *Journal of the Acoustical Society of America*, *82*, 1608–1614.

Gray, L. (1990a). Activity level and auditory responsiveness in neonatal chickens. *Developmental Psychobiology*, *23*, 297–308.

Gray, L. (1990b). Development of temporal integration in newborn chickens. *Hearing Research*, *45*, 169–177.

Gray, L. (1992a). An auditory psychometric function from newborn chicks. *Journal of the Acoustical Society of America*, *91*, 1608–1615.

Gray, L. (1992b). Simultaneous masking in newborn chickens. *Association for Research in Otolaryngology Abstracts*, *15*, 50.

Gray, L. (in press). Developmental changes in chickens' masked thresholds. *Developmental Psychobiology*.

Gray, L., & Jahrsdoerfer, R. (1986). Naturalistic psychophysics: Thresholds of ducklings (*Anas platyrynchos*) and chicks (*Gallus gallus*) to tones that resemble mallard calls. *Journal of Comparative Psychology*, *100*, 91–94.

Gray, L., & Rubel, E. W. (1981). Development of responsiveness to suprathreshold acoustic stimulation in chickens. *Journal of Comparative and Physiological Psychology*, *95*, 188–198.

Gray, L., & Rubel, E. W. (1985). Development of absolute thresholds in chickens. *Journal of the Acoustical Society of America*, *77*, 1162–1172.

Green, D. (1990). Stimulus selection in adaptive psychophysical procedures. *Journal of the Acoustical Society of America*, *87*, 2662–2674.

Green, D., & Swets, J. (1974). *Signal detection theory and psychophysics*. Huntington, NY: Kreiger. (Original work published 1966)

Hawkins, J. E., Jr., & Stevens, S. S. (1950). The masking of pure tones and of speech by white noise. *Journal of the Acoustical Society of America*, *22*, 6–13.

Kerr, L., Ostapoff, E., & Rubel, E. W. (1979). Influence of acoustic experience on the ontogeny of frequency generalization gradients in chickens. *Journal of Experimental Psychology: Animal Behavior Processes*, *5*, 97–115.

Lippe, W. R. (1976). Innate and experiential factors in the development of the visual system: Historical basis of current controversy. In G. Gottlieb (Ed.), *Neural and behavioral specificity: Vol. 3. Studies on the development of behavior and the nervous system* (pp. 3–24). San Diego, CA: Academic Press.

Miller, D. (1983). Alarm call responsivity of mallard ducklings: II. Perceptual specificity along an acoustical dimension affecting behavioral inhibition. *Developmental Psychobiology*, *16*, 195–205.

Morgan, D. E., & Zimmerman, M. C. (1987). Auditory brain stem evoked response characteristics in the full-term newborn infant. *Annals of Otology, Rhinology, and Laryngology*, *96*, 142–151.

Neff, D., & Callaghan, P. (1988). Effective properties of multicomponent simultaneous maskers under conditions of uncertainty. *Journal of the Acoustical Society of America*, *83*, 1833–1845.

Olsho, L. W., & Halpin, C. F. (1987). Gap detection thresholds of 3-, 6-, and 12-month-old human infants. *Association for Research in Otolaryngology: Abstracts, 10*, 91.

Olsho, L. W., & Marean, G. C. (1988). Infant thresholds for short duration tone bursts. *Journal of the Acoustical Society of America*, *84*(Suppl. 1), s144

Philbin, M. K., Ballweg, D., & Gray, L. (1992). *Neonatal intensive care unit sounds alter habituation in neonatal chicks*. Manuscript in preparation.

Saunders, J. C., Gates, G. R., & Coles, R. B. (1974). Brain-stem evoked responses as an index of hearing thresholds in one-day-old chicks and ducklings. *Journal of Comparative and Physiological Psychology*, *86*, 426–431

Scharf, B. (1970). Critical bands. In J. V. Tobias (Ed.), *Foundations of modern auditory theory* (Vol. 1, pp. 159–202). San Diego, CA: Academic Press.

Severns, M., Gray, L., & Rubel, E. W. (1985). An avian vocalization detector. *Physiology and Behavior*, *34*, 843–845.

Spitzer, H., Desimone, R., & Moran, J. (1988). Increased attention enhances both behavioral and neuronal performance. *Science*, *240*, 338–340.

Thorpe, L. A., & Schneider, B. A. (1987). Temporal integration in infant audition. *Abstracts of the Society for Research in Child Development*, *6*, 273.

Tomiak, G., Mullennix, J., & Sawusch, J. (1987). Integral processing of phonemes: Evidence for a phonetic mode of perception. *Journal of the Acoustical Society of America*, *81*, 755–764.

Trehub, S. E., Schneider, B. A., & Endman, M. (1980). Developmental changes in infant sensitivity to octave band noises. *Journal of Experimental Child Psychology*, *29*, 282–293.

Viemeister, N. F., & Wakefield, G. H. (1991). Temporal integration and multiple looks. *Journal of the Acoustical Society of America*, *90*, 858–865.

Watson, C. S. (1963). Masking of tones by noise for the cat. *Journal of the Acoustical Society of America*, *35*, 167–172.

Watson, C. S., & Nichols, T. L. (1976). Detectability of auditory signals presented without defined observation intervals. *Journal of the Acoustical Society of America*, *59*, 655–668.

Watson, C. S., Rilling, M. E., & Bourbon, W. T. (1964). Receiver-operating characteristics determined by a mechanical analog to the rating scale. *Journal of the Acoustical Society of America*, *36*, 283–288.

Werner, L., & Bargones, J. (1991). Sources of auditory masking in infants: Distraction effects. *Perception & Psychophysics*, *50*, 405–412.

Werner, L., & Bargones, J. (in press). Psychoacoustic development of human infants. In C. Rovee-Collier & L. Lipsitt (Eds.), *Advances in infancy research* (Vol. 7). Norwood, NJ: Ablex.

Werner, L., & Gillenwater, J. M. (1990). Pure-tone sensitivity of 2- to 5-week old infants. *Infant Behavior and Development*, *13*, 355–375.

Wilson, W. R., & Thompson, G. (1984). Behavioral audiometry. In J. Jerger (Ed.), *Pediatric audiology: Current trends* (pp. 1–24). San Diego, CA: College-Hill.

CHAPTER 4

Individual Differences in Auditory Capability Among Preschool Children

Frederic Wightman and Prudence Allen

There is increasing evidence that the auditory processing skills of preschool children are considerably less well developed than those of adults. Masked thresholds are higher (Schneider, Trehub, Morrongiello, & Thorpe, 1989); intensity, frequency, and duration discrimination are poorer (Jensen, Neff, & Callaghan, 1987); spectral and temporal resolving power are lower (Allen, Wightman, Kistler, & Dolan, 1989; Wightman, Allen, Dolan, Kistler, & Jamieson, 1989); and spectral pattern recognition is not as acute (Allen & Wightman, in press). Given the importance of hearing to normal intellectual development it is imperative that we understand why normally developing children seem to have diminished auditory capabilities.

It is difficult to know whether the observed differences in auditory skills between children and adults reflect structural or functional immaturities in the

The authors gratefully acknowledge the contributions to this work made by Dr. Doris Kistler and Ms. Ramona Agrawal, and the financial support provided by the NIH-NICHD (R01-HD23333). Prudence Allen is currently affiliated with the University of Western Ontario.

peripheral auditory system or the influence of central factors such as attention, memory, or motivation. While there is some evidence that the auditory nervous system is still developing after birth, the extent to which that development continues into the preschool years is questionable. There seems to be general agreement that the nonsensory central factors can be important, but there have been few empirical measurements of their effects. Recent experiments from our laboratory and others (Allen, 1991; Litovsky, 1991) indicate that the effects can be large.

One factor that complicates interpretation of adult–child differences in auditory abilities is the different methods that are used to measure those abilities in the two groups. In typical adult auditory experiments, a small number of subjects is tested repeatedly, in paradigms that often involve sessions of several hours in duration and hundreds of trials. Individual differences are usually not large, and the multiple testing sessions and large numbers of trials produce very precise measurements. In most studies of hearing in children, all the data from an individual subject are obtained in one or two short sessions. In such paradigms, each of a large number of children contributes a small number of observations, and performance is typically expressed as an average of the responses of all the children in a certain age group. These might be called "group performance" paradigms. For example, in the recent study of masked detection in children, Schneider et al. (1989) reported group psychometric functions for seven age groups and six frequencies. Each of the 209 children who participated in the study heard each intensity–frequency combination only once, for a total of 30 trials of testing.

The group performance paradigm is well suited to the limited attention spans of young children, and avoids the logistical difficulties of multiple testing sessions. However, such a paradigm conceals individual differences. If individual differences are large, group performance functions are not especially informative, and can be misleading.

Our approach, which is inspired by the adult psychophysical methods, is to test a relatively small number of children repeatedly, often over the course of months, in order to obtain stable estimates of both between- and within-subject variability. Results from the four or five studies we have completed to date suggest that the between-subject variability is so great that averages and group performance functions must be interpreted with great caution. In this chapter we will give a few examples of the large between-subject variability, or individual differences, that we have encountered in our own work. In addition, we will present the results of some simulations of the impact of nonsensory factors such as inattention or forgetting.

Methods

Before discussing specific results, a brief review of our psychophysical methods would seem appropriate. The details are published (Allen & Wightman, in press; Allen et al., 1989; Wightman et al., 1989), so only an outline is presented here. All of the studies involve the same basic procedure, with minor modifications that will be described where appropriate.

Subjects

All of our subjects were children from the Waisman Early Childhood Program (an in-house preschool) or a local elementary school. As far as we know, the children were developing normally, as there were no parent or teacher reports of learning difficulties or other related problems. We categorized the children on the basis of chronological age; no intelligence tests or other measures of intellectual development were administered. Hearing was within normal sensitivity limits, as was verified by traditional audiometry before testing began. We also conducted a tympanometric screening before each test session if a middle ear problem was suspected. No data were taken from a child with a detectable middle ear problem.

Psychophysical Procedure

Our experiments required the children to detect a target sound or to discriminate between two sounds, and we used traditional forced-choice paradigms to quantify detectability or discriminability. We have tried several variations of two-interval and three-interval, forced-choice paradigms, and while we sometimes found that one procedure worked better than the others in a given experiment, no consistent differences emerged. In each case, the forced-choice trials (roughly 30 trials per block) were embedded in a type of video game. The video-game animation, which was presented on a TV monitor in front of a child wearing headphones, was used to define the listening intervals on each trial, to provide correct answer feedback, and, in general, to keep the child on task.

We used both adaptive and nonadaptive techniques to quantify detectability and discriminability. The adaptive procedure we favor uses the common "two-down, one-up" rule that tracks 70.7% correct. The nonadaptive procedures include one in which the stimulus is fixed for an entire block of trials, and another in which stimulus level is varied from trial-to-trial in an up-down staircase fashion, so that performance is measured at several levels during each block of trials.

Results

The general trends and age effects revealed by our studies are consistent with nearly all the available literature on the auditory abilities of preschool children. Average discrimination and detection thresholds are higher (i.e., poorer performance) than those obtained from adult listeners, and variability (especially from subject to subject) is higher. However, analyses of the data obtained within individual trial blocks suggests that the quality of the data from the children is generally quite adultlike. There are no indications, for example, of significant interval biases in the forced-choice paradigms, and there is no evidence in the adaptive tracks of lack of attention or motivation. The average number of reversals per block and the distributions of reversal points are virtually the same as from the adult subjects whom we have tested in comparable conditions. Clearly the most striking difference between the adult and child data is the dramatically increased range of performance among the children.

Temporal Resolution

In one of our experiments, 20 children from 3 to 7 years of age and 5 adults were asked to detect the presence of a brief temporal gap in a 400-ms sample of half-octave noise (Wightman et al., 1989). An adaptive three-alternative, forced-choice paradigm was used in 20-trial blocks to estimate the minimum detectable gap at the noise band center frequencies of 400 Hz and 2,000 Hz. Three usable threshold estimates at each center frequency were obtained from each subject. Trial blocks in which fewer than four reversals were obtained (usually as a result of a poor choice of starting gap size) were discarded. Less than 10% of the blocks were discarded.

The results were characterized by large between- and within-subject variability. Figure 1 illustrates the within-subject variability. This figure shows the adaptive tracks (gap width vs. trial number) from a single 4-year-old in the 400-

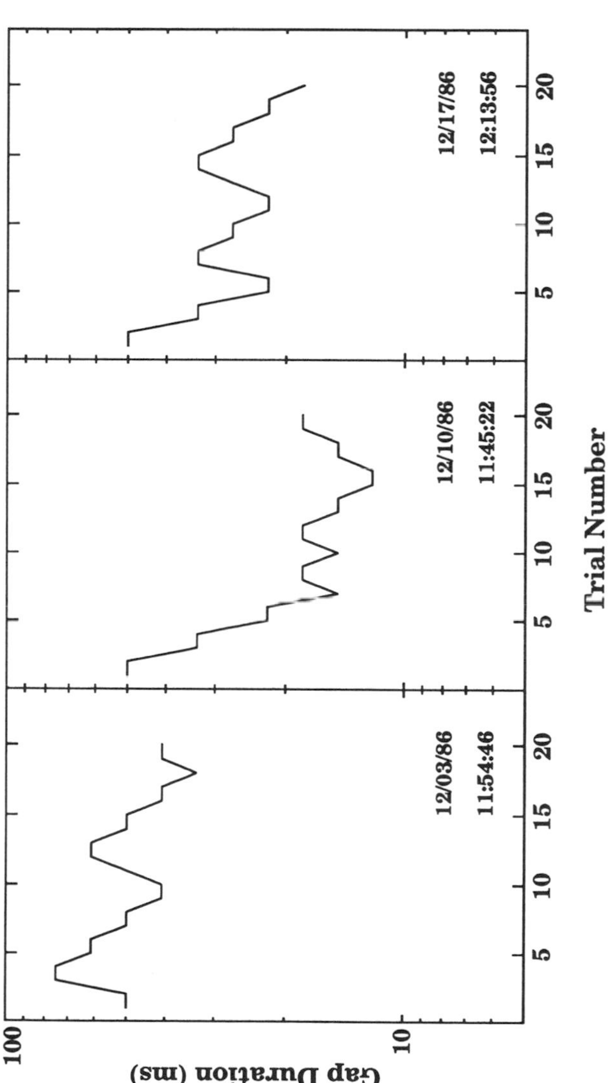

FIGURE 1 Raw data from one child (age 4 years) on three adaptive runs obtained on 3 separate days. Each panel displays the change in gap width, which is a function of correct and incorrect responses. Reversals in direction occurred when a series of correct responses ended with an incorrect response or vice-versa. The track tends to seek that gap width at which the child scores 71% correct. From "Temporal Resolution in Children" by F. Wightman, P. Allen, T. Dolan, D. Kistler, and D. Jamieson, 1989, *Child Development, 60,* p. 619. Copyright 1989 by the Society for Research in Child Development, Inc. Adapted by permission.

Hz condition on 3 separate days. Note that while each adaptive track is well behaved (no late-run deviations from the apparent midpoint), the specific gap duration that is tracked varies from about 45 ms (first day) to about 15 ms (second day). This three-fold range in the performance of a single subject (our most variable subject) is roughly the same as the range of performance between subjects in a given age group. It is also about the same size as the age effect, the difference in average gap threshold between the youngest and oldest subjects. Figure 2 illustrates the latter two points.

In Figure 2 we plotted the mean of each subject's three gap threshold estimates in each condition. Data from the 400-Hz condition and 2,000-Hz condition are plotted in separate panels. Thus, each data point in a given panel represents the mean of three threshold estimates from a single subject. Note that at 400 Hz, the average gap threshold across all subjects within a 1-year age range (asterisks connected by solid lines) varies from about 40 ms for the 3-year-olds to about 15 ms for the adults; at 2,000 Hz the comparable range is from 15 ms to about 7 ms. Note also that this age effect is not substantially changed if we analyze each subject's "best" (i.e., lowest) gap threshold (points connected by dashed lines), assuming that on other blocks the subjects were not paying attention. Thus, while the within-subject variability is large, it neither enlarges nor masks what appears to be a real age effect.

As Figure 2 shows, the between-subject variability in gap threshold is sufficiently large enough to complicate any simple interpretation of the age effect. The problem is particularly clear in the 400-Hz condition. Note that there are individual children in each age group with mean gap thresholds well within the adult range. What distinguishes the high- and low-gap-threshold children is not obvious. It seems unlikely that such differences could be traced to peripheral or central auditory system immaturities. We will argue later in this chapter that at least some of the differences can be explained by the influence of nonsensory factors such as memory or attention.

Frequency Resolution

The aim of one of our experiments was to measure the frequency resolution capabilities of young children (Allen et al., 1989). A variation on the common notched-noise procedure was used, in which pure-tone detection thresholds were measured in two masking conditions: In one, the masker was a flat-spectrum noise, and in the other the masker was a noise with a half-octave-wide, 50-dB-

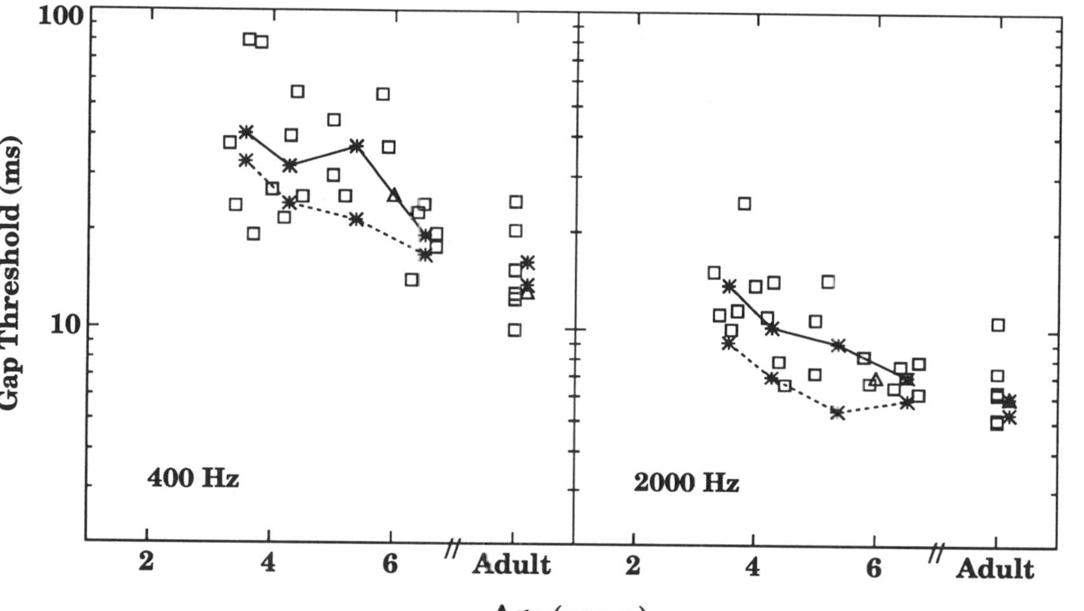

FIGURE 2 Mean gap-width thresholds from individual subjects. Each open square represents the mean of three threshold determinations. The solid lines connect the means of the subjects in each age group. The dotted lines connect the means of each subject's lowest threshold. The noise center frequency is indicated in each panel. From "Temporal Resolution in Children" by F. Wightman, P. Allen, T. Dolan, D. Kistler, and D. Jamieson, 1989, *Child Development, 60*, p. 620. Copyright 1989 by the Society for Research in Child Development, Inc. Adapted by permission.

deep spectral notch, centered at the signal frequency (500 Hz, 2,000 Hz, or 4,000 Hz). The difference in masked threshold between the two conditions was our measure of frequency resolution. Large differences would indicate better resolution and small differences poorer resolution. A three-alternative, forced-choice adaptive paradigm (25-trial blocks) was used to measure the masked thresholds of 24 children, aged 3 to 9 years old, and 7 adults. Each subject's thresholds were measured twice.

Figure 3 shows the main results of the frequency resolution experiment. The mean results show clear age effects in that thresholds decrease systematically with increasing age. Moreover, the decrease is greater in the notched-noise condition. This can be interpreted to suggest that frequency resolution is poorer in children than in adults. However, as in the temporal resolution study discussed previously, the between-subject variability is quite large, so mean data should be interpreted with some caution. Note that for readability only group means are plotted in Figure 3, and that the error bars represent standard error intervals. Since there are more than 4 subjects in each group, the range of individual mean thresholds can be expected to be at least 4 times the size of the standard error interval. Thus, while there are large age effects in terms of mean performance, especially in the notched-noise conditions, individual subjects in each age group (except, perhaps, the youngest) produced thresholds in the adult range.

Spectral Pattern Discrimination

A series of experiments assessed the ability of children to discriminate among sounds on the basis of spectral shape, in much the same way as we imagine some speech sounds to be discriminated (Allen & Wightman, in press). One experiment required subjects to discriminate between two tonal complexes with rippled power spectra. The spectral ripples were wider (i.e., peaks farther apart in frequency) in one complex than in the other. The depth of the ripple (peak-to-valley ratio in dB) was varied adaptively to determine the minimum ripple depth for threshold discrimination. In order to focus the listeners' attention on spectral shape, the overall level of the complexes was randomized both between and within trials over a 20 dB range. Discriminability was measured in quiet and in two noise conditions in which the level of a wideband noise background was set so that the tonal complexes were approximately 15 dB and 5 dB above the average adult masked threshold (SL). A modified two-alternative, forced-choice pro-

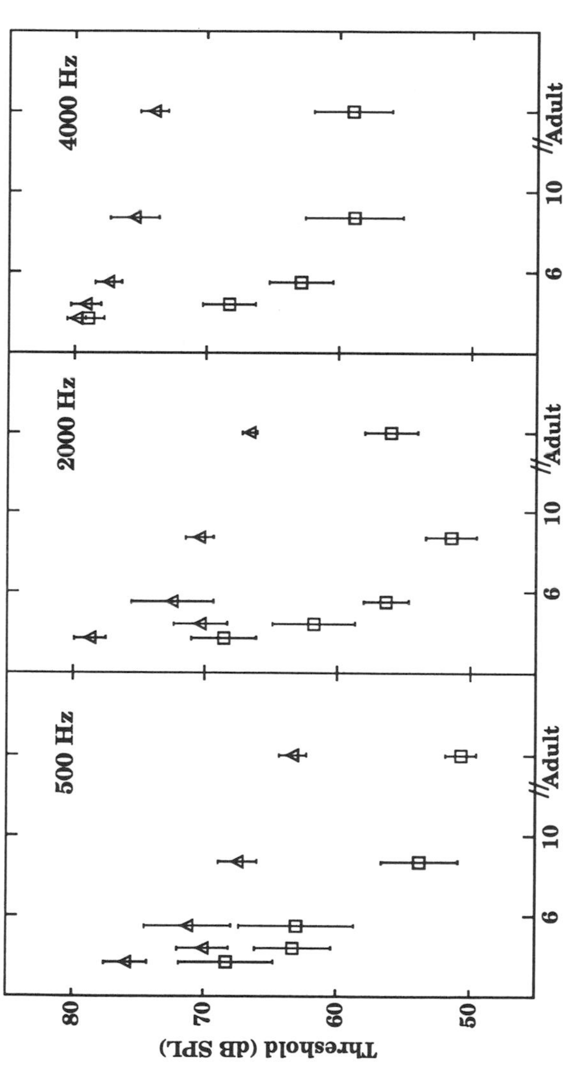

FIGURE 3 Mean masked pure-tone thresholds from the subjects in each group. The error bars indicate ±1 standard error. The open triangles indicate the thresholds in the flat-spectrum masking condition. The open squares indicate the thresholds in the notched-spectrum masking condition. The signal frequency is indicated in each panel. From "Frequency Resolution in Children" by P. Allen, F. Wightman, D. Kistler, and T. Dolan, 1989, *Journal of Speech and Hearing Research, 32*, p. 321. Copyright 1989 by the American Speech-Language-Hearing Association. Adapted by permission.

cedure was used to measure threshold. The modification consisted of the presentation, before the two observation intervals, of a standard stimulus. The subjects' task was to select the observation interval in which the stimulus matched the standard. Each of the 30 children (aged 5 to 9 years old) and 10 adults contributed at least two threshold estimates (35-trial adaptive runs) in each condition.

Figure 4 shows the results of the spectral pattern discrimination experiment. There are clear age effects in all three conditions. The mean threshold ripple depth is higher for the children than for the adults. However, the large between-subject variability, which is characteristic of all our studies but especially prominent here, confounds such a simple conclusion. At each age tested, some subjects produced mean thresholds that were indistinguishable from the adult thresholds. Other children produced thresholds that were 20 dB or more higher.

Pure-Tone Detection

With the hope of gaining a better understanding of the possible sources of the large individual differences in children's performance on auditory tasks, we have recently conducted a series of studies of pure-tone detection (Allen, 1991). This represented a deliberate retreat from our studies of complex auditory processing (spectral and temporal resolution and spectral pattern discrimination) to what is generally considered the simplest of all auditory tasks. It was motivated in part by the large body of data on adult pure-tone detection, which shows that individual differences in adult performance are quite small. We felt that if large individual differences persisted in the performance of the children in such a simple task they could less easily be ascribed to the demands of the task, and the difficulties some children may have understanding them.

In one of the experiments, psychometric functions for detection of a tone (501 Hz, 1,000 Hz, and 2,818 Hz) masked by wideband noise were measured in 18 children, aged 3 to 5 years old, and 14 adults. A traditional two-alternative, forced-choice paradigm was used to measure detection performance at each of at least four signal levels in the three conditions. Signal level was varied from trial to trial in a nonadaptive, up-down staircase fashion, with 10 dB steps, so that within a block of 24 trials, 4 trials were presented at the highest and lowest levels, and 8 trials at the intermediate levels. After several practice trials, each subject completed 3 blocks of trials in each condition. The resulting data were fit with a logistic function using a maximum-likelihood procedure (Allen, 1991). In

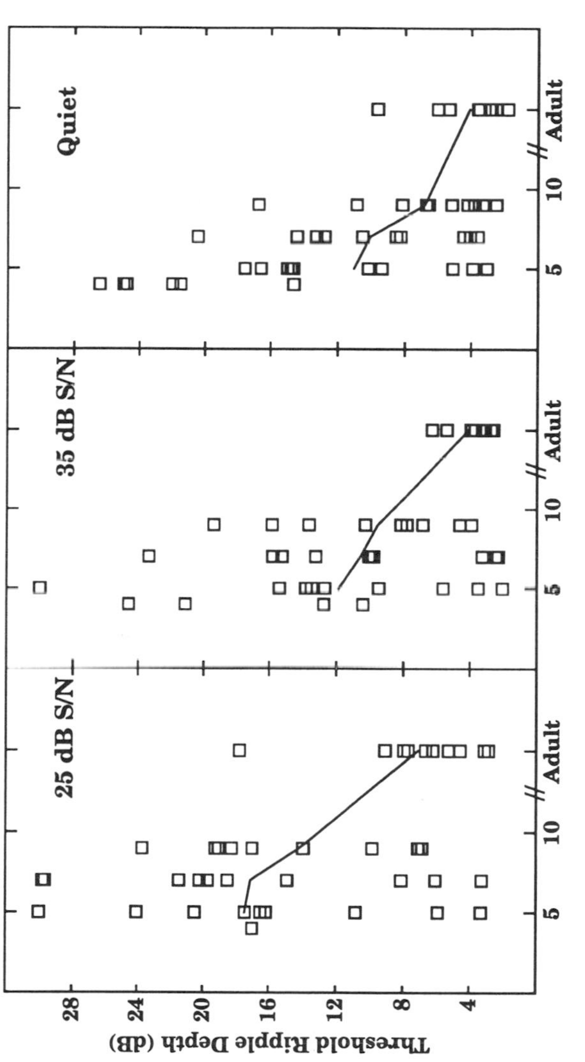

FIGURE 4 Individual spectral pattern discrimination thresholds (ripple depth required for 71% correct discrimination) at three different signal-to-noise (S/N) ratios (indicated in each panel). The solid lines connect the means of each age group. From "Spectral Pattern Discrimination by Children" by P. Allen and F. Wightman, 1992, *Journal of Speech and Hearing Research, 35*, pp. 222–233. Copyright 1992 by the American Speech–Language–Hearing Association. Adapted by permission.

addition, we used a bootstrapping procedure (Maloney, 1990) to estimate the 95% confidence intervals for the two parameters (threshold, or 75% correct point, and slope, in dB from 75% to 95%) of the logistic.

Figure 5 shows psychometric functions for detection of a 1,000-Hz tone obtained from two adults and two children. Data obtained at the other two frequencies parallel the 1,000-Hz data, so in the interest of brevity only the 1,000-Hz data will be discussed here. The examples in Figure 5 have been chosen to represent the extremes of performance in the two groups. Note that while the two adults have generally steeper psychometric functions and lower thresholds than the two children, there is some overlap of the functions from the adults and children when the 95% confidence limits on both parameters are considered. Thus, even in this simple task, individual differences in performance, especially among the children, are sufficiently large enough to show that some children are performing at adult levels.

It is important to emphasize the fact that when only group performance functions are considered, a very different picture of children's auditory skills emerges. Figure 6 shows the 1,000-Hz psychometric functions that result when all of the data from the adults and all of the data from the children are combined into two composite functions. The composite functions suggest no overlap between groups, with the children showing thresholds over 15 dB higher, and much shallower slopes. There is no hint in the group data that some children perform just as well as some adults.

We do not feel that the individual differences in children's pure-tone detection performance reflect simple error variance. A hierarchical cluster analysis of the thresholds and psychometric function slopes obtained from all subjects (adults and children) in all conditions (501 Hz, 1,000 Hz, 2,818 Hz) revealed five distinct groups. All of the adults were placed in one group, and the two children who rarely scored above chance at any level and frequency were placed in another group. The remaining children were distributed among three groups, distinguished by the characteristics of the psychometric functions their members produced (e.g., low slope, high threshold; high slope, low threshold; etc.). A similar cluster analysis conducted after the entire experiment was repeated several months later revealed nearly identical clusters of subjects. The only exceptions were a few children who moved to more "mature" groups. For example, after the

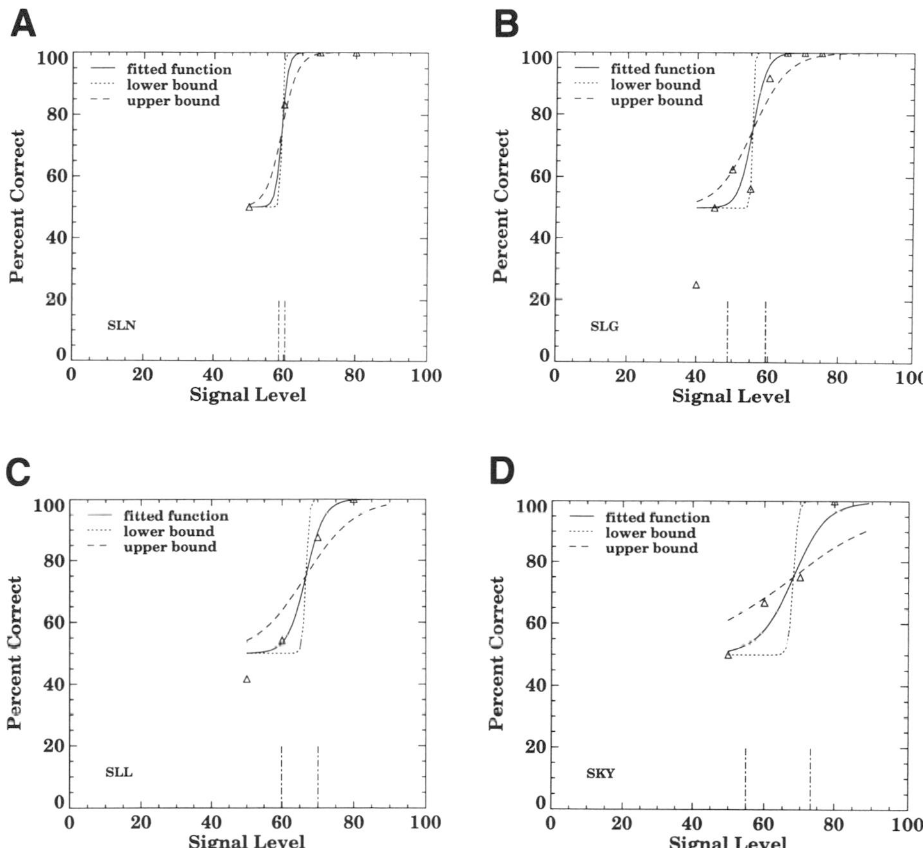

FIGURE 5 Psychometric functions for detection of a 1,000-Hz pure tone masked by wideband noise. Each panel shows the actual data (open triangles) and the maximum-likelihood logistic fit to those data (solid curve). The fitting algorithm compensates for the fact that points at the extreme levels are based on fewer trials. Also shown in the figure are lines depicting the 95% confidence limits for the slope (dotted and dashed lines) and 75% point (dot-dash lines) of the psychometric function. (*A*) and (*B*) show data from two adults, and (*C*) and (*D*) show data from two children. From *Children's Detection of Auditory Signals* by P. Allen, 1991. Copyright 1991 by Prudence Allen. Reprinted by permission.

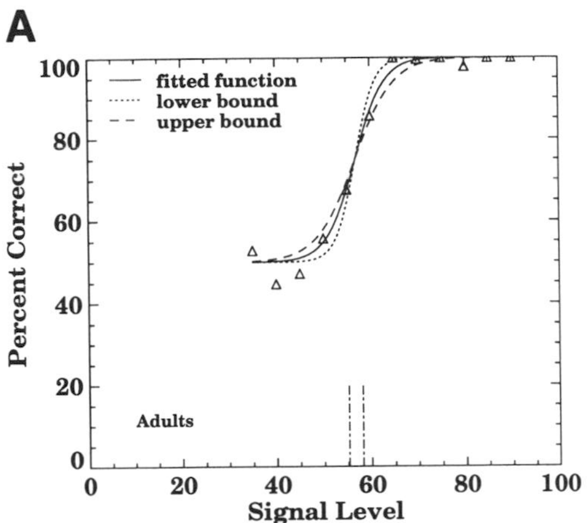

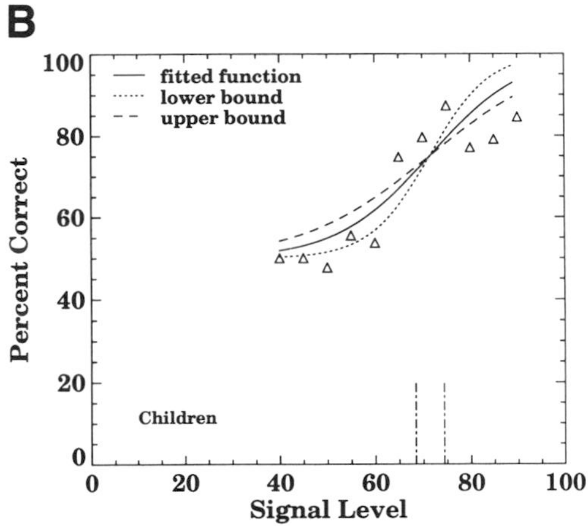

FIGURE 6 Psychometric functions for detection of a 1,000-Hz pure tone masked by wideband noise. Each panel shows the actual data (open triangles) and the maximum-likelihood logistic fit to those data (solid curve). The fitting algorithm compensates for the fact that points at the extreme levels are based on fewer trials. Also shown in the figure are lines depicting the 95% confidence limits for the slope (dotted and dashed lines) and 75% point (dot–dash lines) of the psychometric function. (*A*) and (*B*) show composite psychometric functions formed by combining all of the data from the adults (*A*) and all of the data from the children (*B*). From *Children's Detection of Auditory Signals* by P. Allen, 1991. Copyright 1991 by Prudence Allen. Reprinted by permission.

replication, two children were actually placed in the adult group by the clustering algorithm.

Simulations of the Influence of Nonsensory Factors

There is little, if any, evidence of either a peripheral or central auditory system origin for the generally inferior auditory processing skills manifested by children and the large individual differences in auditory performance among children of the same age. However, the differences between adult and child auditory performance and the individual differences among children are real, and it will be important to understand the sources of these differences in order to deal effectively with the complex auditory processing difficulties demonstrated by some children. Because some progress is almost always made by following an extreme hypothesis to its limits, we have adopted the working hypothesis that the differences arise entirely from nonsensory, cognitive factors such as attention, memory, motivation, and others.

The methods we use to obtain auditory performance data from children control for some of the more obvious nonsensory factors. Response bias and criterion differences are effectively controlled through the use of forced-choice paradigms. Moreover, we use elaborate animated displays and short trial blocks to maintain motivation, and initiate a trial only when the child appears to be attentive. However, the task involves listening, and thus, while a child may appear to be attentive, we can never know for sure. It seems quite reasonable to us that on a certain fraction of the trials, some children may not be fully attentive, may be confused, or may have forgotten the instructions, and that these momentary lapses might be the source of some of the individual differences we observe.

To assess the potential impact of nonsensory factors on the detection and discrimination thresholds we have been measuring, we conducted a series of Monte-Carlo simulations. These are similar to some we have described before (Wightman et al., 1989) and the reader is referred there for further details if necessary. The conditions we simulated were intended to match those used in the experiments described previously. Thus, we simulated both adaptive and nonadaptive psychophysical procedures.

For convenience, and to facilitate comparisons between simulations of adaptive and nonadaptive paradigms, and among those involving very different stimulus dimensions (gap width, signal level, ripple depth, etc.), all simulations assumed a two-interval, forced-choice paradigm, with the value of the independent variable (the "signal value") expressed in normalized units, similar to the z-units of statistics. In each case, the hypothesized underlying psychometric function (which gives the percent correct for the ideal listener as a function of the value of the signal) was a logistic, offset, and scaled to run from 50% to 100%, with a threshold (75% correct point) of 0 z-units and a slope (75%–94%) of 1.0 z-units.

Adaptive Tasks

These were simulations of 35-trial adaptive runs, using the two-down, one-up tracking rule that we have used in all of our work. For the simulated runs, the initial stimulus level was 1.0, about 94% correct for the ideal listener, and the step size was 0.5. On each simulated run (as in our experiments), threshold was estimated by averaging the stimulus values at all reversal points except the first two. Since we collected data on a large number (1,000) of simulated adaptive runs, we were able to produce reconstructed psychometric functions by computing overall percent correct at each level visited.

Figure 7A shows the results of simulating an ideal listener's performance in the adaptive task. Note first that the reconstructed psychometric function (dotted curve) is nearly identical to the underlying psychometric function (solid curve). Note also that the distribution of threshold estimates (the histogram at the bottom of the figure) is slightly asymmetric around a signal value of 0, reflecting the fact that the adaptive rule converges to 70.7% correct, and a signal value of 0 corresponds to 75% correct.

Figures 7B and 7C show the results of simulating an inattentive or confused listener. This listener is assumed to ignore the auditory stimulus altogether on a certain proportion of the trials, and simply guess which interval was correct. In other words, on guessing trials, the actual percent correct is 50%, regardless of the value of the stimulus. Figure 7B shows the impact of guessing on 25% of the trials, and Figure 7C shows the effect of guessing on 50% of the trials. Two effects are evident. First, note that guessing lowers the upper asymptote of the psychometric function to 1.0 minus half the guessing proportion. Thus, with a 50% guessing rate, the function asymptotes at 75% correct. Since the adaptive rule seeks 71%, the lowered upper asymptote causes a dramatic broadening of the distribution of threshold estimates and a shift in the mean of this distribution by over 1.0. The higher thresholds and greater within-subject variability which we

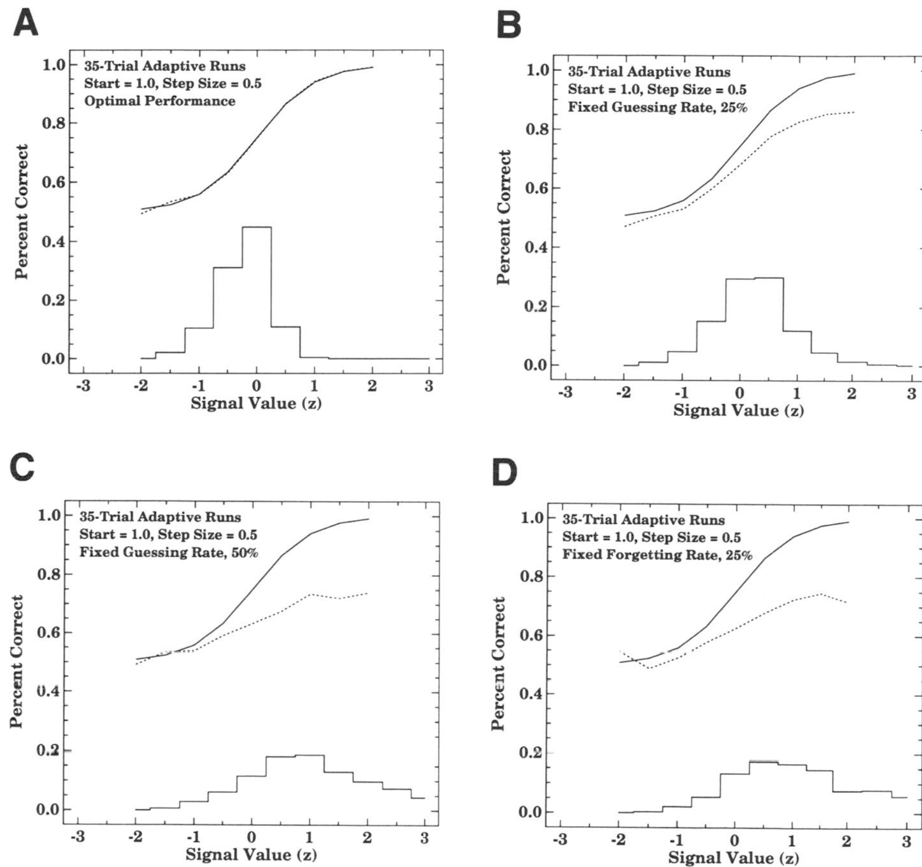

FIGURE 7 Results from simulations of the impact of guessing and forgetting on adaptive threshold estimates are shown. Each panel shows the results from 1,000 simulated 35-trial adaptive two-alternative, forced-choice runs, using the two-down, one-up adaptive rule. Signal values are expressed in *z*-units, so that 1.0 *z*-unit corresponds roughly to 1 *SD* of the approximated cumulative normal function. The assumed underlying logistic function is shown as the solid curve in each panel. The dotted curve shows the psychometric function reconstructed by computing the percent correct at each stimulus level visited by the adaptive tracks. The histogram at the bottom of each panel shows the distribution of threshold estimates from the 1,000 adaptive runs. (*A*) shows a simulation of "optimal" performance. (*B*) and (*C*) show the effect of guessing on 25% and 50% of the trials. (*D*) shows the effect of forgetting on 25% of the trials.

observed in the data from the gap-detection experiment (described earlier) are qualitatively consistent with the effects of guessing that are shown in Figures 7B and 7C.

Figure 7D shows the influence of a nonsensory effect with a slightly different manifestation. In this case, the simulated listener is assumed on a fraction of the trials to "forget" what distinguishes the "signal" interval from the "nonsignal" interval, and respond opposite to what would be correct. Thus, on forgetting trials with signals presented with values sufficiently high to indicate 100% correct performance, this listener would actually score 0% correct, since consistent opposite responses would be made. It is as if the listener simply forgets whether the correct interval contains the louder or the softer sound, the higher or the lower pitch. Since we can never access the subjective dimension on which listeners base their decisions, and since children may have greater difficulty than adults remembering the characteristics of those dimensions, such forgetting seems quite plausible. A comparison of Figures 7C and 7D shows that the impact of forgetting on 25% of the trials is the same as the effect of guessing on 50% of the trials.

Nonadaptive Tasks

Next we considered the simulated impact of guessing and forgetting on performance in a nonadaptive task such as that used in our study of children's pure-tone detection. For these simulations, we assumed that for one block of trials, 24 trials are presented at each of 15 signal levels, 0.25 z-units apart (in the actual experiment 24 trials were presented at the two middle signal levels, and 12 trials were presented at the highest and lowest level). While many more signal levels are used in the simulations than in the actual experiments (to produce a smoother representation of the psychometric function), only the number of presentations per block at each signal level is relevant, since the responses at each level are independent. Each simulation consisted of 1,000 blocks of trials (24 trials at each of 15 levels).

Figure 8 shows the results. Figure 8A shows the simulated data obtained from an ideal listener. As before, the reconstructed psychometric function (mean percent correct over the 1,000 blocks at each of the 15 levels) is nearly identical to the underlying psychometric function. The percent-correct scores at each level on each trial block are shown as dots. The solid curve at the bottom shows the standard deviation of the percent-correct scores at each level. In the case of the ideal listener, this standard deviation is very close to the standard error pre-

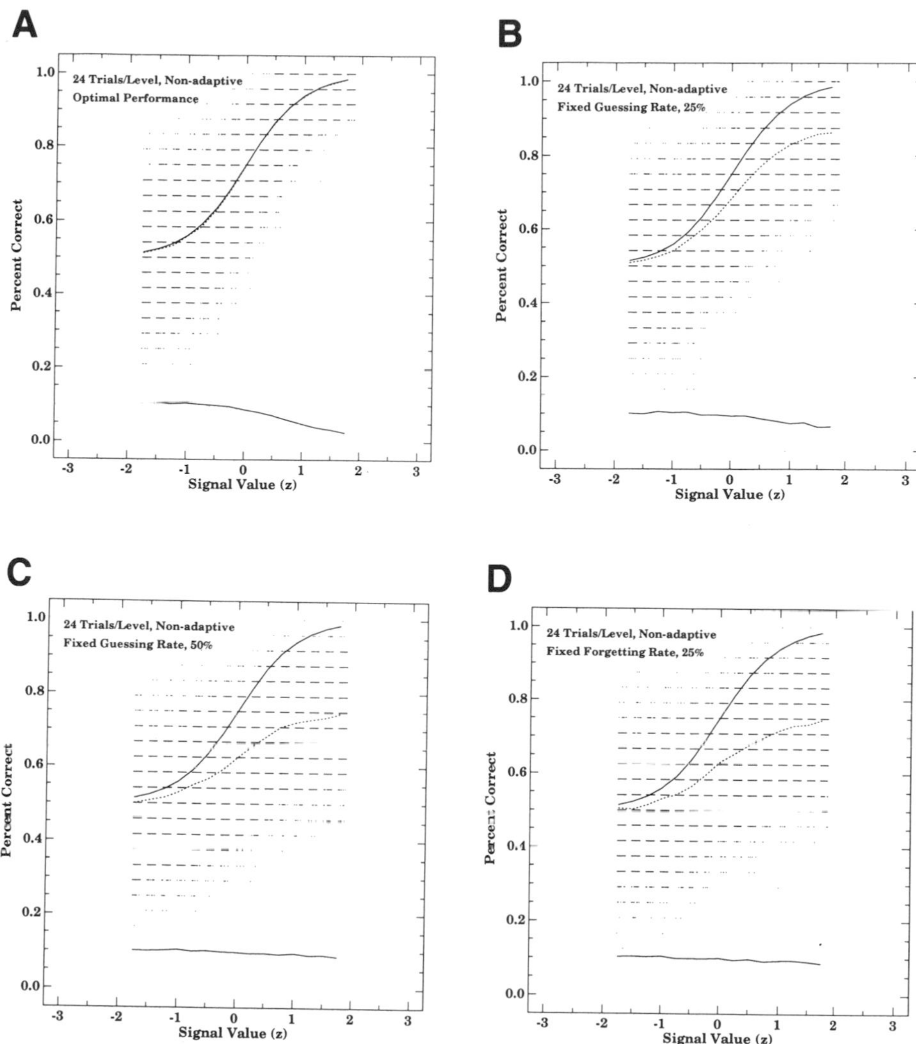

FIGURE 8 Results from simulations of guessing and forgetting on nonadaptive threshold estimates. In these simulations, each of the 1,000 runs is assumed to consist of 24 presentations at each of 15 signal levels, spaced at intervals of .25 *z*-units. The columns of dots represent percent correct at each signal level on individual runs. Thus, there are 1,000 dots in each column. The solid line represents the underlying logistic function, and the dotted line represents the mean percent correct at each signal level. The solid curve at the bottom is the standard deviation of the percent correct values at each signal level. (*A*) shows a simulation of optimal performance. (*B*) and (*C*) show the effect of guessing on 25% and 50% of the trials. (*D*) shows the effect of forgetting on 25% of the trials.

dicted by assuming proportions are binomially distributed. Thus, with an expected percent correct of 50% (lower asymptote of psychometric function), the binomial standard error is $(p^*q/n)^{1/2}$ or $(.5^*.5/24)^{1/2}$ or about 10%. With an expected percent correct of 90%, the binomial standard error is $(.9^*.1/24)^{1/2}$ or 6%.

Figures 8B and 8C show the effects of guessing. The impact on the shape of the psychometric function is identical to that observed in the simulated adaptive runs (Figure 7). The upper asymptote is lowered, and the threshold point is shifted to higher signal values. With a 50% guessing rate, the shift in threshold is about 1.5 z-units, similar to what was observed in the adaptive simulations. Figure 8D shows the effects of forgetting. As before, the impact of a 25% forgetting rate is the same as that of a 50% guessing rate.

The simulations suggest that such nonsensory factors as memory and attention can produce effects that are qualitatively consistent with typical adult–child differences in auditory performance. Estimated thresholds are higher and psychometric function slopes are shallower. In order to determine the extent to which the simulations might agree quantitatively with our data on pure-tone detection, we assumed the children guessed on 50% of the trials (Figure 8C). If we also assume that adults listen optimally, then the solid curve of Figure 8C can be used to represent adult performance, and the dotted curve the predicted child performance. On the normalized abscissa, the solid curve has a threshold value of 0 z-units and a slope (75%–94%) of 1.0 z-units. The dotted curve, after being fit with a logistic exactly as we routinely fit our psychophysical data, has a threshold of 1.5 z-units and a slope (75%–94%) of 2.3 z-units. The average adult threshold at 1,000 Hz in our study was 57 dB SPL, and the slope was 6 dB (Allen, 1991). Using these values we predicted that a child who was guessing on 50% of the trials, but who was like an adult in terms of underlying auditory sensitivity (psychometric function), would produce a threshold of 66 dB SPL (57 + 1.5*6) and a slope of 14 dB (2.3*6). In fact, the average child threshold in our study was 68 dB SPL, and the average slope was 13 dB (Allen, 1991). Given that the 95% confidence limits in that study were ±3 dB around the average threshold and ±2 dB around the average slope, we cannot reject the hypothesis that a guessing rate of 50% can account for the entire adult–child difference in detection performance in that study.

Complete psychometric functions were not obtained in our earlier studies (Allen & Wightman, in press; Allen et al., 1989; Wightman et al., 1989), so it is more difficult to make quantitative predictions about the impact of guessing in those studies. However, a preliminary analysis suggests that a 50% guessing rate could also account for most, if not all, of the observed adult–child differences in performance in those studies as well.

Conclusions

Our simulations represent a first step toward understanding the sources of the apparently diminished auditory capabilities of young children. They also demonstrate that the apparent differences between adults and children in auditory skills may reflect nothing more than the influence of nonsensory factors such as memory and attention. This does not diminish the importance of the adult–child differences, of course, but it does lead us to consider adopting research paradigms with a focus that is somewhat different than before in order to explain the differences more fully.

References

Allen, P. (1991). *Children's detection of auditory signals.* Unpublished doctoral dissertation, University of Wisconsin, Madison.

Allen, P., & Wightman, F. (1992). Spectral pattern discrimination by children. *Journal of Speech and Hearing Research, 35*, 222–233.

Allen, P., Wightman, F., Kistler, D., & Dolan, T. (1989). Frequency resolution in children. *Journal of Speech and Hearing Research, 32*, 317–322.

Jensen, J. K., Neff, D. L., & Callaghan, B. P. (1987). Frequency, intensity, and duration discrimination in young children. *Asha, 29*, 88.

Litovsky, R. Y. (1991). *Developmental changes in sound localization precision under conditions of the precedence effect.* Unpublished doctoral dissertation, University of Massachusetts, Amherst.

Maloney, L. T. (1990). Confidence intervals for the parameters of psychometric functions. *Perception & Psychophysics, 47*, 127–134.

Schneider, B. A., Trehub, S. E., Morrongiello, B. A., & Thorpe, L. A. (1989). Developmental changes in masked thresholds. *Journal of the Acoustical Society of America, 86*, 1733–1741.

Wightman, F., Allen, P., Dolan, T., Kistler, D., & Jamieson, D. (1989). Temporal resolution in children. *Child Development, 60*, 611–624.

CHAPTER 5

The Development of Spatial Hearing in Human Infants

Rachel K. Clifton

An important aspect of spatial hearing is how an organism uses sound to infer certain properties about the immediate environment. What is making the sound? Where is the sound? What is the sound's distance and direction in relation to the observer? For some animals such information is vital for survival, and their skill is legendary. For example, the barn owl uses sound to detect both distance and direction of a mouse's movement on the ground so that it can gauge its dive and orient its talons. But what can we expect from the human infant? Here is an organism capable of responding to sound during the last 2 months of gestation, but this sensory maturity is coupled with extreme motoric immaturity. The former encourages us to expect that the infant will be able to localize and

This research was supported by grants from NIH (DC00362 and HD27714) and a Research Scientist Award from NIMH (MH00332).

I gratefully acknowledge the help of Marsha Clarkson, Eve Perris, Daniel Ashmead, Darwin Muir, Andre Bullinger, Philippe Rochat, Irina Swain, and Ruth Litovsky for their collaboration on various aspects of the research reported.

discriminate sounds at a fairly young age, whereas the latter warns us that it may be difficult to find unambiguous expressions of these perceptual abilities.

Auditory localization is achieved through the complex processing of a multitude of sound cues (Blauert, 1983; Kuhn, 1987). Some are due to structural features of the head itself, such as interaural time difference, interaural intensity difference, and pinna cues, while others arise from the way sound interacts with the environment before it reaches the ear, such as echoes from reflective surfaces or a drop in sound pressure level (SPL) as the wave travels away from the source. What do we know about an infant's sensitivity to any of these available cues? Also, if the infant is sensitive to localization cues, are these cues interpreted in terms of direction and distance in order to locate the object in space? The infant may be capable of discriminating certain interaural differences, but may not be able to use this information to orient its head or body toward a sound's location. This distinction brings us back to the motor issue, and the special nonsensory considerations that must be taken when studying infants' auditory behavior—a theme that runs through many of the presentations in this volume.

Prior to 1980 we had almost no information on spatial hearing in human infants. The 1980s witnessed varied research on this topic. This chapter will present an overview of four main areas of this work:

1. newborn head orientation—the earliest sign of directional discrimination of sound;
2. developmental studies of precision in localization, as indicated by discrimination of angular displacement;
3. developmental studies of the precedence effect, a phenomenon that affects auditory localization in enclosed spaces; and
4. auditory distance discrimination in infants, with particular reference to how acoustic distance information functions to guide the infant's motor behavior.

Newborn Head Orientation Toward Sound

A newborn, tested only a few hours after birth, will turn toward an off-center sound; this is the earliest sign that humans respond to the directionality of sound. Behavioral orienting can be observed in most young mammals soon after the auditory system becomes responsive to sound (Kelly, 1986), underscoring that this response is basic to hearing. The recognition of head orienting toward sound as a reliable newborn behavior took almost 20 years to establish. Wertheimer's original observation was published in *Science* in 1961 but was controversial because it involved a single infant and an experimenter who knew which side the sound was on. Two attempts to replicate this report in the 1970s failed (Butterworth & Castillo, 1976; McGurk, Turnure, & Creighton, 1977). The problem in replicating lay primarily with the stimulus. McGurk et al. used a single click, and Butterworth and Castillo used a 500-ms tone, both of which we now know are too brief to elicit a response in newborns. In 1979, Muir and Field presented newborns with a long duration (20 s) stimulus modeled after the rattle sound used as part of the Brazelton Scale (Brazelton, 1973). After this initial demonstration other labs successfully used newborn head orienting to explore stimulus variations (Clifton, Morrongiello, Kulig, & Dowd, 1981a) as well as habituation and orienting (Zelazo, Brody, & Chaika, 1984). While many aspects of Muir and Field's procedure were critical, including postural support provided for the infant's head and body and the infant's arousal state (see Muir & Clifton, 1985, for discussion), it is the stimulus characteristics that have been explored most extensively. Bandwidth and frequency composition are influential, with a broader bandwidth and higher frequencies (above 3,000 Hz) being more effective (Morrongiello & Clifton, 1984). Like the rattle sound, human speech contains high frequencies and is a pulsed, fairly broadband signal. It too is extremely effective in eliciting head turns (Swain, 1987; Swain, Clifton, & Clarkson, 1989; Weiss, Zelazo, & Swain, 1988). Conspecific sounds have often proved to be the optimal stimulus for eliciting responses in young animals, such as chicks (Gottlieb, 1981), guinea pigs (Clements & Kelly, 1978), and kittens (Olmstead & Villablanca, 1980). Human infants appear to share this tendency.

Another stimulus characteristic, duration, has been studied extensively in our lab. Initially we thought newborns tracked the direction of the ongoing sound, and would be unable to turn correctly if the sound terminated before the turn began or during execution of the movement. This proved to be wrong. In a series of studies we found that a continuous sound that lasts at least 1 s (note that this is longer than either McGurk et al.'s [1977] or Butterworth & Castillo's [1976] stimulus) will elicit a head turn toward it, but that shortening the duration to 500 ms or less leads to nonresponsiveness (Clarkson, Clifton, & Morrongiello, 1985; Clarkson, Clifton, Swain, & Perris, 1989). However, a brief stimulus of a few milliseconds, rapidly repeated (no slower than 2/s), is effective (Clarkson et al., 1985). Clarkson, Swain, Clifton, and Cohen (1991) recently reported on the complex interaction of rate, duration, and number of stimulus bursts. This work has been extensively reviewed in Clarkson and Clifton (1991) and will not be discussed here.

In addition to indicating the infant's perception of a sound's direction, head orienting can also reflect the newborn's memory for a specific sound across a 24-hour span (Swain, 1987). After neonates were habituated on Day 1 (mean age 47 hours) to a repeating word (either "beagle" or "tinder"), they were given either the same word or a different word on Day 2 (mean age 71 hours). These groups were compared with a control group who were tested for the first time on Day 2. The group who heard the same word on Day 2 showed significantly less head orienting toward the sound compared with the same-age control group, while the group who heard a new word on Day 2 responded in-between. Perhaps more significant, the group who continued to experience the same word on Day 2 began turning *away* from the sound source. Repeated exposure to the same sound, presented equally often from left and right, elicited an initial orienting response appropriate to the sound's direction, followed by an active turning away. This report joins others (Engen, Lipsitt, & Kaye, 1963; Pomerleau-Malcuit, Malcuit, & Clifton, 1975) that found that infants turn their heads away from negative stimuli such as unpleasant odors or tactile stimulation. Studies of habituation to sound have reported that head-turns away come to dominate head-turns toward eventually (Weiss et al., 1988; Zelazo, Weiss, Randolph, Swain, & Moore, 1987). But Swain (1987) is unique in showing that a once-attractive auditory stimulus became less desirable (perhaps even noxious) through repetition, even when this repetition was spread over 2 days. That memory over 24 hours for particular sounds was shown soon after birth is not surprising in light of DeCasper, Fifer, and colleagues who have reported remarkable retention for the sound of the mother's voice across the prenatal–postnatal boundary (DeCasper & Fifer, 1980; DeCasper & Spence, 1986; Moon & Fifer, 1990). Because the auditory system is functioning well before birth and at birth is remarkably mature compared with visual or motor systems, a concentrated effort to reveal the full range of discriminatory powers as well as memory for sounds is warranted. Directional responding of the head holds promise as an appropriate response to explore these issues (for discussion see Zelazo, Weiss, & Tarquino, 1991).

When infants beyond the newborn period were tested on head orienting to sound, a mysterious result surfaced: They stopped turning around 6–8 weeks of age. First Muir and colleagues tested infants longitudinally with the rattle sound (Field, Muir, Pilon, Sinclair, & Dodwell, 1980; Muir, Abraham, Forbes, & Harris, 1979) and discovered that they were unable to elicit the head turn that had proved so reliable in the newborn period. Clifton and colleagues (Clifton, Morrongiello, & Dowd, 1984) found that the stimulus was critical at this age as well as during the newborn period. At 8 weeks of age, a click train was totally ineffective, but a female voice speaking "baby talk" managed to get a response rate above chance. Recently, a detailed study was run in which infants from birth to 7 months were tested at monthly intervals in cross-sectional groups (Muir, Clifton, & Clarkson, 1989). At birth infants turned toward the correct side on 75% of trials, but this fell to 52% and 55% at 1 and 2 months, respectively. By 3 months responding was back up to 78% correct. Throughout this period incorrect responding remained about the same, around 20% or less, but the incidence of failure to respond at all caused performance to deteriorate at 1 and 2 months. Not only was there a dip in frequency of head turning, but the morphology of the head movement changed as well. Head turns during the dip had longer latency and less amplitude than turns during either the newborn period or later. This decrease in head turning around 6–8 weeks probably has little to do with the infant's sensitivity to interaural cues; rather, it may reflect a difficulty in organizing auditory space and coordinating this with appropriate motor behavior. Muir and Clifton (1985) interpreted these developmental changes in terms of a maturational shift in locus of control from subcortical to cortical structures. Behaviors other than head orienting to sound show a similar decline around the same age. The 2-month age is well-known in infancy for being a transitional period when many neonatal behaviors drop out and new behaviors have not yet become well-organized. When the head-orienting response reappears around 3–4 months of age, it is accompanied by visual search. This new behavior may signify the beginning of true spatial hearing in infancy.

To summarize, newborns reliably orient in the direction of a sound soon after birth, but the response is fragile. Both the infant's state and the stimulus must meet certain conditions or the response will not be observed. On the other hand, if these conditions are met, the behavior is robust enough to be used as an indicator of habituation, learning, and memory. Questions remaining include whether the newborn actually localizes the sound outside the head in space, or is responding to interaural differences based on brainstem activity. We will return to this issue in the last section of this chapter. A second unresolved question is whether the newborn is capable of only a hemifield distinction when turning toward sound. Muir (1985) reported that newborns do not align their heads in the correct orientation when presented with an array of loudspeakers. However, there was a tendency to make a smaller head turn when the loudspeaker was located at 45° rather than 90°. This issue is important because animal work has made a distinction concerning discrimination between hemifields and discrimination within a hemifield. Jenkins and Masterton (1982) reported that cats with unilateral lesions of the auditory cortex failed to discriminate among several sound positions within the hemifield contralateral to the lesion, but continued to correctly choose the appropriate hemifield in a two-choice situation. A parallel may be found in infant behavior such that the newborn distinguishes directionality only to the left and right of midline, and refinement within a hemifield is a later development. However, the motor system rather than perceptual abilities could be the limiting factor here, in that poor control of head movement may prevent expression of a more precise behavioral response.

Developmental Studies of Precision in Localization

The newborn head-turning data suggest that infants are born with some sensitivity to binaural cues that are important for directional discrimination, such as interaural differences in intensity and time of arrival. However, we do not know the limits of this sensitivity, nor do we know if intensity, time, or a combination of these are being used. These cues are confounded in the head-orienting research because sound was delivered in a sound field over loudspeakers. To date, only two earphone studies have attempted to disentangle the localization information mixed in the loudspeaker signals. The initial study by Bundy (1980), who presented infants with only one token from each interaural parameter, concluded that 8- and 16-week-olds could discriminate a large interaural time difference of 300 μs, but only the older infants responded to an intensity difference of 6 dB. The latter finding should be viewed with caution because it has been questioned on methodological grounds (Clifton, Morrongiello, Kulig, & Dowd, 1981b), and has never been followed up. A second study by Ashmead, Davis, Whalen, and Odom (1991) concentrated on interaural time differences, establishing thresholds with an adaptive psychophysical procedure for infants 16- to 28-weeks-old. They reported that all ages could discriminate interaural time differences in the range of 50–75 μs. We can conclude from this that at an early age (16 weeks), infants are sensitive to time of arrival differences that should enable them to distinguish small changes in the spatial position of sounds.

How might this binaural cue function to give the infant knowledge of a sound's location in space? To be able to discriminate an interaural time difference (ITD) is one thing, but to use it to locate a sound implies much more complex processing. Some sort of mapping process must take place where binaural differences get translated into auditory space. We know from the extensive work of Knudsen and his colleagues on barn owls that mapping takes place very early in life for this species, that it is influenced by auditory and visual experience, and that plasticity in coordinating audition with vision ends at a definite point in development (Knudsen & Knudsen, 1985). While we do not understand how the neural code for auditory localization develops in young humans, we do know that considerable plasticity must exist in infancy because changing head size affects interaural cues quite dramatically over the first year of life. Clifton, Gwiazda, Bauer, Clarkson, & Held (1988) graphed theoretical interaural time differences based on Woodworth's formula (1938) for head size at three ages, with sound sources located between azimuths of midline (0°) and 90° (see Figure 1). To illustrate the potential change in mapping of interaural time differences onto space, compare the same ITD across ages. Newborns would experience an ITD of 411 μs at 90°, which would be the ITD near 65° for 22-week-olds and 47° for adults. Considering changes in ITD over age, between birth and 22 weeks the ITDs shift upward by roughly 100 μs for a sound located at 90°. This changing ITD would not be a problem for an organism that used visual and sensorimotor experience to constantly recalibrate auditory space. Data from both normal adults (Held, 1955) and clinical patients (Gray & Jarsdoerfer, 1986) indicate that this is the case for humans. The parallel case for recalibration in vision due to growth of head and eyes has been shown elegantly by Banks (1988).

Apparently discriminative sensitivity also outstrips performance on tasks that test functioning of binaural cues involved in discrimination of angular displacement. The subject's task is to detect the smallest change in a sound's loca-

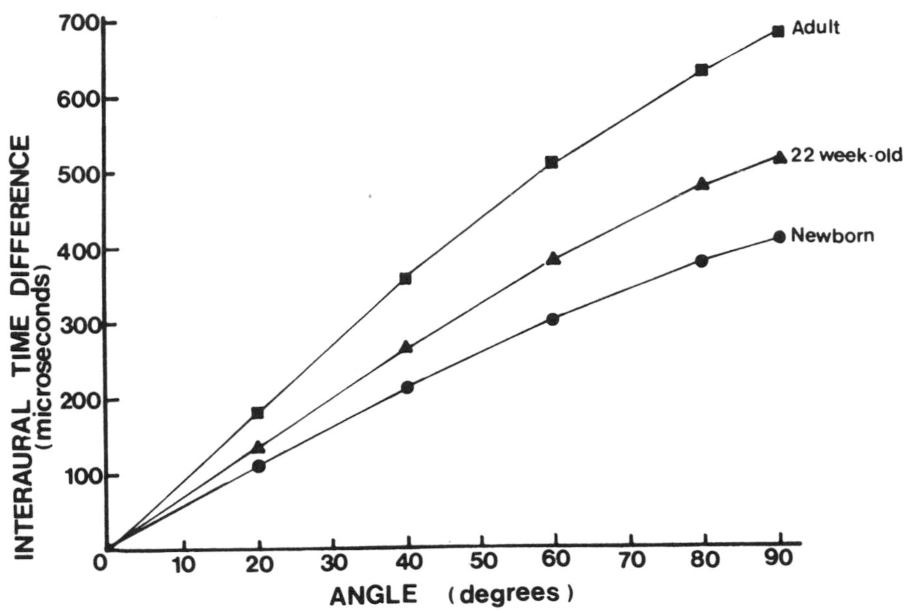

FIGURE 1 Estimates of interaural time-of-arrival differences from sound sources located at angles between midline and 90° horizontal eccentricity at three ages. From Clifton, Gwiazda, Bauer, Clarkson, and Held (1988). Copyright 1988 by the American Psychological Association. Reprinted by permission.

tion, a procedure that yields a threshold called the minimal audible angle (MAA). By 6 months of age, infants can be easily conditioned to make a head turn in the direction of a sound, and this behavior can be exploited to force a left/right discrimination of a sound moving off-midline. Ashmead, Clifton, and Perris (1987) were the first to use an adaptive procedure with infants based on the adult MAA. They found that 6-month-olds distinguished a change in a sound's location of 19° left and right off-midline. Morrongiello, Fenwick, and Chance (1990) tested younger ages, using an observer-based procedure that does not require head turns, combined with the method of constant stimuli. They reported that MAA was around 27° in the youngest age tested (8 weeks), and steadily fell to 18° at 24 weeks. The 18° MAA was limited because these infants were only presented with stimuli at 18°, 24°, and 30°. These data agree with Ashmead et al. (1991), who used an adaptive procedure and spanned a similar age range. Earlier Morrongiello (1988) had tested the age range between 6 and 18 months. Six-month-olds had an estimated MAA of 12°, which fell to 8° by 12 months and to 4° by 18 months. Litovsky (1991) reported a slightly higher threshold of 6° for 18-month-olds, which was significantly different from her adult subjects; her 5-year-olds were not different from adults. Figure 2 presents a composite of these data, illustrating how MAA changes across infancy and early childhood. We can conclude that during infancy there is rapid improvement in localization acuity, that precision in localization approaches adult performance by 18 months and is not different from an adult's by 5 years of age. Moreover, Ashmead et al. (1991) pointed out that the limiting factor during early infancy is probably not binaural sensitiv-

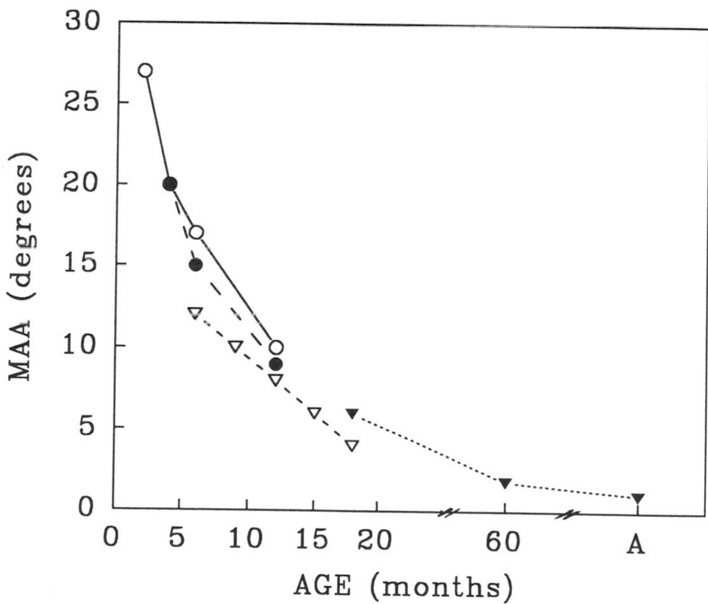

FIGURE 2 Minimal audible angle (MAA) data as a function of age, replotted from several studies that used different methodologies. See text for full description. Data represented by ● from Ashmead, Davis, Whalen, and Odom (1991, copyright 1991 by the Society for Research in Child Development); by ▼ from Litovsky (1991, copyright 1991 by Litovsky); by ▽ from Morrongiello (1988, copyright 1988 by the American Psychological Association); and by ○ from Morrongiello, Fenwick, and Chance (1990, copyright 1990 by the American Psychological Association). Adapted by permission.

ity, but the integration process that coordinates binaural differences with other localization cues (e.g., those arising from head movement) and changing head size. This conclusion was based on their finding that thresholds for ITD were around 50–75 μs for infants as young as 4 months, whereas thresholds for discrimination of angular displacement, as exemplified in the data plotted in Figure 2, translated to ITDs around 120–130 μs at this age. For adults, ITD discrimination from earphone studies predicts MAA performance in the sound field fairly well (Mills, 1972). The fact that this does not hold for infants suggests that factors other than binaural sensitivity are at work (see Ashmead et al., 1991, for more detailed discussion).

Developmental Studies of the Precedence Effect

Under normal room conditions we localize a sound at its source, while failing to localize or even recognize the presence of numerous echoes or reflections from surrounding surfaces. The echoes enhance and enrich the original sound, but their directional information is suppressed to the extent that they are not heard as separate sounds. These echoes, if it were not for the precedence effect, would produce "acoustic bedlam" in Mills' words (1972, p. 341), and make localization of the true source of sound very difficult. To produce the precedence effect in the laboratory two identical sounds are delivered from two loudspeakers, located to the listener's right and left, with the onset of one leading the other by a few milliseconds. The listener localizes the sound solely at the leading loudspeaker, and is unaware of the sound from the lagging loudspeaker, even though sound was produced at the *same* intensity through both sources. By increasing the time delay between onsets, the echo threshold is reached and the lagging sound (or echo) is heard at its location, along with the leading sound at its location. The precedence effect is due to the nervous system's active suppression of the echoes rather than a failure to resolve temporal delays, because the delays between loudspeaker onsets are well within the auditory system's capabilities for discriminating interaural differences. The precedence effect has been recognized as an important aspect of sound localization for more than 100 years (see Gardner, 1968, for historical review), with great relevance for the theories of binaural hearing as well as having practical significance for the design of auditoria and other rooms.

The interest in working with the precedence effect developmentally grew out of a series of studies in which cats with unilateral lesions of the auditory cortex were shown to be impaired in their localization of precedence-effect stimuli, while their localization of single-source stimuli from one loudspeaker was maintained at normal levels (Whitfield, 1978; Whitfield, Cranford, Ravizza, & Diamond, 1972; Whitfield, Diamond, Chiveralls, & Williamson, 1978). In addition, work with epileptic children with foci in the temporal region indicated impaired localization of precedence-effect sounds when compared with their performance with single-source sounds (Hochster & Kelly, 1981). Both the animal and clinical data suggested that localization of precedence-effect stimuli involved the auditory cortex. We predicted that human newborns would fail to turn toward a precedence-effect stimulus, but would turn toward that same sound when it was presented without a delayed echo because their auditory cortex is still quite immature. In Clifton et al. (1981a) each newborn was presented with an equal number of three trial types: single source from a single loudspeaker (SS), precedence effect from two loudspeakers with one leading by 7 ms (PE), and two speakers with simultaneous onset as a control (Control). (See the left side of Figure 3 labeled "Newborn".) There was head turning toward single-source sounds on about 50% of the trials, with a few contralateral turns, and many trials when no turn occurred at all. During the precedence-effect trials, the infants almost never turned, and when they did they were as likely to turn away from the sound as toward it; they behaved similarly on the simultaneous control trials. To the adult, the simultaneous onset appears to come from midline. We concluded that newborns did not inhibit the echo sound, and were thus unable to distinguish between the leading and lagging sides.

Following this study a number of studies sought to determine when infants would begin to respond to the precedence effect. We tested 6- to 8-week-olds and 5- to 6-month-olds (Clifton et al., 1984), and found that the younger infants did not respond to the precedence effect but by 6 months they did (see the right side of Figure 3). When more intermediate ages were tested, we found that the first reliable response to the precedence effect comes around 4 months, about 1 month after the reappearance of single-source responding, on average (Muir et al., 1989). However, in a longitudinal study we found that 3 infants, tested on a weekly basis between 8 and 24 weeks, began responding again to single-source sounds in the *same session* that they first began turning toward the leading side

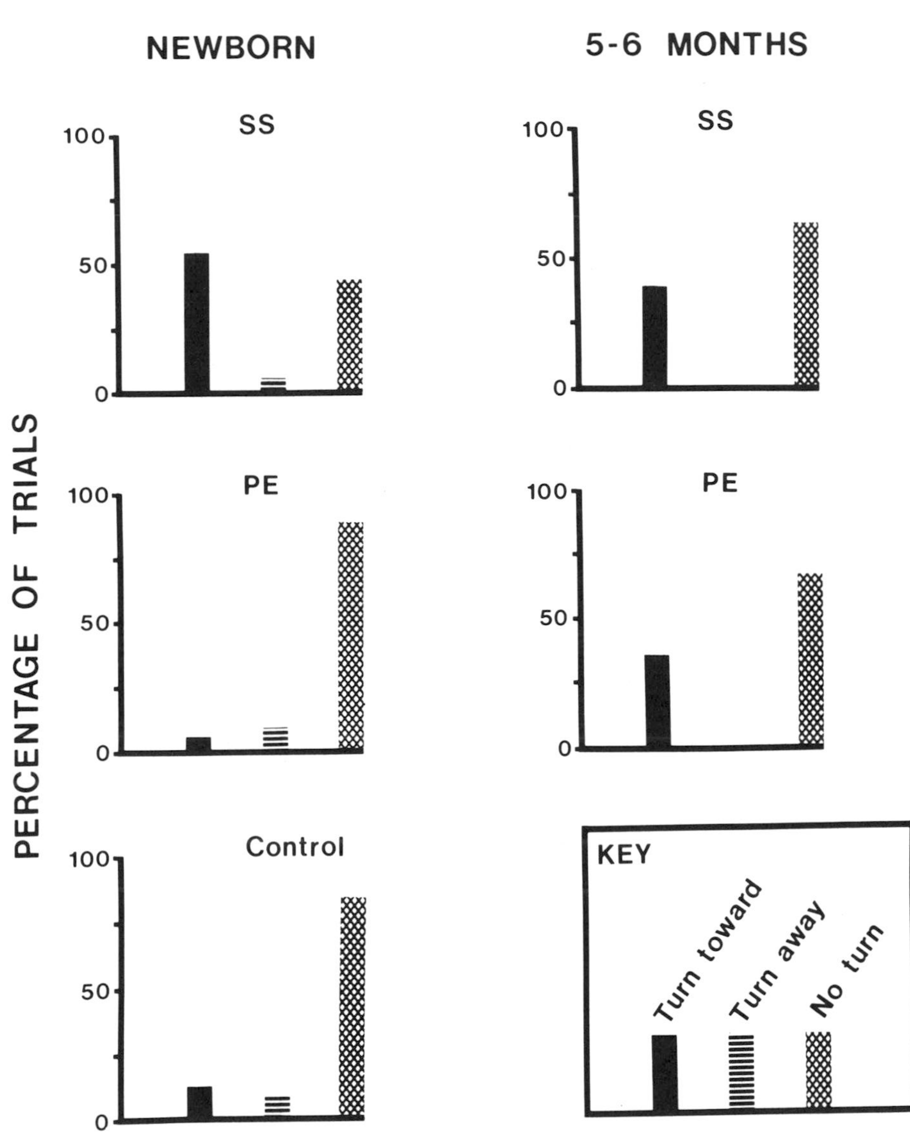

FIGURE 3 Percentage of trials in which infants turned toward (solid bars), turned away (striped bars), or made no turn (cross-hatched bars) to three conditions: sounds from a single loudspeaker (SS), two loudspeakers with one leading to produce the precedence effect (PE), and simultaneous onset (control). Data for newborns are plotted on the left. From Clifton, Morrongiello, Kulig, and Dowd (1981a). Copyright 1981 by the Society for Research in Child Development. Adapted by permission. Data for 5- to-6-month-olds are plotted on the right. From Clifton, Morrongiello, and Dowd (1984). Copyright 1984 by John Wiley and Sons. Adapted by permission.

of the precedence-effect sound. A fourth infant had a 1-week difference in these two behaviors. Thus in some infants these behaviors were extremely coordinated, while in other infants onset of response to the precedence effect lagged several days or weeks behind the reappearance of reliable head orienting toward single-source sounds. What is clear from these data is that the *initial* head turning to single-source sound was present at birth and preceded head turning to the leading side of precedence-effect sounds by 4–5 months, suggesting that localization of these two types of sounds arises from two different processes that have different maturational courses.

We believed that this developmental sequence for single-source and precedence-effect responses occurred in most mammals. We chose dogs to test this hypothesis (largely for convenience—we had available a litter of 12 German shepherd puppies). Head orienting to sound is not present at birth in dogs (or kittens for that matter), but develops within 2 weeks. We tested the puppies daily from about 7 days to 39 days; head orienting to sound appeared to the tape recording of conspecific sounds (barking, whining) at 16 days of age for the sound delivered from a single loudspeaker, but the pups did not respond to the leading side of the precedence-effect recording even at 39 days, the oldest testing age (Ashmead, Clifton, & Reese, 1986). Adult dogs did respond to the leading side, so we know that at some point after 40 days, the pups would show the onset of the precedence effect. We concluded that in both dogs and humans, there is a developmental sequence in which head orienting is elicited to single-source sounds soon after birth, but orienting to the precedence effect is delayed for several weeks or months, depending on the species.

After human infants begin to respond to the precedence effect, their echo threshold continues to change with age. Echo threshold is defined as the shortest time delay between onsets at which subjects respond reliably to the echo as a separate sound coming from a location different from the leading sound. Infants' echo threshold is higher than preschoolers' or adults', while 5-year-olds' echo threshold appears to be the same as adults' for some sounds, like clicks, but higher for more complex sounds, like a continuously shaken rattle (Clifton, 1985; Morrongiello, Kulig, & Clifton, 1984). Litovsky (1991) has recently tested the effect of the echo on the leading sound's location in an MAA procedure that featured single-source sounds and precedence-effect sounds. She found that younger subjects (18 months and 5 years old) were more influenced by the lagging sound than were adults, with far greater minimal audible angles to precedence-effect stimuli than to single-source stimuli.

The echo suppression required in perceiving the precedence effect is complex and multifaceted. Adults' perception and suppression of the echo undergo systematic changes as a function of ongoing sound (Clifton, 1987; Clifton & Freyman, 1989; Freyman, Clifton, & Litovsky, 1991). There is a buildup in echo suppression, such that threshold rises by several milliseconds as sound continues. Hafter, Buell, and Richards (1988) saw a strong cognitive role in adults' perception of the precedence effect, and our data support this view. Clifton et al. (1981b; 1984) hypothesized that the newborns' immature auditory cortex was the limiting factor in their processing of lead and lag sounds. They attributed the onset of echo suppression in older infants to basic neuronal maturation. While this hypothesis may be correct, it cannot be the whole story because adult research points to transient influence of stimulation in the acoustic environment on perception of the echo, as in the buildup process. We do not know if infants would experience similar dynamic changes in their echo thresholds as a function of buildup, because this has never been tested. If so, this would indicate a more sophisticated processing of temporally complex stimuli than has been shown before, and would open the door to cognitive considerations in what has been regarded as basically a perceptual task.

Auditory Distance Discrimination

The issue of whether an infant can discriminate auditory distance is more than a question of sensory discrimination of distance cues. It encompasses the problem of an infant's representation of space and object location in space—a topic well studied by those interested in infants' visual development, but one hardly touched by those working with the auditory sense. Space is specified by audition as well as by vision. When you hear a sound, that sound is experienced as being out in space (unless you're wearing headphones or suffering from tinnitis). Head orienting, the response used in all studies described up to this point, proved inadequate to evaluate spatial differentiation. The morphology of the head-orienting response limits it to indicating *direction*, not depth, a limitation pointed out by those studying visual depth cues (Yonas & Granrud, 1985). The binaural cues underlying localization, such as interaural differences in time and intensity, are present to some extent in the newborn, enabling the head turn toward sound, and are quite refined by around 3–4 months, as demonstrated by discrimination over earphones (Ashmead et al., 1991; Bundy, 1980). However, the question of whether this processing of binaural cues is integrated in a way to produce outside-the-head sensations at these ages is unknown. Certainly, we should not infer such sensations from the head-orienting response, as this response also occurs to lateralized earphone stimulation that produces sound location within the head. Are infants born with some differentiation of inside-the-head versus outside-the-head sound? Do they have to learn to associate interaural difference information with spatial locations of sounds? These questions must await further experimentation with regard to newborns, but we can give a definitive answer for older infants. By 6 months of age infants are adept at reaching for objects, with a strong tendency to reach when objects are placed within reach and a reluctance when objects are placed beyond reach. This behavior has been exploited by Yonas and colleagues to study infants' sensitivity to visual depth cues (for review, see Yonas & Granrud, 1985). Using the same technique, we have studied infants' perception of auditory distance by turning out the lights, presenting sounding objects in the dark at various angles and distances, and video tape recording their behavior with infrared cameras.

In the first study distance was not manipulated because we were unsure whether infants would reach at all for sounding objects they could not see, and secondly, whether they would be accurate if they did reach. The sounding object was a finger puppet (replica of Big Bird from Sesame Street®) attached with Velcro® to a rattle. Infants were allowed to see and handle this stimulus before trials in the dark. The sounding object was presented at five different locations in the dark: midline, 30° and 60° left and right. Six-month-olds were willing to reach for this unseen, sounding object, and could accurately grasp this toy at every location (Perris & Clifton, 1988). In two subsequent studies distance was manipulated by presenting the object within the infant's reach in half of the trials and beyond reach in the remaining trials, keeping the same orientation of 30° for both distances (Clifton, Perris, & Bullinger, 1991). The results of one study are shown in Figure 4. In this study half of the infants received the block of trials in which the object was within reach first, while the other half received the block of trials in which the object was beyond reach first. Infants in both groups reached significantly more often when the toy was within reach than

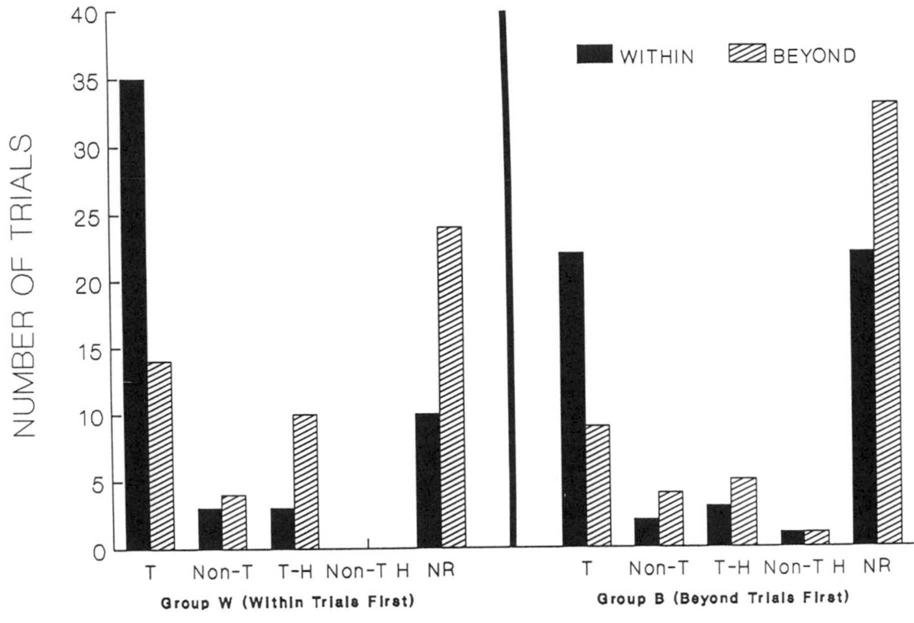

FIGURE 4 The number of trials in the dark in which either hand entered the specified area on within- and beyond-reach trials. (T = target area, scored the same for within- and beyond-reach trials, but occupied by the object only on within-reach trials; Non-T = target area on the opposite side of the apparatus; T-H = hemifield containing the target area; Non-T H = hemifield containing the non-target area; NR = trials with no reaching.) From Clifton, Perris, and Bullinger (1991). Copyright 1991 by the American Psychological Association. Reprinted by permission.

when it was out of reach. When the object was within reach, infants reached correctly for the object on the majority of trials (designated as T in Figure 4), with a few errors either in the target's hemifield (designated as T-H) or in the empty target area on the opposite side of the apparatus (designated as Non-T). When the object was beyond reach, infants usually did not reach at all (NR in the figure). If they did reach, they often reached into the space that the object *would* have occupied if within reach (the 30° orientation, labeled T in Figure 4) or somewhere in that hemifield. These results were true for both groups, but were more clearly expressed in the group having the block of trials with the object within reach first.

Although we have shown that 6-month-olds can discriminate distance in at least a dichotomous sense relative to their bodies (within vs. beyond reach), we do not know what cues they used to make this discrimination. We have manipulated the most obvious cue—sound pressure level—by having a group who received within-reach trials at one sound pressure level, with a natural drop in SPL of 6–7 dB when the sounding object was presented 1 m away (beyond reach). A second group had sounding objects presented at the same locations, but with SPL uncoordinated with distance, so that responding would be random with respect to distance if infants relied on SPL change as the cue. Adult groups were run under these same conditions. In both age groups within-reach and beyond-reach trials were randomly intermixed. Adults were completely fooled by this manipulation and judged distance on the basis of SPL, but infants were not fooled. They reached more often for the near object than the far object, regardless of which SPL was present (Litovsky & Clifton, 1992). This study does not prove that infants either cannot or do not use SPL as a cue for distance. Rather, it suggests that when SPL is not a reliable cue infants are able to use other distance cues, such as spectral changes due to diffraction of sound waves around the head or the ratio of direct to reverberant sound. Changes in sound pressure level appear to be the dominant distance cue for adults, but they can use other cues under conditions of training where SPL has been randomized with respect to distance (Ashmead, LeRoy, & Odom, 1990; Mershon & King, 1975).

A complete picture of infants' auditory localization should include their ability to identify the sound source itself, that is, *what* object is producing the sound. In evolutionary terms the issue of what is making a sound is surely as important as where the sound is coming from. This question extends beyond the organism's ability to respond to binaural cues and asks how auditory localization functions to guide subsequent behavior. Should the sounding object be approached or avoided? Does it evoke interest or is it to be ignored? Infants appear to recognize correspondences between some visual events and auditory events. Spelke and colleagues (for review, see Spelke, 1985) found that 4-month-olds presented with two videotapes will look longer at the one showing an object whose action corresponds to a soundtrack located centrally between the displays. Walker-Andrews and Lennon (1985) found that 5-month-olds looked longer at a videotape of an automobile approaching (or receding) when the soundtrack matched the visual event. This correspondence between sound and object extends to the situation of unseen objects. Clifton, Rochat, Litovsky, and Perris (1991) found that 6-month-olds could use sound to identify the object making the sound. Two different-sized objects had a sounding device (either rattle or bell) attached to them. The type of sound was counterbalanced with size of object so that half of the infants had the bell on the big object and rattle on the small object, with the reverse for the other half. Infants were exposed to both sound-making objects several times in the light, then were tested in the dark. Motor behavior was affected by object size in that infants reached for the larger object ("steering wheel") with a bimanual reach and for the smaller object (doughnut) with one hand. This differential reaching behavior was present both in the light and subsequently in the dark, indicating that the infants remembered which sound was attached to which object, and adjusted their manual behavior accordingly in the dark. This study suggests that infants use sound to evaluate environmental events and objects at a very young age, integrating this auditory information with their motor activity and cognitive functioning.

To briefly summarize the major points on the development of spatial hearing in infants:

1. At birth humans are sensitive to direction of sound, but special stimulus characteristics are needed to support the behavior. It remains unclear whether this directional sensitivity is truly spatial hearing, or reflects a limited binaural cue discrimination.
2. Sensitivity to binaural time cues is well-developed by 4 months of age; sensitivity to binaural intensity differences has not been well studied, so definitive conclusions must await further research. Behavioral tasks such as minimal audible angle reveal a steep rise in acuity during the first year of life, with a small improvement between 18 months and 5 years, when acuity closely approaches adult performance.
3. Perception of the precedence effect first becomes evident around 4–6 months. The developmental trend of head orienting toward sound from a single source earlier than orienting toward the leading side of precedence-effect sound is present in other mammalian species (dogs) as well as humans. Temporal parameters affecting the precedence effect continue to change through the preschool years. Work with young children on more cognitive aspects of the

precedence effect may reveal new complexities of echo-inhibition effects on spatial hearing.

4. By 6 months infants appear to appreciate auditory space, shown by their sensitivity to distance of auditory events. Which distance cues are critical is unclear, although sound pressure level changes do not appear to be necessary. Finally, infants can use sound to identify an unseen object, expressing this cognitive activity through differential motor behavior based on sound.

References

Ashmead, D., Clifton, R., & Perris, E. (1987). Precision of auditory localization in human infants. *Developmental Psychology*, *23*, 641–647.

Ashmead, D., Clifton, R., & Reese, E. (1986). Development of auditory localization in dogs: Single source and precedence effect sounds. *Developmental Psychobiology*, *19*, 91–104.

Ashmead, D., LeRoy, D., & Odom, R. (1990). Perception of the relative distances of nearby sound sources. *Perception & Psychophysics*, *47*, 326–331.

Ashmead, D., Davis, D., Whalen, T., & Odom, R. (1991). Sound localization and sensitivity to interaural time differences in human infants. *Child Development*, *62*, 1211–1226.

Banks, M. (1988). Visual recalibration and the development of contrast and optical flow peception. In A. Yonas (Ed.), *Perceptual development in infancy: The Minnesota Symposia on Child Psychology: Vol. 20* (pp. 145–196). Hillsdale, NJ: Lawrence Erlbaum Associates.

Blauert, J. (1983). *Spatial hearing*. Cambridge, MA: MIT Press.

Brazelton, T. B. (1973). *Neonatal behavioral assessment scale*. London: Spastics International Medical Publications.

Bundy, R. (1980). Discrimination of sound localization cues in young infants. *Child Development*, *51*, 292–294.

Butterworth, G., & Castillo, M. (1976). Coordination of auditory visual space in newborn human infants. *Perception*, *5*, 155–160.

Clarkson, M., & Clifton, R. (1991). Acoustic determinants of newborn orienting. In M. J. S. Weiss & P. R. Zelazo (Eds.), *Newborn attention: Biological constraints and the influence of experience* (pp. 99–119). Norwood, NJ: Ablex.

Clarkson, M., Clifton, R., & Morrongiello, B. (1985). The effects of sound duration on newborns' head orientation. *Journal of Experimental Child Psychology*, *39*, 20–36.

Clarkson, M., Clifton, R., Swain, I., & Perris, E. (1989). Stimulus duration and repetition rate influence newborns' head orientation toward sound. *Developmental Psychobiology*, *22*, 683–705.

Clarkson, M., Swain, I., Clifton, R., & Cohen, K. (1991). Newborns' head orientation toward trains of brief sounds. *Journal of the Acoustical Society of America*, *89*, 2411–2420.

Clements, M., & Kelly, J. (1978). Auditory spatial responses of young guinea pigs (*Cavia porcellus*) during and after ear-blocking. *Journal of Comparative & Physiological Psychology, 92*, 34–44.

Clifton, R. (1985). The precedence effect: Its implications for developmental questions. In S. E. Trehub & B. A. Schneider (Eds.), *Auditory development in infancy* (pp. 85–99). New York: Plenum Press.

Clifton, R. (1987). Breakdown of echo suppression in the precedence effect. *Journal of the Acoustical Society of America, 82*, 1834–1835.

Clifton, R., & Freyman, R. (1989). Effect of click rate and delay on breakdown of the precedence effect. *Perception & Psychophysics, 46*, 139–145.

Clifton, R., Gwiazda, J., Bauer, J., Clarkson, M., & Held, R. (1988). Growth in head size during infancy: Implications for sound localization. *Developmental Psychology, 24*, 477–483.

Clifton, R., Morrongiello, B., & Dowd, J. (1984). A developmental look at an auditory illusion: The precedence effect. *Developmental Psychobiology, 17*, 519–536.

Clifton, R., Morrongiello, B., Kulig, J., & Dowd, J. (1981a). Auditory localization of the newborn infant: Its relevance for cortical development. *Child Development, 52*, 833–838.

Clifton, R., Morrongiello, B., Kulig, J., & Dowd, J. (1981b). Developmental changes in auditory localization in infancy. In R. Aslin, J. Alberts, & M. Petersen (Eds.), *Development of perception: Psychobiological perspectives: Vol. 1: Audition, somatic perception, and the chemical senses* (pp. 141–160). New York: Academic Press.

Clifton, R., Perris, E., & Bullinger, A. (1991). Infants' perception of auditory space. *Developmental Psychology, 27*, 187–197.

Clifton, R., Rochat, P., Litovsky, R., & Perris, E. (1991). Object representation guides infants' reaching in the dark. *Journal of Experimental Psychology: Human Perception & Performance, 17*, 323–329.

DeCasper, A., & Fifer, W. (1980). Of human bonding: Newborns prefer their mother's voice. *Science, 208*, 1174–1176.

DeCasper, A., & Spence, M. (1986). Prenatal maternal speech influences newborns' perception of speech sounds. *Infant Behavior and Development, 9*, 113–150.

Engen, T., Lipsitt, L., & Kaye, H. (1963). Olfactory responses and adaptation in the human neonate. *Journal of Comparative & Physiological Psychology, 56*, 73–77.

Field, J., Muir, D., Pilon, R., Sinclair, M., & Dodwell, P. (1980). Infants' orientation to lateral sounds from birth to three months. *Child Development, 51*, 295–298.

Freyman, R., Clifton, R., & Litovsky, R. (1991). Dynamic processes in the precedence effect. *Journal of the Acoustical Society of America, 90*, 874–884.

Gardner, M. D. (1968). Historical background of the Haas and/or precedence effect. *Journal of the Acoustical Society of America, 43*, 1243–1248.

Gottlieb, G. (1981). Roles of early experience in species-specific perceptual development. In R. Aslin, J. Alberts, & M. Petersen (Eds.), *Development of perception: Psychobiological perspectives: Vol. 1: Audition, somatic perception, and the chemical senses* (pp. 5–44). New York: Academic Press.

Gray, L., & Jarsdoerfer, R. (1986). Effects of congenital aural atresia on the ability to localize sounds. *Otolaryngology—Head and Neck Surgery, 94* (August Special Issue), 46.

Hafter, E., Buell, T., & Richards, V. (1988). Onset-coding in lateralization: Its form, site, and function. In G. M. Edelman, W. E. Gall, & W. M. Cowan (Eds.), *Auditory function: Neurobiological bases of hearing* (pp. 647–676). New York: John Wiley & Sons.

Held, R. (1955). Shifts in binaural localization after prolonged exposures to atypical combinations of stimuli. *American Journal of Psychology, 68*, 526–548.

Hochster, M., & Kelly, J. (1981). The precedence effect and sound localization by children with temporal lobe epilepsy. *Neuropsychologia, 19*, 49–55.

Jenkins, W., & Masterton, B. (1982). Sound localization: Effects of unilateral lesions in central auditory system. *Journal of Neurophysiology, 47*, 987–1016.

Kelly, J. (1986). The development of sound localization of auditory processing in mammals. In R. N. Aslin (Ed.), *Advances in neural and behavioral development: Vol. 2.* (pp. 202–234). Norwood, NJ: Ablex.

Knudsen, E., & Knudsen, P. (1985). Vision guides the adjustment of auditory localization in young barn owls. *Science, 230*, 545–548.

Kuhn, G. (1987). Physical acoustics and measurements pertaining to directional hearing. In W. A. Yost & G. Gourevitch (Eds.), *Directional hearing* (pp. 3–25). New York: Springer.

Litovsky, R. (1991). *Developmental changes in sound localization precision under conditions of the precedence effect.* Unpublished doctoral dissertation, University of Massachusetts, Amherst.

Litovsky, R., & Clifton, R. (1992). Use of sound pressure level in auditory distance discrimination by 6-month-old infants and adults. *Journal of the Acoustical Society of America, 92*(1).

McGurk, H., Turnure, C., & Creighton, S. (1977). Auditory-visual coordination in neonates. *Child Development, 48*, 138–143.

Mershon, D., & King, L. (1975). Intensity and reverberation as factors in the auditory perception of egocentric distance. *Perception & Psychophysics, 18*, 409–415.

Mills, A. (1972). Auditory localization. In J. V. Tobias (Ed.), *Foundations of modern auditory theory: Vol. 2* (pp. 301–345). New York: Academic Press.

Moon, C., & Fifer, W. (1990). *Newborns prefer a prenatal version of mother's voice.* Poster presented at the International Conference on Infant Studies, Montreal, Quebec, Canada.

Morrongiello, B. (1988). Infants' localization of sounds in the horizontal plane: Estimates of minimum audible angle. *Developmental Psychology, 24*, 8–13.

Morrongiello, B., & Clifton, R. (1984). Effects of sound frequency on behavioral and cardiac orienting in newborn and five-month-infants. *Journal of Experimental Child Psychology, 38*, 429–446.

Morrongiello, B., Fenwick, K., & Chance, G. (1990). Sound localization acuity in very young infants: An observer-based testing procedure. *Developmental Psychology, 26*, 75–84.

Morrongiello, B., Kulig, J., & Clifton, R. (1984). Developmental changes in auditory temporal perception. *Child Development, 55*, 461–471.

Muir, D. (1985). The development of infants' auditory spatial sensitivity. In S. E. Trehub & B. Schneider (Eds.), *Auditory development in infancy* (pp. 51–83). New York: Plenum Press.

Muir, D., Abraham, W., Forbes, B., & Harris, L. (1979). The ontogenesis of an auditory localization response from birth to four months of age. *Canadian Journal of Psychology*, *33*, 320–333.

Muir, D., & Clifton, R. (1985). Infants' orientation to the localization of sound sources. In G. Gottlieb & N. Krasnegor (Eds.), *The measurement of audition and vision during the first year of postnatal life: A methodological overview* (pp. 171–194). Norwood, NJ: Ablex.

Muir, D., Clifton, R., & Clarkson, M. (1989). The development of a human auditory localization response: A U-shaped function. *Canadian Journal of Psychology*, *43*, 199–216.

Muir, D., & Field, J. (1979). Newborn infants orient to sounds. *Child Development*, *50*, 431–436.

Olmstead, C. E., & Villablanca, J. R. (1980). Development of behavioral audition in the kitten. *Physiology and Behavior*, *24*, 705–712.

Perris, E., & Clifton, R. (1988). Reaching in the dark toward sound as a measure of auditory localization in infants. *Infant Behavior and Development*, *11*, 473–491.

Pomerleau-Malcuit, A., Malcuit, G., & Clifton, R. (1975). An attempt to elicit cardiac orienting and defense responses in the newborn to two types of facial stimulation. *Psychophysiology*, *12*, 527–535.

Spelke, E. (1985). Preferential-looking methods as tools for the study of cognition in infancy. In G. Gottlieb & N. Krasnegor (Eds.), *Measurement of audition and vision in the first year of postnatal life: A methodological overview* (pp. 323–363). Norwood, NJ: Ablex.

Swain, I. U. (1987). *Newborn longterm retention of speech sounds*. Unpublished master's thesis, University of Massachusetts, Amherst.

Swain, I., Clifton, R., & Clarkson, M. (1989). *Change in stimulus location influences newborns' head orientation to sound*. Poster presented at the Society for Research in Child Development, Kansas City, MO.

Walker-Andrews, A., & Lennon, E. (1985). Auditory-visual perception of changing distance by human infants. *Child Development*, *56*, 544–548.

Weiss, M., Zelazo, P., & Swain, I. (1988). Newborn response to auditory stimulus discrepancy. *Child Development*, *59*, 1530–1541.

Wertheimer, M. (1961). Psychomotor coordination of auditory and visual space at birth. *Science*, *134*, 1692.

Whitfield, I. (1978). Auditory cortical lesions and the precedence effect in a four-choice situation. *Journal of Physiology*, *289*, 81.

Whitfield, I., Cranford, J., Ravizza, R., & Diamond, I. (1972). Effects of unilateral ablation of auditory cortex in cat on complex sound localization. *Journal of Neurophysiology*, *35*, 718–731.

Whitfield, I., Diamond, I., Chiveralls, K., & Williamson, T. (1978). Some further observations on the effects of unilateral cortical ablation on sound localization. *Experimental Brain Research*, *31*, 221–234.

Woodworth, R. S. (1938). *Experimental psychology*. New York: Holt.

Yonas, A., & Granrud, C. (1985). Reaching as a measure of infants' spatial perception. In G. Gottlieb & N. Krasnegor (Eds.), *Measurement of audition and vision during the first year of postnatal life: A methodological overview* (pp. 301–322). Norwood, NJ: Ablex.

Zelazo, P., Brody, L., & Chaika, H. (1984). Neonatal habituation and dishabituation of headturning to rattle sounds. *Infant Behavior and Development*, *7*, 311–321.

Zelazo, P., Weiss, M., Randolph, M., Swain, I., & Moore, D. (1987). The effect of delay on neonatal retention of habituated head-turning. *Infant Behavior and Development*, *10*, 417–434.

Zelazo, P., Weiss, M., & Tarquino, N. (1991). Habituation and recovery of neonatal orienting to auditory stimuli. In M. J. S. Weiss & P. R. Zelazo (Eds.), *Newborn attention: Biological constraints and the influence of experience* (pp. 120–141). Norwood, NJ: Ablex.

CHAPTER 6

Infants' Perception of Low Pitch

Marsha G. Clarkson

The field of psychoacoustics has traditionally emphasized the processing of simple, pure tones, which formed the basis for many existing models of auditory processing (cf. Wever, 1949). However, in daily life, such pure tones rarely occur; instead people encounter a variety of complex spectra, including human voices, musical instruments, car horns, and slamming doors. Because complex spectra so dominate the auditory environment, any attempt to understand auditory perception must explain abilities to detect, identify, and gather information from them. Likewise, developmental psychoacoustics must address these issues. In recent years, interest in the perception of complex acoustic signals has increased, in part, due to the availability of digital computers that permit production, control, and measurement of complex signals. Researchers are beginning to understand the nature of complex auditory processing in adults, but knowledge of this processing in infants lags far behind.

This research was funded by grants from the National Science Foundation (BNS8103541 and BNS8304419) to M. G. Clarkson and R. K. Clifton and from the National Institutes of Health (HD16480) to M. G. Clarkson.

Rather than the single frequency that characterizes a pure tone, complex tones are composites of two or more components. Each component has a frequency, an amplitude, and a phase relative to other components. Tonal complexes that repeat themselves are called periodic. They contain a fundamental frequency as well as a number of components or partials, termed *harmonics*, that are multiples of the fundamental frequency. Most "natural" communicative sounds such as the purrs of mammals, the calls of birds, and the voiced elements of human speech are periodic sounds. The multiple partials in a tonal complex elicit not the perception of many different frequencies, but rather a percept of a unitary signal having a distinctive pitch, quality (or timbre), and loudness. Listeners must attach meaning to these complex signals based on those attributes. For example, the young infant must distinguish periodic from aperiodic background sounds, glean relevant information from the signals in the auditory world, and learn appropriate behaviors in response to that information.

Of the three attributes of complex spectra—pitch, timbre, and loudness—the processing of pitch is best understood in both adults and infants. An extensive empirical literature describes adults' synthesis of pitch from complex signals, and a number of theories have emerged to explain pitch perception. Nonetheless, the mechanisms underlying pitch perception are not completely understood. Although our knowledge of pitch perception in infants is less extensive than that in adults, it is beginning to expand. The goals of the present chapter are to consider what researchers know about infants' pitch perception and to relate that work to critical issues in adults' pitch perception.

Critical Issues in Adult Pitch Perception

Pitch is the attribute of a sound that allows a listener to judge one sound as higher or lower than another. It provides the information that conveys the musical message in a melody. Periodic sounds, such as those produced by human voices and musical instruments, evoke the perception of a pitch equivalent to their fundamental frequency. Although experimental conditions and theoretical biases have led to many designations for the pitch of complex signals, I shall adopt Plomp's (1975), theoretically neutral term *low pitch*. The psychoacoustics literature contains many extensive reviews of low-pitch perception, which have evaluated whether pitch perception relies upon the spectral characteristics of signals or upon temporal features of the waveform (e.g., de Boer, 1976; Plomp, 1976). Rather than duplicate those reviews here, I shall briefly summarize some critical issues and current theories of pitch perception, which must guide this study of infant pitch perception.

The Fundamental Frequency Is Not Necessary for Pitch Perception

While low pitch is typically equivalent to the fundamental frequency of a periodic, complex signal, that frequency need not be present in the signal for its pitch to be heard (Fletcher, 1924). In 1841, Seebeck (described in de Boer, 1976), using a simple device called an acoustic siren, first demonstrated that signals with only a weak fundamental component evoke a strong pitch equivalent to the fundamental—much stronger than the spectral energy at the fundamental appeared to justify. Nearly a century after Seebeck's demonstration, the Dutch scientist J. F. Schouten (1938) extended that work. He showed not only that the low pitch of complex signals is equivalent to the fundamental frequency but also that the fundamental frequency is *not* reconstituted by nonlinear distortions as claimed by staunch "place" theorists.

Subsequent masking experiments confirmed that the fundamental frequency is not introduced into the listener's internal spectrum (Licklider, 1954; Patterson, 1969; Small & Campbell, 1961). For example, Patterson (1969) compared the effectiveness of noise in masking changes in both the frequency of a sinusoid and the low pitch of a complex signal. Although the sinusoids and complex signals conveyed the same pitches, their masking patterns were quite different. Listeners could not detect a change in the pitch of the sinusoid in the presence of a noise band of comparable frequency, but the low pitch of a complex signal did not disappear when the frequency region of the fundamental was masked by a band of noise. Rather, a band of noise spanning the higher component frequencies eliminated the perception of the pitch of the missing fundamental (Patterson, 1969). If nonlinear distortion products provide a basis for low-pitch perception, the low-frequency noise should have masked the pitch of the missing fundamental. These findings confirmed the importance of the higher partials in a complex for determining the perceived low pitch.

Low Pitch Remains Constant in the Presence of Spectral Variations

If the higher partials of a signal are the critical ones, how do they relate to low pitch? Is there a one-to-one correspondence between the partials and the pitch of complex spectra? To address this question, one need only consider the musicians in an orchestra tuning their instruments to the same pitch. Listeners in this situation can easily distinguish the instruments in the orchestra: An oboe clearly sounds different from a clarinet. Despite these differences, listeners can recognize that the various instruments are all sounding the same pitch as they tune.

In the laboratory, Patterson (1973) found that complex signals having differing numbers of partials (6 vs. 12 components) and differing phase relations among those partials (random vs. cosine phase) evoked the same low pitch as long as the spectra had the same lowest component. Across a variety of studies, the number of components in complex spectra evoking "common" low pitches has ranged from 2 (Smoorenburg, 1970) to 12 (e.g., Patterson, 1973). The low pitch of the signal remains that of the fundamental frequency, but its salience decreases with very small numbers of components. Thus, sounds having vastly different physical properties can produce the same low pitch. Rather than a one-to-one correspondence between the spectrum and pitch, a many-to-one correspondence exists. This pitch invariance, often termed perceptual constancy, suggests that listeners will tolerate considerable spectral variability in assigning low pitch.

Ambiguity of Pitch Occurs for Inharmonic Signals

While signals having different spectra can elicit the perception of equivalent low pitches, in some circumstances exactly the opposite can happen. In other words, a single spectrum can evoke the perception of more than one pitch. For harmonic tonal complexes, the pitch of a signal is equivalent to its fundamental frequency, which in turn equals the simple difference frequency separating the harmonics. If the frequencies of all components of a harmonic tonal complex are shifted upward (or downward), the signal becomes inharmonic. The frequency difference separating the components remains the same, but the perceived low pitch of the signal changes in the direction of the frequency shifts (de Boer, 1976; Schouten, Ritsma, & Cardozo, 1962). For very slight degrees of inharmonicity (i.e., slight changes in the component frequencies), the signal sounds almost as tonal as harmonic signals. As the degree of inharmonicity increases, the signal becomes increasingly atonal, and its low pitch becomes less salient. When the shift in the partials approaches half the difference frequency, two possible pitches can be heard. The single spectrum gives rise to a truly ambiguous pitch.

Low Pitch Is Derived From Spectrally Resolvable Partials

The low pitch of complex spectra certainly depends upon their higher frequency partials—in some instances evoking perceptual constancy for pitch in the presence of spectral variations, and in other instances evoking competing pitches from a single spectrum. But which partials in a complex signal actually mediate the perception of low pitch? The answer to this question first emerged when Ritsma (1962) demonstrated that a listener perceives a tonal low pitch only when the fundamental frequency and harmonic numbers are within certain limits. The so-called existence region for pitch was restricted to relatively low fundamental frequencies (below 800 Hz) and to relatively low-frequency, spectrally resolvable partials. No low pitch is detected when all partials in a complex signal are above the tenth harmonic (Ritsma, 1962). Ritsma (1967) and, independently, Plomp (1967) showed that the dominant spectral region conveying low pitch lies between the third and fifth harmonics. The low pitch conveyed by these spectrally resolvable partials is even dominant over the fundamental frequency.

Synthesis of Low Pitch Involves a Central Process

Granted that spectrally resolvable components determine low pitch, how and where is the information from those components integrated into a singular percept of pitch? Although the how of pitch synthesis remains in question, most investigators agree that the processing occurs at central levels of the nervous system. An elegant demonstration by Houtsma and Goldstein (1972) provided the initial impetus to place the pitch processor at a central level. Subjects identified musical intervals produced by the low pitches of two-component, tonal complexes. These intervals were reliably identified even when the two components in each complex were presented dichotically (i.e., one component to each ear). Houtsma and Goldstein (1972) argued that a fundamental period in the cochlear output is not necessary for the perception of low pitch and that the synthesis of spectral information must occur centrally. The central origin of low pitch was confirmed neurophysiologically by Whitfield and his colleagues. Heffner and Whitfield (1976) showed that cats can synthesize the low pitch of complex spectra, but perception of the missing fundamental was impaired following cortical ablation (Whitfield, 1980). Under this circumstance, animals responded to the frequencies of the partials. Thus, cortical ablation appears to impair the central processing of pitch while the peripheral analysis of complex spectra remains intact. Similar findings have been reported for damage to the auditory cortex in humans (Zartorre, 1988).

Spectral Cues Are More Salient Than Are Temporal Cues

Most of the findings described above suggest a strong spectral basis for the perception of low pitch, but signals lacking such information can sometimes evoke pitch sensations. For example, the spectrum of amplitude-modulated (AM), wideband noise remains constant with changes in modulation frequency. Nonetheless, this signal does have pitchlike properties (Burns & Viemeister, 1976). Listeners can identify simple melodies and musical intervals when the "notes" correspond to different modulation frequencies. Although these flat spectra evoke a perception of low pitch, their pitch is less salient than that of pure tones or tonal complexes. Pitch sensations can also emerge as a result of binaural interactions of noise signals (Fourcin, 1970; Huggins & Cramer, 1958). For example, Huggins and Cramer (1958) reported that a faint low pitch was produced by interaural differences in the phase spectrum of a white-noise signal. Once more, the pitch percept was less salient than that evoked by tonal complexes. Both the AM results and the binaural results indicate that some temporal process must contribute to pitch perception.

Modern Theories of Pitch Perception

A number of theories of pitch perception address the importance of low-frequency partials (Goldstein, 1973; Terhardt, 1974; Wightman, 1973). These theories posit two stages in the perception of low pitch. Each theory suggests that a peripheral analyzer, having limited spectral resolution, extracts the spectral components of a complex signal in a Fourier-like fashion. Then a central, synthetic stage, whose action differs for the theories, transforms the results of the spectral analysis into an estimate of low pitch.

In Wightman's (1973) pattern-transformation model, peripheral neural activity reflects the power spectrum of the signal, and a central Fourier-type analysis of the power spectrum determines low pitch from the location of the spectrum's maximum. Goldstein (1973), on the other hand, describes a statistical theory wherein a central processor uses information from noisily represented, aurally resolvable components of a signal. The processor recognizes pitch by matching the input to a stored pattern via a maximum likelihood estimation. Terhardt (1974) suggests that the components of a signal are transformed at the periphery into spectral pitch cues. Low pitch, as well as pure-tone pitch, is derived from those spectral pitch cues by matching to a best-fitting set of subharmonics previously stored in a neural matrix. Both Goldstein and Terhardt posit a template-matching process, but only Terhardt specifies the origin of the templates by suggesting that the matrix is built up from experience with harmonically related speech elements. Attempts to evaluate these models quantitatively indicate that both the pattern-transformation theory and Terhardt's theory cannot account for some of the data (e.g., Hall & Soderquist, 1982; Houtsma, 1979, 1981).

While most theorists advocate a strong spectral basis for the perception of low pitch, instances of flat spectra producing pitch sensations (e.g., Burns & Viemeister, 1976) are not easily reconciled with spectral models. More recent, "spectro-temporal" models posit a role for temporal information provided by firing patterns of the auditory nerve (Patterson, 1987; Srulovicz & Goldstein, 1983). This temporal information supplements spectral cues in the calculation of pitch.

Critical Issues for Infant Pitch Perception

The extensive literature on adults' pitch perception identifies many critical aspects of the process. To understand the nature of infants' pitch perception requires that the same phenomena be evaluated in infants. At a general level, it is necessary to know whether infants can synthesize the low pitch of complex spectra and whether their perception follows the same rules defined for adults. More specifically, the adult literature raises many interesting questions about the development of auditory processing.

The first, most obvious, and perhaps most critical issue that arises is whether infants are capable of the central processing required to perceive the pitch of the missing fundamental. Is some experience or learning required, as posited by Terhardt (1974)? The perception of the missing fundamental is the essential finding in the adult literature that separates the analytic processing of frequency from the synthetic processing of pitch. Whenever signals contain the fundamental frequency, infants could rely on analytic processing of that component in their perception. To assess central processing of pitch, infants must be tested with missing fundamental signals. If infants cannot synthesize the low pitch of those signals, then their perception must be limited by the physical energy in signals. Infants' perception of the pitch of the missing fundamental would argue in favor of central processing on their part and lead to a host of other questions regarding the nature of pitch synthesis.

One critical issue is whether infants' pitch perception depends upon the spectra of signals in a manner similar to that of adults. Perceptual constancy for pitch addresses one part of this issue. Do infants show perceptual constancy for pitch in the presence of spectral variations, and across what variations do they show it? Evidence of perceptual constancy would suggest that infants are responding not to the precise spectral content of signals but rather to their underlying pitches. Because theories of adult pitch perception assume invariance of pitch across certain spectral variations, that same invariance must be evaluated in infants.

The synthesis of low pitch from inharmonic tonal complexes permits evaluation of another part of the spectral-dependence issue. Does the decreased salience of pitch for inharmonic tonal complexes render them harder for infants to process, and is infants' difficulty a function of the degree of inharmonicity? If they process pitch like adults, infants should have increasing difficulty synthesizing low pitch as signals become increasingly inharmonic. With sufficient inharmonicity, a single spectrum should give rise to an ambiguous pitch.

Infants' processing of inharmonic signals would also address the importance of auditory nonlinearities in pitch perception. For example, if infants base their perception upon simple difference tones, then their performance with inharmonic signals should not deteriorate. Difference tones are no less salient in inharmonic than in harmonic signals. In any event, once infants' perception of low pitch is established, nonlinearities must be eliminated as a basis for their performance. Is the fundamental frequency reintroduced into the infant's internal spectrum? To the extent that infants' pitch processing is inherently the same as adults', one would expect a negative answer to this question.

A final part of the spectral-dependence issue relates to the partials necessary for the synthesis of low pitch. Do infants rely upon low-frequency, spectrally resolvable partials? Do infants have an existence region for tonal low pitch and is their existence region comparable to that of adults? Are harmonics 3–5 dominant in infants' perception of low pitch? All theories of adult pitch perception incorporate the existence and dominance data into their explanations of low pitch, so answers to these questions will be critical to any understanding of infants' pitch perception. If infants' synthetic processing is similar to adults', one would expect them to evidence both an existence region and a dominance region.

One aspect of peripheral auditory processing, infants' spectral resolution, is relevant to the existence region questions. Any developmental differences in peripheral resolution should change the existence-region for pitch across age. Although Olsho (1985) reported that infants' frequency-tuning curves are virtually equivalent to adults', other measures of frequency resolution show continuing development into the early school years (Allen, Wightman, Kistler, & Dolan, 1989; Irwin, Stillman, & Shade, 1986). The developmental course of this peripheral coding should impact the existence region over which infants synthesize low pitch.

Although many questions surround the spectral coding of pitch, recent spectro-temporal theories dictate that we must also look at temporal cues for pitch. Can infants use both spectral and temporal information to perceive low pitch? For example, might amplitude-modulated noise generate a percept of pitch? Evaluating these nonspectral pitches may prove difficult because even adults report them as quite faint. Infants' failure to synthesize low pitch from temporal cues could result simply from the decreased salience of the percept. Nonetheless, the question of whether infants can perceive nonspectral pitch will have important bearing on the theories applied to their pitch perception.

Beyond the initial question of whether infants can perceive the low pitch of complex spectra, each of the developmental questions posed addresses the "how" of pitch perception. If infants assign pitch in a similar way to adults, using the same acoustic cues, adult models can be generalized to infants. Any differences in these critical issues will indicate qualitative differences in the pitch perception process for infants and adults. Separate models of infant pitch perception will be required and a description of the transition to adultlike processing must follow. In recent years, our laboratory has begun to address some of the critical issues in infant pitch perception.

Studies of Infant Pitch Perception

Synthesis of Low Pitch From Harmonic Tonal Complexes

We first asked whether infants can synthesize the low pitch of complex spectra. Because harmonic tonal complexes provide the clearest, most easily matched pitch for adults, we started with such signals. To address the question of infant pitch perception, we attempted to demonstrate two of the basic phenomena related to pitch perception: perceptual constancy for pitch and perception of the pitch of the missing fundamental.

Perceptual constancy for pitch can be demonstrated by having infants categorize spectrally different signals according to their pitches. Research on infant speech perception reveals that infants can recognize the perceptual constancy of vowels despite variations in talker and intonation (e.g., Kuhl, 1979). Likewise, infants can categorize speech signals according to the sex of the talker (Miller, Younger, & Morse, 1982). Hence, we anticipated that infants would recognize the perceptual constancy of pitch.

Demonstrating perception of the pitch of the missing fundamental is requisite to the conclusion that infants actually synthesize the low pitch of complex signals. If we accept the neurophysiological evidence of cortical involvement in synthesizing the pitch of the missing fundamental, we might anticipate developmental changes in pitch perception abilities. Perception of the precedence effect, another auditory phenomenon for which the cortex has been implicated, changes developmentally such that before about 5 months of age infants cannot locate the source of those sounds (Clifton, Morrongiello, Kulig, & Dowd, 1981). After 5 months, infants readily locate the source of precedence effect signals (e.g., Muir, Clifton, & Clarkson, 1989; also see chapter 5 in this volume). Based on the localization data, we can predict that very young infants would have difficulty synthesizing low pitch but that older infants, such as those tested in the experiments to be reported here, would perceive the pitch of the missing fundamental.

Normally developing, 7-month-old infants, who were healthy at the time of testing with no ear infections or colds, participated in all the research to be described. Infants were tested in an adaptation of a conditioned head-turning procedure developed as an audiometric test for infants (Wilson, Moore, & Thompson, 1976) and commonly used to assess auditory sensitivity and discrimination (Kuhl, 1985). In this simple operant procedure, the infant sat on a parent's lap (see Figure 1) across from an experimenter who entertained her with silent toys. Sounds (each lasting 500 ms) from a background-pitch category were played repeatedly at sound pressure levels of 45 to 60 dB(A) from a loudspeaker located to one side of the infant. The infant learned to turn toward the sound when a change in the pitch of the sounds occurred. If the infant turned during a change in stimulation (i.e., a signal trial), she or he was credited with a "hit," and an animated toy was illuminated and activated. Turns at other times during the background and on no-signal trials (i.e., false alarms) were not reinforced. Complete details of the testing procedures can be found in Clarkson and Clifton (1985).

With complex spectra, determining the basis for responding is difficult, as many different cues are available. This problem is heightened for nonverbal subjects, such as infants, because they cannot be asked how they performed the task. Rather, stimuli must force the infant to attend to particular stimulus attri-

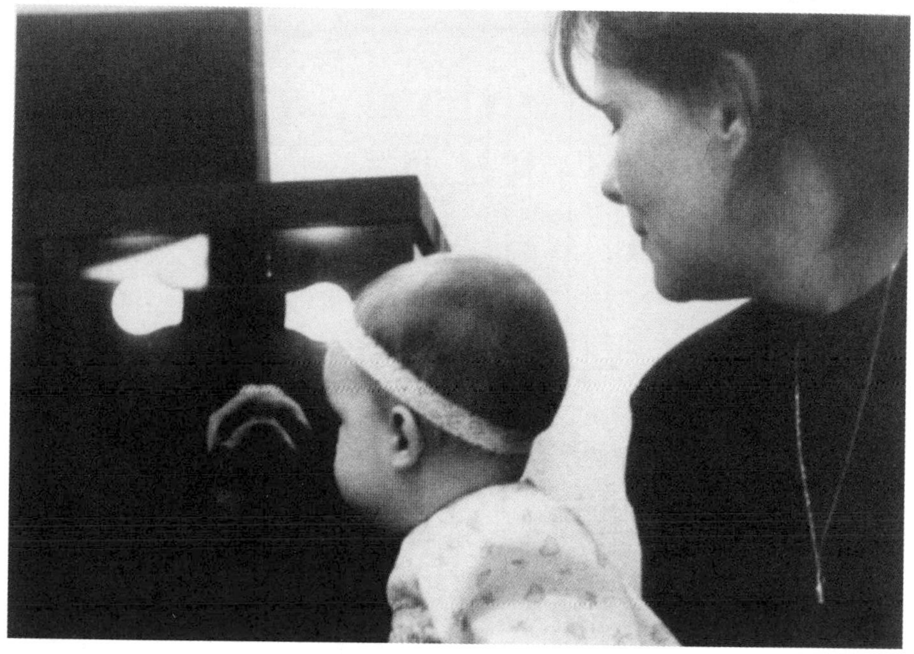

FIGURE 1 Experimental arrangement for conditioned head-turning procedure.

butes. To determine what acoustic information in complex spectra infants could use, we employed a transfer-of-learning format wherein infants progressed through several experimental stages. The infants' task remained the same throughout the experiment—to turn when the pitch category of the sounds changed. However, the exemplars representing each pitch category varied across stages to limit the effective strategies for solving the task. Restricting the acoustic cues available to infants allowed us to draw inferences about the bases of their responding. Failure in later stages of the experiment suggests that infants need the acoustic cues available in the preceding stage(s).

At the start of the session, infants learned to discriminate two harmonic tonal complexes (HTCs) differing in pitch: 160 Hz versus 200 Hz, 200 Hz versus 160 Hz, or 200 Hz versus 240 Hz. Each signal contained the fundamental frequency and eight, equal-amplitude harmonics of the fundamental (see Figure 2). Initially, infants received only signal trials, and when they made unassisted turns on three consecutive trials, testing proceeded to a discrimination stage.

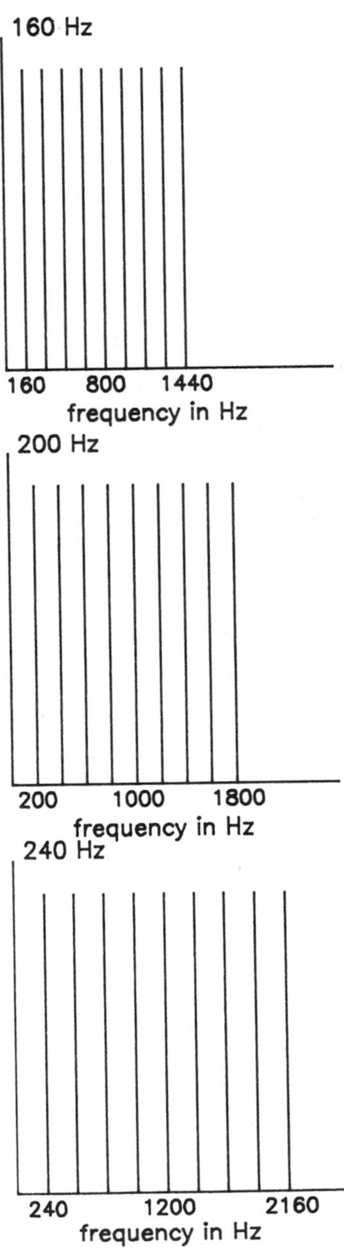

FIGURE 2 Line spectra of the three harmonic tonal complexes presented in the discrimination stage. The frequency of components (in hertz) is shown along the horizontal axis, and the amplitude of each component (in arbitrary units) is indicated by the vertical extent of the component.

The discrimination stage presented the same task to the infants, but procedural changes assured that they responded on the basis of pitch changes. To control for spontaneous turning, the pitch category did not change on half the trials (i.e., no-signal trials). In this and remaining stages, the experimenter and parent listened to music over headphones so they could not cue the infant when a signal trial occurred. Infants were tested for 30 trials or until they reached a criterion of correct responding on five of six trials. Infants who successfully completed this stage showed that they could discriminate the HTCs on the basis of one of the following: (a) the fundamental frequency; (b) the frequencies of the partials; (c) a combination of those cues; or even (d) the low pitches of the complexes. To narrow these bases of responding, successful infants proceeded to a second stage.

The procedures for this perceptual constancy stage followed those of the discrimination stage except that three HTCs constituted each pitch category. Each exemplar contained the fundamental frequency and six consecutive harmonics of the fundamental (see Figure 3 for representative line spectra). Although the frequencies comprising the exemplars within a pitch category differed, the range of frequencies for the two pitch categories overlapped considerably. This overlap minimized the availability of specific frequencies or frequency regions for solving the task. During the background and for no-signal trials, three background exemplars were presented in a random sequence, and a random presentation of change exemplars occurred on signal trials. The infant's task was to ignore the constant changes in the quality of the signals and to turn only when the pitch category also changed. Infants who passed this stage recognized some commonality in the signals for each category, most likely the fundamental frequency. Because infants could isolate the fundamental frequency in this stage, subjects who met criterion here proceeded to a final experimental stage.

The pitch categories for the low-pitch stage remained the same as in the preceding stages, but each exemplar contained only six consecutive harmonics of a missing fundamental (see Figure 4 for representative line spectra). Because the frequency ranges for the two pitch categories overlapped, the simplest strategy for categorizing the signals was to synthesize the pitch of the missing fundamental.

While the transfer-of-learning format permits inferences about the acoustic cues that infants use, the procedure has its drawbacks. It is time consuming with up to 30 or more trials in each stage. Furthermore, the most interesting informa-

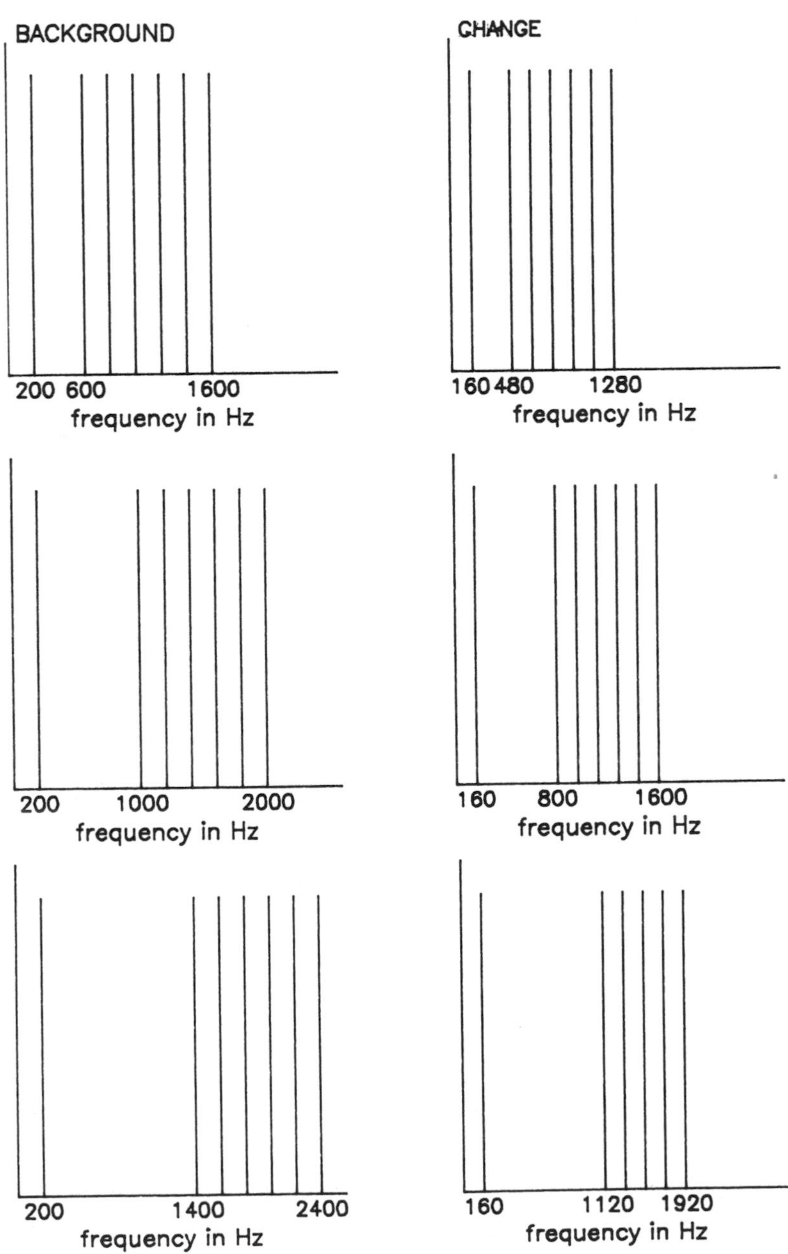

FIGURE 3 Line spectra of the harmonic tonal complexes presented in the perceptual constancy stage for an infant receiving a 200-Hz background-pitch category and a 160-Hz change-pitch category. The frequency of components (in hertz) is shown along the horizontal axis, and the amplitude of each component (in arbitrary units) is indicated by the vertical extent of the component.

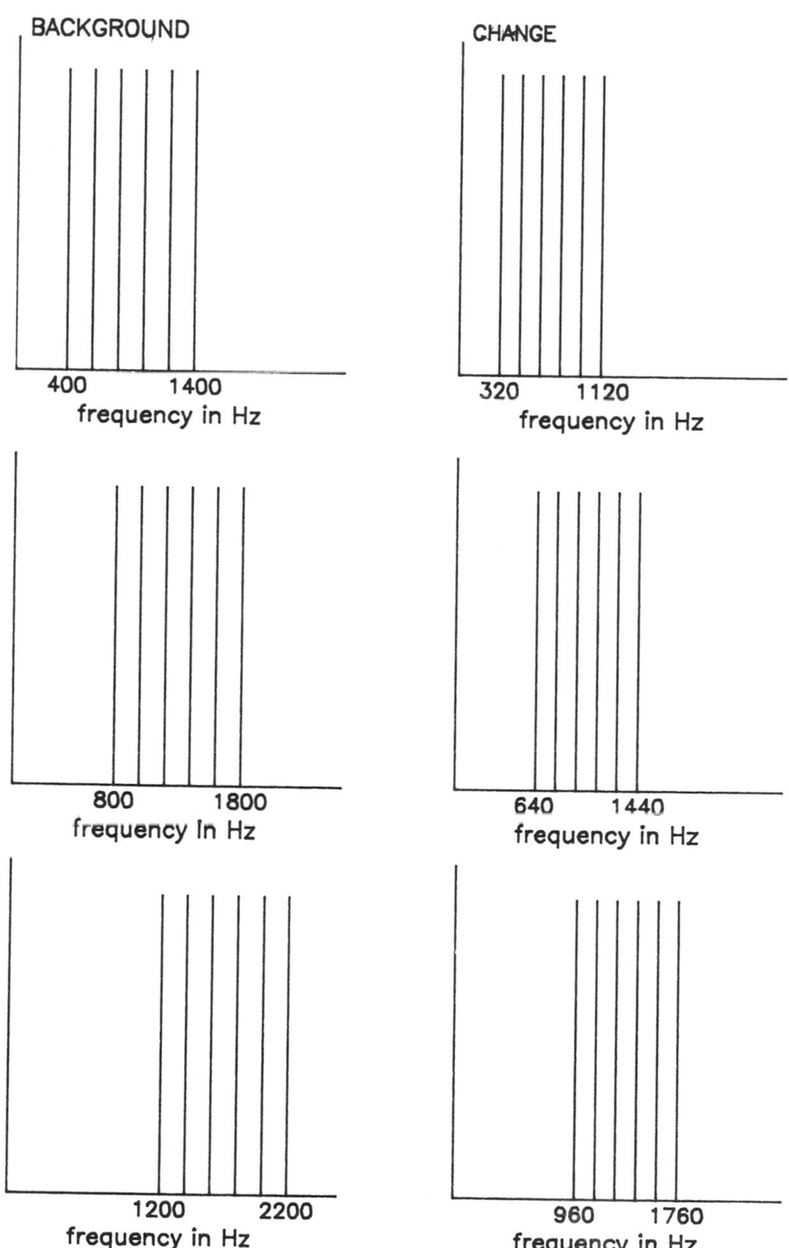

FIGURE 4 Line spectra of the harmonic tonal complexes presented in the low-pitch stage for an infant receiving a 200-Hz background-pitch category and a 160-Hz change-pitch category. The frequency of components (in hertz) is shown along the horizontal axis, and the amplitude of each component (in arbitrary units) is indicated by the vertical extent of the component.

tion emerges from the later stages of the experiment. How do we know that failure to synthesize the pitch of the missing fundamental might have occurred simply because an infant was sleepy, bored, or hungry? Might the introduction of multiple tokens confuse infants so that they make mistakes and stop playing the game?

We introduced a priming procedure to assure that infants remained aware of the game and were willing to play it. If infants get tired or confused in the later stages of the experiment, they should either stop turning altogether or turn all the time. Therefore, when infants did not turn on four consecutive signal trials or turned on two of three consecutive no-signal trials, they went back to the immediately preceding stage of the experiment to be reminded of the game. Because infants had already completed this stage, they were expected to quickly reorient to the task. Infants received up to 10 priming trials to reach a criterion of correct responding on 3 of 4 trials. Criterion performance in priming indicated that the infant knew what to do and would still play the game. When the infant met criterion in priming, testing resumed in the relevant experimental stage. If the infant failed priming, testing ended for the day. Because the infant was not performing with stimuli for which she or he had already been successful, we concluded that she or he was tired or bored, and return visits were scheduled.

During testing, infants received up to four runs through any experimental stage with priming stimuli interspersed between runs. As long as infants continued to meet criterion in priming, testing continued. If infants passed priming three times but still failed to successfully complete the experimental stage, we concluded that they failed the task because of a perceptual difficulty.

The results of this procedure can be viewed at two levels. Group performance permits conclusions about the average infant's perceptual abilities, whereas individual performance reveals the acoustic cues used by each infant and permits comparisons of relative performance with different signals across studies. Figure 5 summarizes group performance at the end of each experimental stage (i.e., for those trials contributing to criterion). The hit rate was significantly higher than the false alarm rate at criterion for each experimental stage ($ps < .05$), suggesting that infants discriminated the HTCs, recognized the perceptual constancy of those signals, and synthesized the pitch of the missing fundamental.

Analyses of the number of trials to criterion revealed no significant differences as a function of experimental stage ($M = 16.19$). Multiple exemplars in

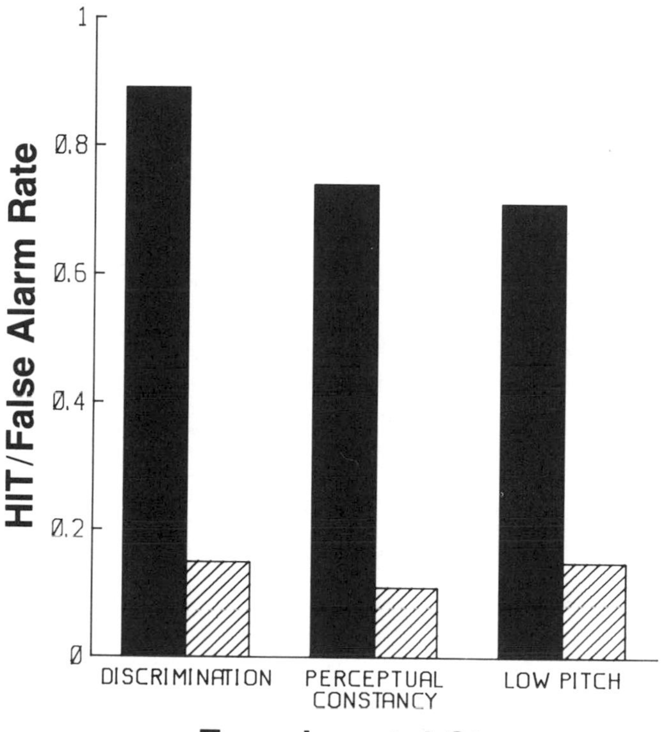

FIGURE 5 Mean hit rates (solid bars) and false-alarm rates (hatched bars) for the trials contributing to criterion performance in each experimental stage.

the perceptual constancy stage and the removal of the missing fundamental in the low pitch stage did not significantly increase the difficulty of the task.

At an individual level, 18 infants met criterion in the discrimination stage, whereas 16 of the 18 infants (88.89%) did so in the perceptual constancy stage. Fourteen of the infants tested with missing-fundamental signals successfully categorized them. Thus, 77.77% of the infants who discriminated two signals in the first experimental stage met categorization criterion in the low-pitch stage. Successful infants apparently synthesized the low pitch of the signals. Because each infant tested in the low-pitch stage successfully categorized the signals in the perceptual constancy stage, those who failed with the low-pitch stimuli probably could not synthesize a low pitch and required the physical presence of the fundamental frequency.

The results of this experiment demonstrate that 7-month-old infants can recognize the constancy of pitch for harmonic tonal complexes having different spectral characteristics and can categorize those sounds consistently with their pitches. The findings for the low-pitch stage provide an affirmative answer to our first question regarding infant pitch perception: Infants can synthesize the low pitch of the missing fundamental. The question of whether that synthesis is adultlike remains. One phenomenon that addresses this question is the perception of inharmonic tonal complexes.

Synthesis of Low Pitch From Inharmonic Tonal Complexes

For adults, the low pitch of inharmonic signals becomes less salient and more difficult to hear as the frequencies of partials are shifted increasingly away from a harmonic relation (cf. de Boer, 1976). If infants also have difficulty synthesizing the low pitch of inharmonic tonal complexes, one might conclude that these signals generate weak pitch cues for infants. Poor performance with inharmonic signals would also suggest that infants do not rely upon peripheral, nonlinear distortion products to perceive low pitch. In two experiments, we asked whether infants can categorize inharmonic tonal complexes in accordance with their low pitches and whether infants' performance is a function of the degree of inharmonicity in the signals.

Pitch synthesis from moderately inharmonic signals

Infants were tested as in the preceding experiment. We wanted to ensure that all infants could learn some discrimination, so they were initially tested with two harmonic tonal complexes, identical to the 160 Hz and 200 Hz HTCs in the preceding experiment except that they lacked energy at the fundamental frequency (see Figure 6). Testing with these signals continued for 30 trials or until infants met criterion: a hit rate of .8 or higher and a false alarm rate of .2 or lower. Successful infants proceeded to an inharmonic-discrimination stage.

For this stage, inharmonic tonal complexes (ITCs) were generated from the HTCs by shifting the frequency of each partial upward by 30 Hz (see Figure 7). Although adult listeners rated these signals to have moderate inharmonicity, they did not report truly ambiguous pitches. In this and the preceding stage, infants could discriminate the signals on the basis of one of the following: (a) their low pitches; (b) their spectral profiles; or (c) their isolated frequency components. Infants who met criterion with these ITCs proceeded to a final stage.

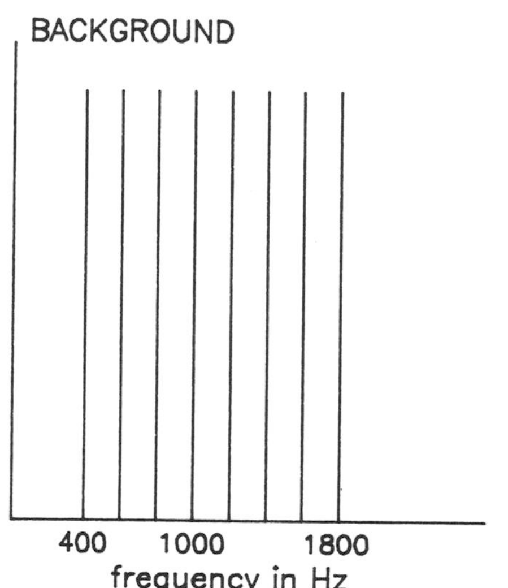

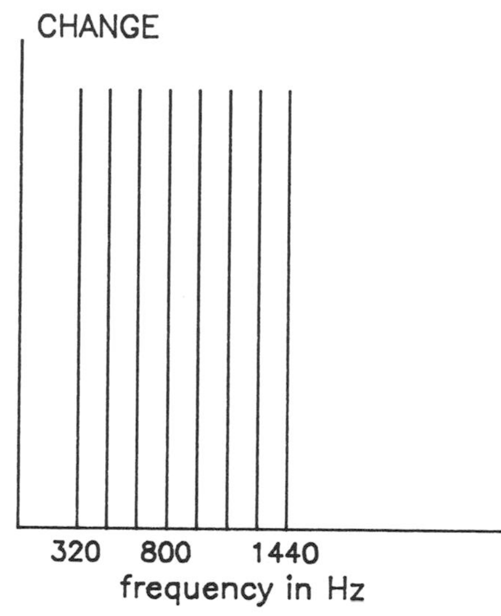

FIGURE 6 Line spectra of the harmonic tonal complexes presented in the harmonic discrimination stage for an infant receiving a high (200 Hz) background-pitch category and a low (160 Hz) change-pitch category. The frequency of components (in hertz) is shown along the horizontal axis, and the amplitude of each component (in arbitrary units) is indicated by the vertical extent of the component.

In the low-pitch stage, infants were asked to categorize spectrally different ITCs according to their low pitches. Each pitch category was represented by three inharmonic exemplars comprised of six consecutive, frequency-shifted partials (see Figure 8). The overlap in the frequency ranges of the exemplars for the two pitch categories minimized the usefulness of spectral profiles for solving the task and forced infants to use low-pitch cues.

The group's mean performance on the trials contributing to criterion is shown in Figure 9. Although the hit rate was significantly greater than the false-alarm rate for each experimental stage (all ps $<.001$), the interaction between experimental stage and response type was also significant ($p <.05$). This interaction reflected a smaller difference between hit and false-alarm rates for the low-pitch stage than for the two discrimination stages. Apparently, the categorization stage was more difficult than the discrimination ones. The number of trials to criterion did not differ across experimental stages ($M = 22.62$), perhaps reflecting the large variability across subjects.

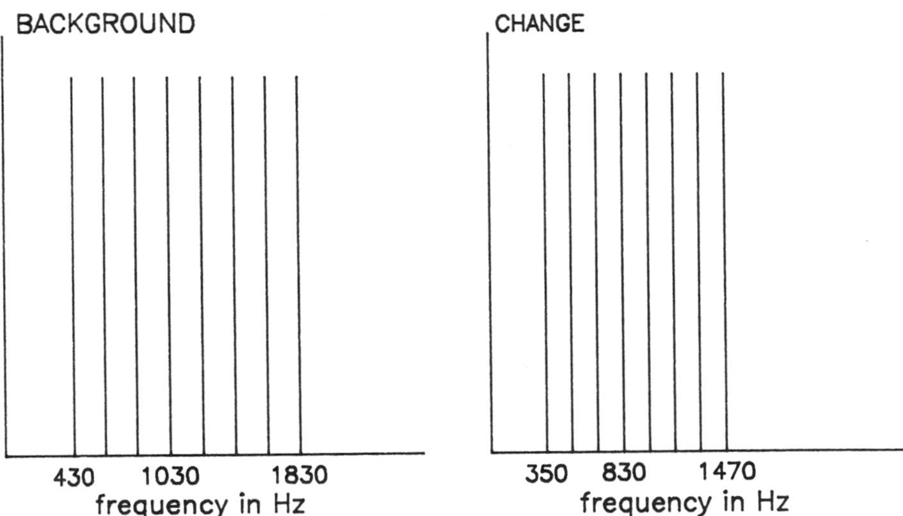

FIGURE 7 Line spectra of the inharmonic tonal complexes presented in the inharmonic discrimination stage for an infant receiving a high background-pitch category and a low change-pitch category. The frequency of components (in hertz) is shown along the horizontal axis, and the amplitude of each component (in arbitrary units) is indicated by the vertical extent of the component.

Nineteen infants met criterion in the harmonic-discrimination stage, whereas 16 (84%) of those infants did so for the inharmonic stimuli. In the low-pitch stage, only 11 of the infants successfully categorized the three ITCs in accordance with their low pitches. Thus, approximately 58% of the infants who discriminated the HTCs were also able to synthesize the low pitch of the ITCs. The relatively poor performance with these signals improved with development. Seven infants, who failed one of the latter two stages of this experiment, were retested at 10 months of age. Each infant passed at least one more stage than she or he had completed 3 months earlier.

The results of this experiment show that, as a group, 7-month-old infants can synthesize the low pitch of ITCs. However, both the group and individual analyses suggest that the inharmonic signals were more difficult than the harmonic ones of the previous experiment. For the group, the difference between hit and false-alarm rates at criterion was smaller for the categorization of inharmonic signals than for the discrimination of either harmonic or inharmonic ones.

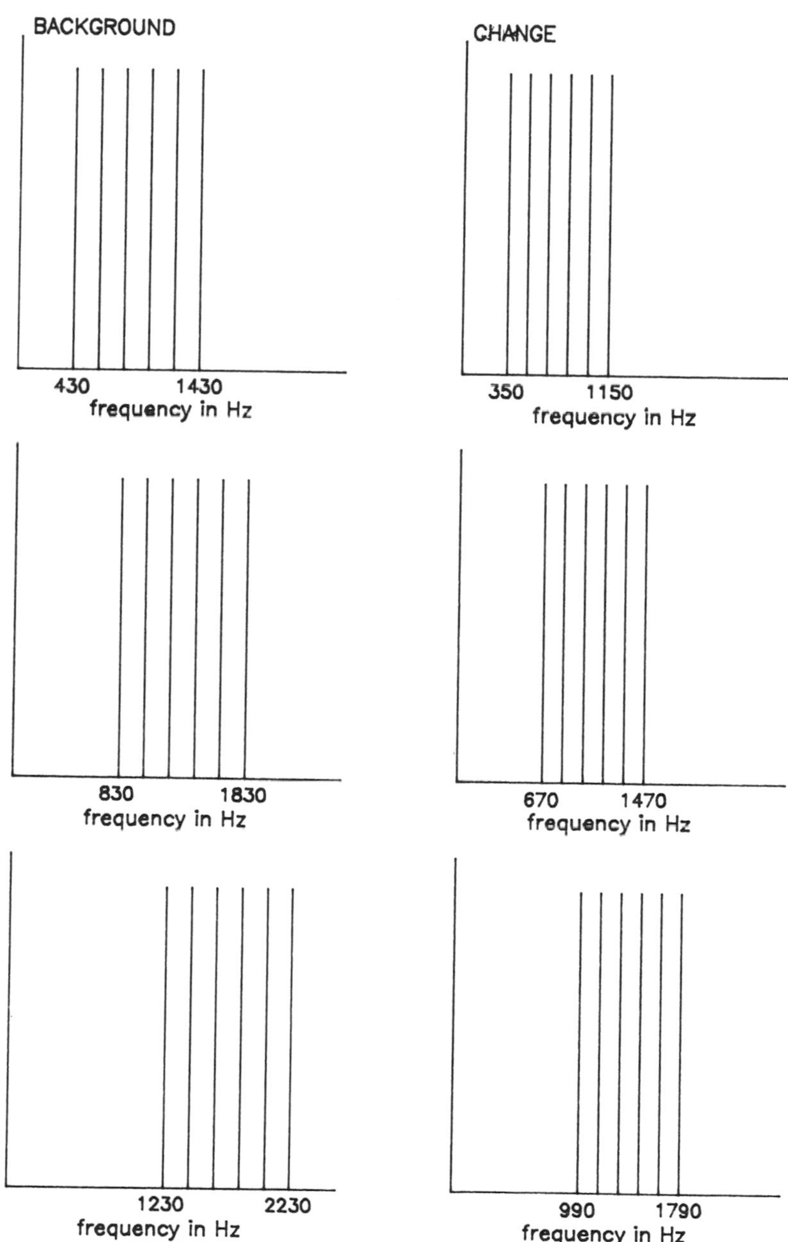

FIGURE 8 Line spectra of the inharmonic tonal complexes presented in the low pitch stage for an infant receiving a high background-pitch category and a low change-pitch category. The frequency of components (in hertz) is shown along the horizontal axis, and the amplitude of each component (in arbitrary units) is indicated by the vertical extent of the component.

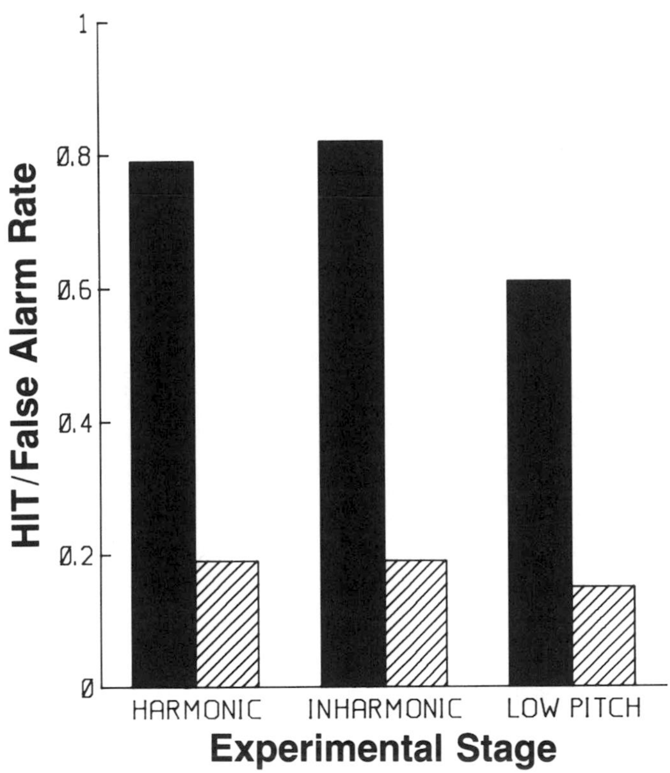

FIGURE 9 Mean hit rates (solid bars) and false-alarm rates (hatched bars) for the trials contributing to criterion performance in each experimental stage.

Infants' performance on HTCs did not differ for categorization and discrimination. Thus, relatively poor performance was limited to low-pitch categorization of inharmonic signals.

At an individual level, the percentage of infants categorizing the ITCs indicates that about half the infants carried the group performance. The percentage of infants synthesizing the low pitch of ITCs (58%) was much lower than the nearly 78% who synthesized the low pitch of HTCs. The relative difficulty infants exhibited with these inharmonic signals agrees with adult data from ITCs and suggests that infants actually synthesized the low pitch of signals in both experiments. With two available data points, infants' perception of low pitch appears to vary with the spectral characteristics of signals. A final experiment provided a third point on this inharmonicity function.

Pitch synthesis from slightly inharmonic signals

Adults judge low pitch to approach the tonality and salience of harmonic signals as the degree of inharmonicity in ITCs decreases (cf. de Boer, 1976). If inharmonicity influences infants' pitch perception in a manner similar to that of adults', lessened inharmonicity should improve the performance of individual infants and perhaps the performance of the group as a whole. This possibility was evaluated with a second set of inharmonic signals.

Infants were tested as in the previous experiment. They first learned to discriminate the same HTCs used in that experiment. This stage established an equivalent level of performance across the two studies, so performance in subsequent stages could be compared. Infants who met criterion with these signals moved on to discriminate inharmonic ones. Inharmonicity was introduced by shifting the frequency of each partial upward by 20 Hz, as depicted in Figure 10. Successful infants proceeded to a final stage in which they attempted to categorize the three ITCs depicted in Figure 11 according to their low pitches.

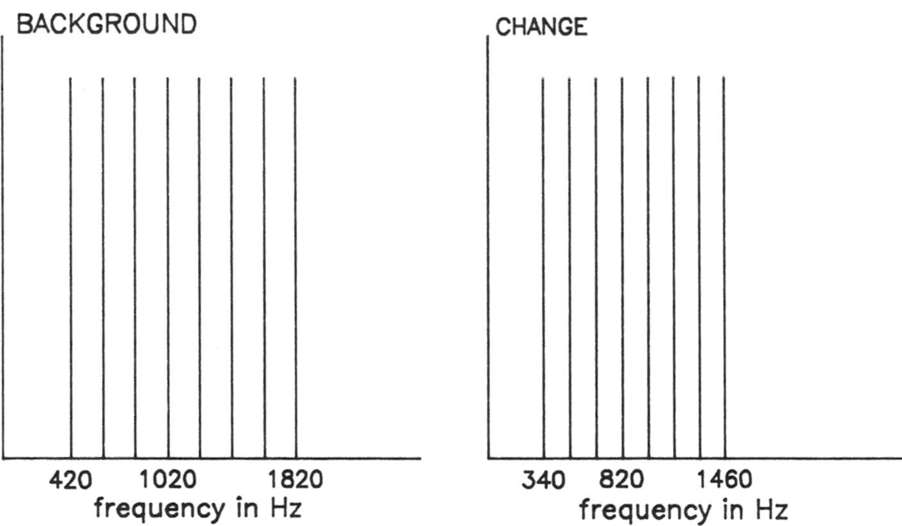

FIGURE 10 Line spectra of the inharmonic tonal complexes presented in the inharmonic discrimination stage for an infant receiving a high background-pitch category and a low change-pitch category. The frequency of components (in hertz) is shown along the horizontal axis, and the amplitude of each component (in arbitrary units) is indicated by the vertical extent of the component.

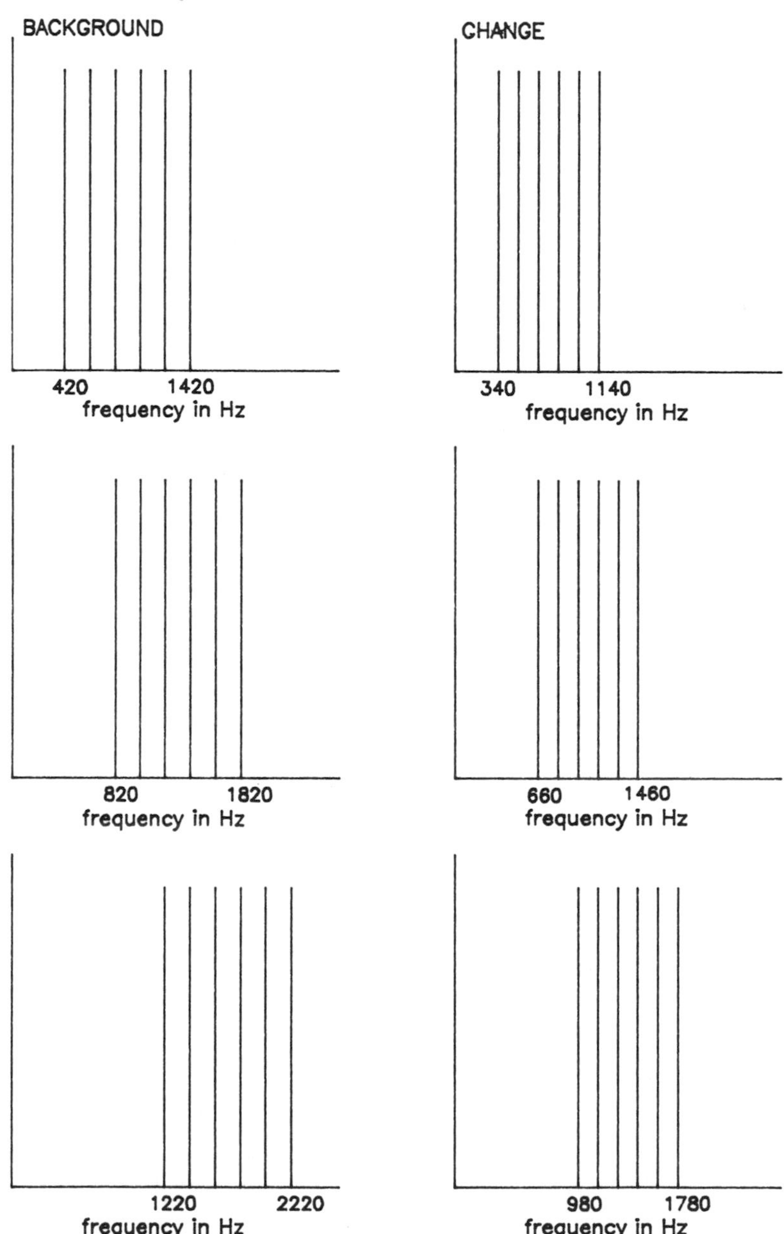

FIGURE 11 Line spectra of the inharmonic tonal complexes presented in the low-pitch stage for an infant receiving a high background-pitch category and a low change-pitch category. The frequency of components (in hertz) is shown along the horizontal axis, and the amplitude of each component (in arbitrary units) is indicated by the vertical extent of the component.

Figure 12 summarizes group performance on the trials contributing to criterion in each stage. Responding did not differ as a function of experimental stage, and the hit rate significantly exceeded the false-alarm rate in each stage ($ps < .0001$). As in the preceding experiment, the number of trials to criterion did not differ as a function of experimental stage ($M = 24.42$).

Individually, 13 infants met criterion in the harmonic discrimination stage, and 10 of those infants (77%) also reliably discriminated the inharmonic signals. In the low-pitch stage, 9 infants met criterion for grouping the signals according to their low pitches. Thus, 70% of those infants who discriminated the HTCs synthesized the low pitch of the ITCs. This compares with 58% for the more strongly inharmonic signals of the preceding experiment.

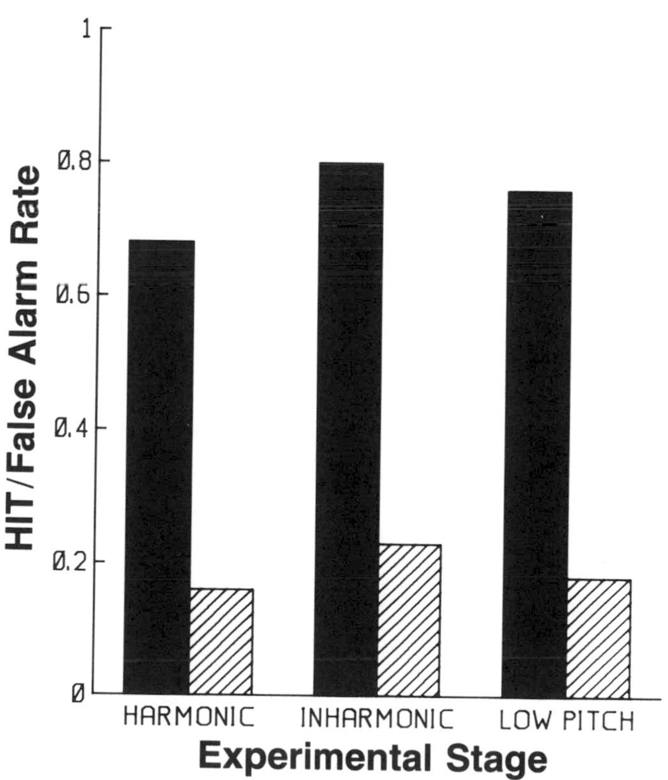

FIGURE 12 Mean hit rates (solid bars) and false-alarm rates (hatched bars) for the trials contributing to criterion performance in each experimental stage.

Conclusions

The results of these experiments provide an initial description of infants' pitch perception. In the first experiment, infants successfully discriminated harmonic tonal complexes. When inharmonic complexes were presented, more than 75% of infants who discriminated HTCs also reliably discriminated those signals. That some infants did not discriminate the inharmonic signals suggests that they might be harder for infants to process than harmonic ones. Nonetheless, the degree of inharmonicity does not appear to influence the discrimination of ITCs.

The categorization stages of these experiments begin to elucidate the bases of infants' pitch perception. The first experiment demonstrated perceptual constancy for pitch with the majority of infants (89%) ignoring the changing spectra of HTCs and recognizing their common fundamental frequency. When the fundamental frequency was removed from the signals, infants (78%) successfully synthesized low pitch. This result indicates that infants are capable of the central processing posited by pitch theories. When infants were asked to categorize inharmonic signals, their success diminished. The worst individual performance (58% success) occurred for the 30-Hz shift off-harmonic, and although performance improved (70% success) for the 20-Hz shift, it remained below that for harmonic signals. At a group level, performance deteriorated significantly only when infants attempted to categorize moderately inharmonic stimuli.

These experiments indicate that infants' pitch perception depends upon the spectral characteristics of signals in a manner similar to that of adults. Low pitch was most easily synthesized for harmonic tonal complexes. As signals became increasingly inharmonic, infants demonstrated increasing difficulty synthesizing low pitch. To the extent that infants' problems reflect the reduced salience of low pitch for inharmonic signals, more strongly inharmonic signals should prove even more difficult.

The inharmonic results also strengthen the interpretation that infants actually synthesized the low pitch in the harmonic study. For adults, the pitch shift for inharmonic signals indicates that low-pitch perception does not result from generation of the fundamental frequency as a distortion product. Infants' difficulty synthesizing the low pitch of inharmonic signals suggests that the same is true for them. If infants had relied upon combination tones in these experiments, their performance should not have deteriorated in the inharmonic tasks.

Developmental research on the processing of pitch has been quite limited. One study concluded that 4-month-old infants may not derive pitch in an adult-like manner (Bundy, Colombo, & Singer, 1982). In a habituation–dishabituation paradigm, infants heard a sequence of harmonic tonal complexes having different pitches. Although the habituation results suggested that infants either did not differentiate the spectrally varying exemplars of each pitch category or categorized them as having the same pitch, infants showed no evidence of discrimination upon dishabituation. Removing the fundamental frequency did not influence performance, but the importance of this finding remains unclear because infants failed to categorize even those signals that contained the fundamental frequency. These results indicate that further investigation of low-pitch perception in 2-to-4-month-old infants is warranted.

Music theory inspired a second, developmental investigation of pitch perception (Demany & Armand, 1984). Some music theories suggest that pitch is a two-dimensional attribute reflecting (a) tone height, a perceptual quality that is monotonically related to frequency, and (b) tone chroma, a quality shared by tones forming an octave interval (cf. Burns & Ward, 1982). Reports that musically trained adults exhibit octave confusions when asked to identify the notes corresponding to complex tones support the notion of an independent, chroma dimension. Because musically naive adults do not show octave generalization, Burns and Ward (1982) have argued that both octave generalization and tone chroma are learned.

Demany and Armand (1984) investigated the role of learning in infants' pitch perception by evaluating octave confusions. They habituated 3-month-old infants' responses to a sequence of tones and then changed the melodic sequence. When two tones in the sequence were shifted in frequency by a seventh or ninth, infants evidenced discrimination, but no discrimination was observed if the tones changed by an octave. The authors concluded that two tones forming an octave interval have some degree of perceptual equivalence for young infants and that perception of tone chroma may not necessitate some form of musical experience.

All the research evaluating infants' pitch perception suggests that infants can identify the pitch of complex signals. To the extent that infants can glean information about pitch from periodic signals in their environments, how might they use this information? One suggestion is that the prosodic cues inherent in the pitch and pitch excursions of speech signals convey communicative intent

(Fernald, 1989). These prosodic cues are typically exaggerated in infant-directed speech, which emphasizes the prosodic information carried by fundamental-frequency excursions over the linguistic content of the speech (Fernald & Kuhl, 1987; Fernald et al., 1989). If the communicative message in infant-directed speech lies in its prosodic cues, pitch may be especially important to the young infant.

The identification of periodic signals in the environment and, for the young infant, the processing of the pitch of these signals may represent critical elements of communication. Our findings that infants can synthesize the low pitch of complex spectra suggests that pitch information is available to the infant. While our understanding of infants' pitch processing remains incomplete, the initial parallels between their performance and that of adults suggest that adult models of pitch perception may generalize to infants. A full understanding of the development of pitch perception abilities must await further investigations of theoretically crucial phenomena and of younger infants than have been tested heretofore. Nonetheless, our initial look at infants' pitch perception promises that we can uncover its nature and perhaps even evaluate the efficacy of adult models from a developmental perspective.

References

Allen, P., Wightman, F., Kistler, D., & Dolan, T. (1989). Frequency resolution in children. *Journal of Speech and Hearing Research*, *32*, 317–322.

Bundy, R. S., Colombo, J., & Singer, J. (1982). Pitch perception in young infants. *Developmental Psychology*, *18*, 10–14.

Burns, E. M., & Viemeister, N. F. (1976). Nonspectral pitch. *Journal of the Acoustical Society of America*, *60*, 863–869.

Burns, E. M., & Ward, W. D. (1982). Intervals, scales, and tuning. In D. Deutsch (Ed.), *The psychology of music* (pp. 241–269). Orlando, FL: Academic Press.

Clarkson, M. G., & Clifton, R. K. (1985). Infant pitch perception: Evidence for responding to pitch categories and the missing fundamental. *Journal of the Acoustical Society of America*, *77*, 1521–1528.

Clifton, R. K., Morrongiello, B. A., Kulig, J. W., & Dowd, J. M. (1981). Newborns' orientation toward sound: Possible implications for cortical development. *Child Development*, *52*, 833–838.

de Boer, E. (1976). On the "residue" and auditory pitch perception. In W. D. Keidel & W. D. Neff (Eds.), *Handbook of sensory physiology* (pp. 479–583). Berlin: Springer.

Demany, L., & Armand, F. (1984). The perceptual reality of tone chroma in early infancy. *Journal of the Acoustical Society of America*, *76*, 57–66.

Fernald, A. (1989). Intonation and communicative intent in mothers' speech to infants: Is the melody the message? *Child Development, 60*, 1497–1510.

Fernald, A., & Kuhl, P. (1987). Acoustic determinants of infant preference for motherese speech. *Infant Behavior and Development, 10*, 279–293.

Fernald, A., Taeschner, T., Dunn, J., Papousek, M., de Boysson-Bardies, B., & Fukui, I. (1989). A cross-language study of prosodic modifications in mothers' and fathers' speech to preverbal infants. *Journal of Child Language, 16*, 477–501.

Fletcher, H. (1924). The physical criterion for determining the pitch of a musical tone. *Physical Review, 23*, 427–437.

Fourcin, A. J. (1970). Central pitch and auditory lateralization. In R. Plomp & G. F. Smoorenburg (Eds.), *Frequency analysis and periodicity detection in hearing* (pp. 319–326). Leiden: Sijthoff.

Goldstein, J. L. (1973). An optimum processor theory for the central formation of the pitch of complex tones. *Journal of the Acoustical Society of America, 63*, 498–510.

Hall, J. L., & Soderquist, D. R. (1982). Transient complex and pure tone pitch changes by adaptation. *Journal of the Acoustical Society of America, 71*, 665–670.

Heffner, H., & Whitfield, I. C. (1976). Perception of the missing fundamental by cats. *Journal of the Acoustical Society of America, 59*, 915–919.

Houtsma, A. J. M. (1979). Musical pitch of two-tone complexes and predictions by modern pitch theories. *Journal of the Acoustical Society of America, 66*, 87–99.

Houtsma, A. J. M. (1981). Noise-induced shifts in the pitch of pure and complex tones. *Journal of the Acoustical Society of America, 70*, 1661–1668.

Houtsma, A. J. M., & Goldstein, J. L. (1972). The central origin of the pitch of complex tones: Evidence from musical recognition. *Journal of the Acoustical Society of America, 51*, 520–529.

Huggins, W. H., & Cramer, E. M. (1958). Creation of pitch through binaural interaction. *Journal of the Acoustical Society of America, 30*, 413–417.

Irwin, R. J., Stillman, J. A., & Shade, A. (1986). The width of the auditory filter in children. *Journal of Experimental Child Psychology, 41*, 429–442.

Kuhl, P. K. (1979). Speech perception in early infancy: Perceptual constancy for spectrally dissimilar vowel categories. *Journal of the Acoustical Society of America, 66*, 1668–1679.

Kuhl, P. K. (1985). Methods in the study of infant speech perception. In G. Gottlieb & N. A. Krasnegor (Eds.), *Measurement of audition and vision in the first year of postnatal life: A methodological overview* (pp. 223–251). Norwood, NJ: Ablex.

Licklider, J. C. R. (1954). Periodicity pitch and place pitch. *Journal of the Acoustical Society of America, 26*, 945A.

Miller, C. L., Younger, B. A., & Morse, P. A. (1982). The categorization of male and female voices in infancy. *Infant Behavior and Development, 5*, 143–149.

Muir, D. W., Clifton, R. K., & Clarkson, M. G. (1989). The development of a human auditory localization response: A U-shaped function. *Canadian Journal of Psychology, 43*, 199–216.

Olsho, L. W. (1985). Infant auditory perception: Tonal masking. *Infant Behavior and Development, 8*, 371–384.

Patterson, R. D. (1969). Noise masking of a change in residue pitch. *Journal of the Acoustical Society of America*, *45*, 1520–1524.

Patterson, R. D. (1973). The effects of relative phase and number of components on residue pitch. *Journal of the Acoustical Society of America*, *53*, 1565–1572.

Patterson, R. D. (1987). A pulse ribbon model of peripheral auditory processing. In W. A. Yost & C. S. Watson (Eds.), *Auditory processing of complex sounds* (pp. 167–179). Hillsdale, NJ: Erlbaum.

Plomp, R. (1967). Pitch of complex tones. *Journal of the Acoustical Society of America*, *41*, 1526–1533.

Plomp, R. (1975). Auditory psychophysics. *Annual Review of Psychology*, *26*, 207–232.

Plomp, R. (1976). *Aspects of tone sensation: A psychophysical study*. London: Academic Press.

Ritsma, R. J. (1962). Existence region of the tonal residue. *Journal of the Acoustical Society of America*, *34*, 1224–1229.

Ritsma, R. J. (1967). Frequencies dominant in the perception of the pitch of complex sounds. *Journal of the Acoustical Society of America*, *42*, 191–198.

Schouten, J. F. (1938). The perception of subjective tones. *Proceedings Koninklijke Nederlandse Akademie Van Wetenschappen*, *41*, 1086–1094.

Schouten, J. F., Ritsma, R. J., & Cardozo, B. L. (1962). Pitch of the residue. *Journal of the Acoustical Society of America*, *34*, 1418–1424.

Small, A. M., & Campbell, R. A. (1961). Masking of pulsed tones by bands of noise. *Journal of the Acoustical Society of America*, *33*, 1570–1576.

Smoorenburg, G. F. (1970). Pitch perception of two-frequency stimuli. *Journal of the Acoustical Society of America*, *48*, 924–941.

Srulovicz, P., & Goldstein, J. L. (1983). A central spectrum model: A synthesis of auditory-nerve timing and place cues in monaural communication of frequency spectrum. *Journal of the Acoustical Society of America*, *73*, 1266–1276.

Terhardt, E. (1974). Pitch, consonance, and harmony. *Journal of the Acoustical Society of America*, *55*, 1061–1069.

Wever, E. G. (1949). *Theory of hearing*. New York: Dover.

Whitfield, I. C. (1980). Auditory cortex and the pitch of complex tones. *Journal of the Acoustical Society of America*, *54*, 407–416.

Wightman, F. L. (1973). The pattern-transformation model of pitch. *Journal of the Acoustical Society of America*, *54*, 407–416.

Wilson, W. R., Moore, J. M., & Thompson, G. (1976, November). *Auditory thresholds of infants utilizing Visual Reinforcement Audiometry (VRA)*. Paper presented at the meeting of the American Speech and Hearing Association, Houston, TX.

Zartorre, R. J. (1988). Pitch perception of complex tones and human temporal lobe function. *Journal of the Acoustical Society of America*, *84*, 566–572.

PART TWO

Interpretative Issues in Developmental Psychoacoustics

CHAPTER 7

Issues in Infant Psychoacoustics

Neal F. Viemeister and Robert S. Schlauch

A primary goal of research in infant psychoacoustics is to describe how the sensory capacity of hearing changes during development. The question repeatedly arises, however, whether such a description is possible using current behavioral techniques. The issue, simply, is whether measures of performance that truly reflect sensory capacity can be obtained from infants, particularly young infants where "stimulus control" can be a major problem. This issue is especially nettlesome when the work using infants is contrasted with that using adults. In adult psychoacoustics, highly trained, experienced, motivated, and homogeneous subjects are typically used. How much confidence can we have in thresholds obtained from infants where the opposite is essentially the case, and where the problem is compounded by the necessary use of few trials and of psychophysical techniques that are compromised for efficiency?

There are several approaches to this issue. At one extreme, there is the position that the problem is so severe that it is essentially useless to study the

We thank Davida Y. Teller for helpful and provocative comments on an earlier version of this chapter.

auditory capacity of infants using behavioral techniques. This is the position of a small, but vocal, minority. In suggesting that infant work should focus on identification rather than threshold measurement, Macmillan (1985) seems to be taking this position. The problem with this position is that there are interesting and important "capacity" questions that would be ignored, and there are clinical applications that simply cannot be (see chapter 13 in this book). An alternative approach is to address capacity questions using nonbehavioral techniques, such as those based upon auditory brainstem responses (ABR) or otoacoustic emissions. These techniques have their own sets of problems, of course, and it is still questionable whether they offer anything but a crude measure of auditory capacity. It also can be questioned whether these techniques really say anything about hearing as a perceptual process.

At nearly the other extreme, there is the position that we should accept the limitations of behavioral measurement and proceed to use such measurement to study auditory development: Research on infants requires compromise and we should simply accept that. In our opinion this is not satisfactory—it is asking us to ignore a very real problem, one that is fundamental to the whole enterprise of infant psychoacoustics. If we question the validity of something as basic as the audibility curve for infants, can we have confidence in other statements about masking, tuning, and so on?

The approach to the validity issue we wish to consider is, essentially, to model the "nonsensory" factors that may be affecting behaviorally measured thresholds. If the effects of such factors are understood then we can better assess the seriousness of their confounding influence and, perhaps, correct for them.

Criterial and Attentional Effects: Theoretical Considerations

In order to explore the effects of nonsensory factors on estimates of thresholds, we must first assume a specific form for the psychometric function. The general form of the function we use is $d' = m\ (E/N_0)^k$, where d' is a "criterion-free" measure of performance (see Egan, 1975; Green & Swets, 1966), E is the energy of the signal, N_0 is the spectral density of the noise, and m and k are constants. This function was first used by Egan, Lindner, and McFadden (1969) to describe the psychometric functions obtained from adult observers detecting pure-tone signals in broadband noise. It has been widely used and appears to provide a satisfactory description of empirical psychometric functions for a wide variety of tasks, including intensity and frequency discrimination (with E replaced by ΔI and ΔF, respectively). For detection of pure tones in quiet and in noise by adults, the exponent (k) typically ranges from 1.0 to 1.4. We will assume that $k = 1$ and that m and N_0 are such that $d' = E$. This assumed psychometric function is similar in form to that predicted by the energy detector (see Green & Swets, 1966). When d' is converted to percent correct [$P(\mathrm{C})$] the psychometric function, with E in linear units, is the upper half of the Gaussian distribution function. When $P(\mathrm{C})$ is plotted as a function of E in decibels (dB), as is typically done, the function appears as shown in Figure 1.

At 0 dB, $P(\mathrm{C})$ is 69.1 ($d' = 1$) and the "slope" of the psychometric function between 70 and 90% correct is approximately 5%/dB. This is considerably steeper than is indicated by the limited data available for young infants (Olsho, Koch, Carter, Halpin, & Spetner, 1988; Trehub, Schneider, Thorpe, & Judge, 1991) and, even in older infants, upper asymptotic performance is frequently less

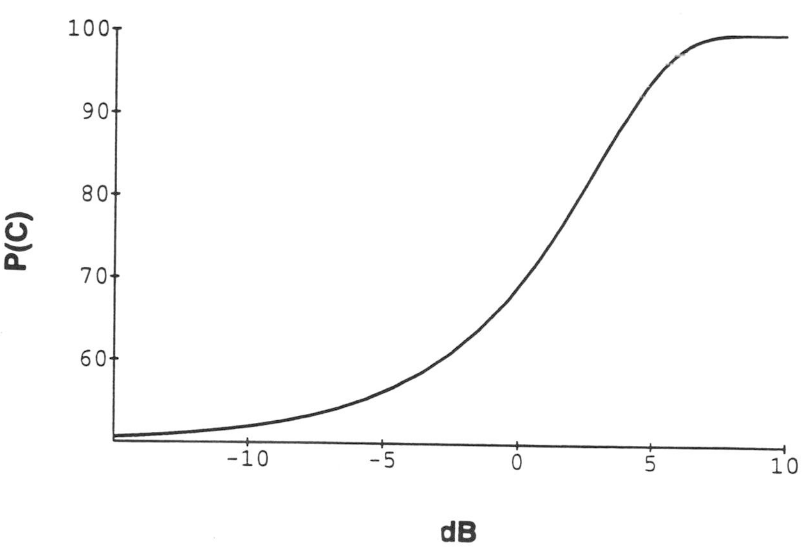

FIGURE 1 Psychometric function (percent-correct function, PCF) described by $d' = E$. dB = decibels.

than perfect (e.g., Nozza, Miller, Rossman, & Bond, 1991; Trehub, Schneider, & Endman, 1980). We assume that the "true" psychometric function for infants is as described above and will consider nonsensory factors that may yield an observed psychometric function that is much less steep.

Criterial Effects

The performance measure d' is criterion-free in the sense that for a given signal level, the same value of d' will be obtained regardless of the criterion adopted by the observer for responding "yes": Changes in this criterion affect both the observed hit and false-alarm rates in such a way that d' is constant. The measure $P(C)$ is, in general, *not* criterion-free: Changes in the hit and false-alarm rates resulting from criterial changes will affect $P(C)$. A $P(C)$ measure that is criterion free is $P(C)_{max}$: This is the value of $P(C)$ that would be observed if the observer adopted a criterion that yields the largest possible $P(C)$ for a given signal level. For equal probabilities of signal and no-signal trials, and assuming that d' is criterion-free, $P(C)_{max}$ is simply the probability of obtaining a Gaussian deviate that is less than $d'/2$. This is the conversion that was used for Figure 1. If d' is criterion-free, as numerous adult studies have shown, then $P(C)$, as computed above, will also be criterion-free. We will use $P(C)$ rather than d' because it is more "natural" for most readers.

To estimate performance in a single-interval psychophysical task, both the hit rate and false-alarm rate must be known: A hit rate of 75% could correspond to chance performance (if the false-alarm rate is also 75%) or to essentially perfect performance (if the false-alarm rate is zero). It is surprisingly common to see published psychophysical experiments using single-interval procedures in which either no estimate of the false-alarm rate is possible or, more commonly, in which the estimated false-alarm rate is not used to compute a measure of performance such as d'. This was true of the literature on adult vision and hearing before techniques based upon signal detection theory became widely used. It is still true of many studies using reaction time, where it is typically reported only that the false-alarm rate was less than some value. It is also true of many psychophysical studies on infants and animals where, presumably for reasons of efficiency, single-interval procedures are often used.

Theoretically, measures of performance and threshold measures that are based only on hit rates tell essentially nothing about true performance or sensitivity. The question is: How important is this in practice? More specifically, how much are threshold estimates likely to be affected by realistic changes in false-alarm rates?

Figure 2A shows a family of hit-rate functions with false-alarm rate as the parameter. These functions are sometimes called "frequency of seeing (hearing) curves" and are typically fitted with an ogival function from which a threshold is estimated. We refer to such a function as a hit-rate function (HRF), in contrast to the percent-correct function (PCF) such as shown in Figure 1. For a given HRF, the threshold is defined as the signal level necessary to achieve a certain hit rate, typically 50%, and a probit procedure (Finney, 1971) is often used to fit the function and estimate this value.

Figure 2B shows a family of HRFs for which the hit rate has been "corrected for guessing." The basis for this correction is a "high threshold" model for sensory detection (Blackwell, 1963): If the signal is above "threshold" the subject always says "yes"; if it is below threshold, the subject is assumed to guess. The notion of a high threshold has been discredited by several studies (see Swets, Tanner, & Birdsall, 1961). Also, the correction for guessing has been shown not to work empirically (Swets et al., 1961). This is illustrated in Figure 2B where the corrected HRFs do not coincide. The appropriate correction is to use the false-alarm and hit rates to compute d'. All the PCFs would be identical, regardless of the false-alarm rate, and, of course, the thresholds would be identical.

As shown in Figures 2A and 2B, a threshold defined as a certain hit rate will increase as the false-alarm rate decreases. Figures 3A and 3B more clearly

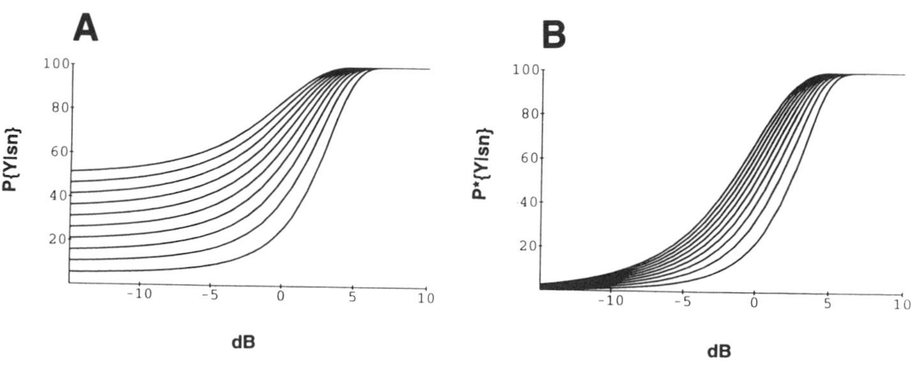

FIGURE 2 (*A*) shows a family of hit-rate functions (HRFs) with false-alarm rate as the parameter. The false-alarm rate varies from .05 to .5 in steps of .05. (*B*) is similar, but the hit rate is corrected for guessing.

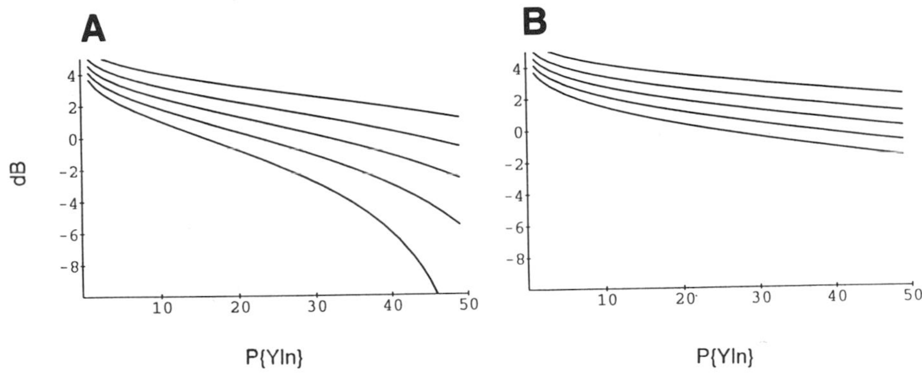

FIGURE 3 (*A*) shows the signal level necessary to achieve a criterion hit rate as a function of the false-alarm rate. The parameter is the criterion rate and varies from .5 to .9 in steps of .1. (*B*) is similar, but the hit rate is corrected for guessing.

illustrate this. Threshold in dB is plotted as a function of false-alarm rate with the threshold hit rate as the parameter. For a given hit rate, the threshold depends upon the false-alarm rate. Not surprisingly, the dependence is less for the corrected hit rate. The important point is that the range of threshold variation is relatively small, at least for this range of false-alarm rates. For example, with a "threshold" hit rate of .8, a change in false-alarm rate from .05 to .4 causes the threshold to decrease by only 3.5 dB. This is a rather large range of false-alarm rates, considerably larger than is generally observed in infant psychophysics.

There are two implications of the finding that the hit-rate threshold is not markedly dependent on the false-alarm rate over a realistic range of false-alarm rates. The first is that comparisons of thresholds across subjects with different, typical, false-alarm rates is likely to be reasonably accurate. Second, for a given subject, the form of a functional relationship, such as an audibility curve, is not likely to be highly distorted due to criterion changes. Criterion changes will be reflected as changes in false-alarm rate; a change in false-alarm rate from .05 to .4 represents a relatively large change in criterion, larger than is likely to occur due to changes in stimulus variables or "spontaneously."

Although ignoring the false-alarm rate appears not to be as heinous as previously thought, it clearly is not recommended. False-alarm rates should be measured—if they are unusually high or low the threshold estimates can be severely in error. Assuming that false-alarm rates are estimated reliably, it usually is straightforward to use this estimate to compute d's and corresponding thresholds.

Attentional Effects

In infant psychoacoustics, a problem more serious than criterion effects appears to be the lack of "stimulus control." Although this can refer to many different uncontrolled behaviors, the common and crucial aspect is presumably the poor control of attention during the observation interval(s) of the psychophysical task. It is intuitively clear that inattention during the observation interval can lead to a degradation in performance. To understand the effects of attention and, possibly, to correct for them, we will consider a specific attentional model. For each observation interval, the probability that the subject "attends" is p_a. If the subject attends, then the decision is sensory based and the observed hit and false-alarm rates are the "true" ones. If the subject does not attend, there is a (low) probability, p_s, of a spontaneous "yes" response. Specifically, the observed hit and false-alarm rates are as follows:

$$P\{\mathrm{Y}|\mathrm{sn}\}_{\mathrm{obs}} = p_a P\{\mathrm{Y}|\mathrm{sn}\} + (1 - p_a)\, p_s \tag{1}$$

$$P\{\mathrm{Y}|\mathrm{n}\}_{\mathrm{obs}} = p_a P\{\mathrm{Y}|\mathrm{n}\} + (1 - p_a)\, p_s. \tag{2}$$

This attentional model is similar to that used by Banks (personal communication, August 23, 1991) and by Wightman and Allen (see chapter 4 in this book). We believe that our version is a considerable oversimplification. It assumes that attention does not depend on signal level (cf. chapter 4) and that attention is an all-or-none process, somewhat similar to the "high sensory threshold" model previously mentioned. The purpose of this analysis, however, is not to develop a model of attention per se, but rather to explore the possible consequences of attention on psychophysical estimates of threshold. The model probably is adequate for that.

The dashed lines in Figure 4 illustrate the predictions of the attentional model on the HRF when $p_s = 0$, that is, when the subject makes no spontaneous responses. These functions are based upon the PCF of Figure 1. A fixed "true" false-alarm rate was assumed (Neyman-Pearson criterion): This is likely to capture the situation when multiple signal levels are used within a block of trials, as in the method of constant stimuli. For the functions shown in Figure 4, $P\{\mathrm{Y}|\mathrm{n}\} = .067$. This value was chosen because it is within the lower end of the range of

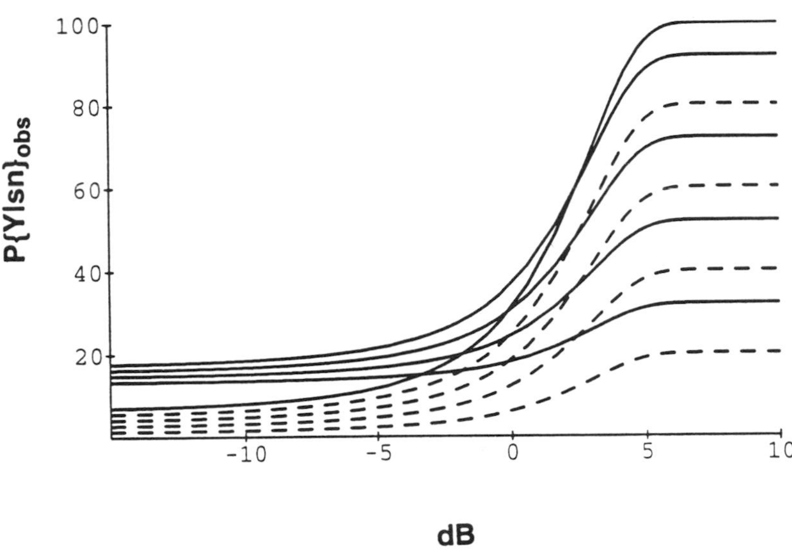

FIGURE 4 Hit-rate functions predicted by the attentional model. Dashed lines: no spontaneous responses and a fixed "true" false-alarm rate of .067. Solid lines: spontaneous response probability (p_s) covaries with attention parameter (p_a) such that observed false-alarm rate is approximately constant. The parameter for both families of functions is p_a and varies from .2 to 1.0 in steps of .2.

false-alarm rates observed for infants (Berg & Smith, 1983; Nozza, Rossman, Bond, & Miller, 1990) and because it will increase when $p_s > 0$. As can be seen in Figure 4, decreases in p_a have the expected effect of decreasing the upper asymptotic hit rate and "flattening" the HRF.

The solid lines in Figure 4 show the family of HRFs when p_s covaries with p_a. Specifically, we assumed that $(1 - p_s)\, p_a = 0.12$. This gives observed false-alarm rates that are fairly constant, independent of p_a and which fall within the range observed in the data from infants.

The functions shown in Figure 4 point to a potentially serious problem when threshold is defined in terms of a criterion hit rate. Depending upon p_a, it is possible that the threshold level of performance is unachievable. The problem this presents in practice is that if there is inattention ($p_a < 1.0$) and one fits the HRF with a function whose upper asymptote is 1.0, then the threshold estimate may be invalid. More specifically, consider the case when one or more of the obtained points on the HRF are in the region of the upper asymptote. Fitting a cumulative Gaussian to such data would yield a function with a low "slope" (large σ) and a threshold estimate that is much larger than that which would have been obtained if $p_a = 1.0$ (cf. chapter 8 in this book). Such fitting procedures are fairly commonly used.

The HRFs under this attentional model can be easily "corrected" for inattention. At sufficiently high signal levels, it is reasonable to assume that the true hit rate approaches 1.0. The upper asymptote of the HRF is thus $p_a + (1 - p_a)\,p_s$. Similarly, assume that at low signal levels or on no-signal trials, the true hit rate (and false-alarm rate) approaches 0. The lower asymptote is then $(1 - p_a)\,p_s$. Under these assumptions, both p_a and p_s can be obtained and used to solve for $P\{\mathrm{Y}|\mathrm{sn}\}$. Specifically,

$$P\{\mathrm{Y}|\mathrm{sn}\} = \frac{P_{\mathrm{obs}}\{\mathrm{Y}|\mathrm{sn}\} - C}{D - C} \tag{3}$$

where C is the lower asymptote and D is the upper asymptote of the HRF. This is essentially Abbot's formula (Abbott, 1925) and is a simple rescaling of the HRF. Applying this rescaling to the functions shown in Figure 4 where the criterion is fixed will collapse the family of functions onto one function.

In a later section we consider how well the correction for attention might work in practice, especially when hit rates are based upon relatively few trials. It is important to note at this point, however, that this correction model is valid only under the assumptions of our simple attentional model. If p_a were to vary with signal level, then the correction would not work. Also, the assumption that the true hit rate or false-alarm rate approaches zero contradicts the assumption, used to present Figure 4, that the criterion is fixed. Essentially, the assumption that the true false-alarm rate is zero (as it must be if the true hit rate is zero) is equivalent to assuming a "high threshold" model for detection. Accordingly, Abbott's formula is simply the familiar "correction for guessing." The practical question, however, is whether these somewhat dubious assumptions will help us to better interpret the data.

Figure 5 shows the predictions of the attentional model on the PCF. Again, the upper asymptotic value decreases with decreases in p_a. As with the HRFs, the "threshold" increases with decreases in p_a and, depending on the value of $P(\mathrm{C})$ defined as threshold performance, the threshold may become indeterminately

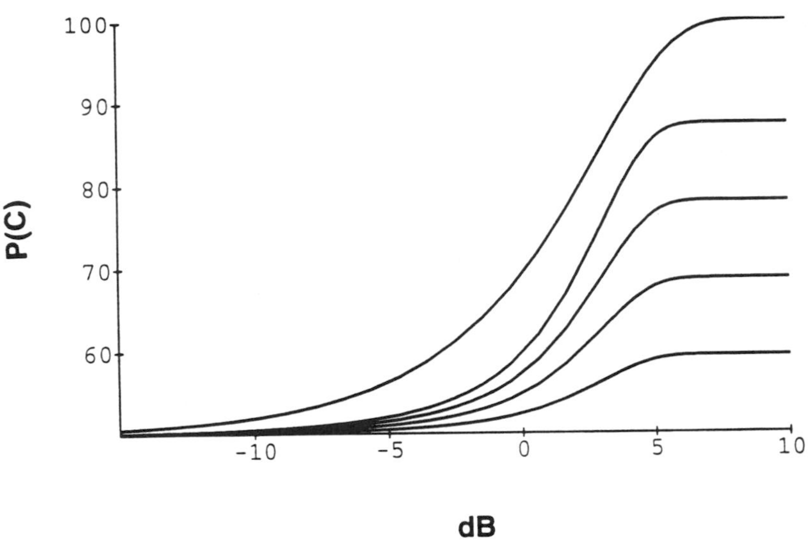

FIGURE 5 Percent-correct functions predicted by the attentional model. The parameter is p_a and varies from .2 to 1.0 in steps of .2.

large. The PCFs, unlike the HRFs, cannot be easily "corrected" to obtain the true $P(C)$. As discussed above, the correction assumes, in effect, that the false alarm rate is 0. In that case, d' is indeterminate, and $P(C)$, as we are using it, is undefined. It is possible, of course, to rescale the functions shown in Figure 5 so that their domain is always 0 to 1. As shown in the following section, this crude method works surprisingly well in removing attention effects.

Attentional and Criterial Effects Combined

We argued earlier that changes in criterion do not produce large changes in the hit-rate threshold, at least over a reasonable range of criteria. There is the possibility, however, that when combined with attentional effects, criterial changes can become much larger and severely affect threshold estimates. Figure 6 shows two families of HRFs. The solid lines are the functions shown also as solid lines in Figure 4: These are based upon the attentional model with a criterion that yields $P\{Y|n\} = .067$. The set of dashed lines in Figure 6 is the same family of functions but with a considerably more lax criterion, one that yields $P\{Y|n\} = .40$. Figure 6 illustrates that within the context of this model, the effects of criterial and attentional changes are complementary: Changes in attention primarily affect

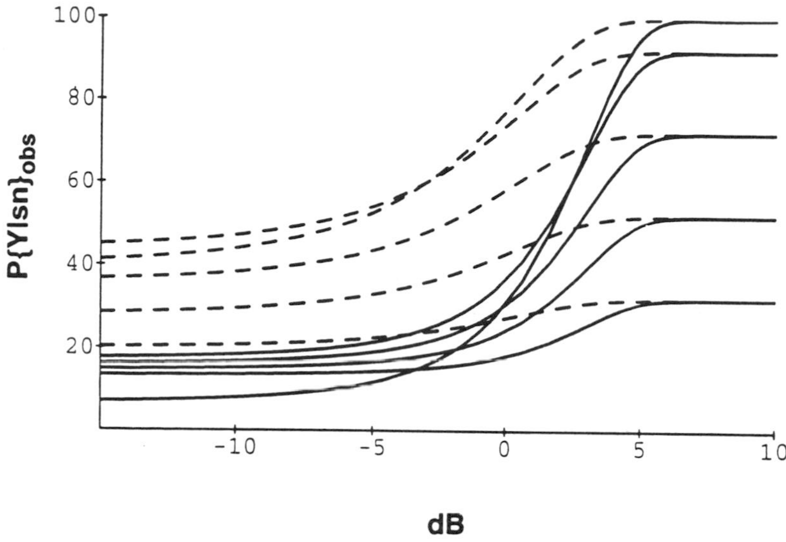

FIGURE 6 Hit-rate functions predicted by the attentional model. The solid lines are replotted from Figure 4 and correspond to a "true" false-alarm rate of .067. The dashed lines correspond to a true false-alarm rate of .4. The parameter for both families of functions is p_a and varies from .2 to 1.0 in steps of .2.

the upper asymptote, changes in criterion primarily the lower asymptote. As a consequence, the choice of a threshold hit rate becomes problematical. If the hit rate is chosen too low, the threshold may become indeterminate due to criterial effects; if it is too high, then the thresholds will be greatly affected by attention.

Figure 7 shows the functions of Figure 6 after applying the correction for attention. All of the functions shown as dashed and as solid lines in Figure 6 collapse onto the dashed and solid lines, respectively, in Figure 7. The correction clearly works, as it must, for attention. It does not, however, remove criterial effects. These effects are small: For a corrected hit rate of .5, the threshold for the stricter criterion is only about 3 dB higher. Somewhat similar results are obtained by rescaling the PCF. In this case, the rescaling does not completely remove either the effects of changing attention or criterion. (Criterial effects are seen, even though d' is being computed, because of the contribution of p_s to the observed false-alarm rate.) Even over this rather wide range of attention and criteria, however, the thresholds at the 50% point are all within approximately 3 dB.

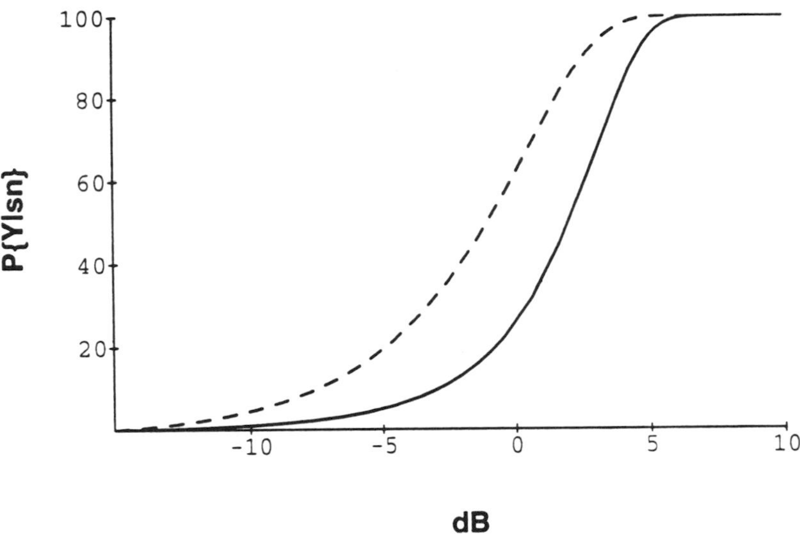

FIGURE 7 Corrected hit-rate functions. All of the functions shown as solid lines in Figure 6 collapse onto the solid line of this figure; similarly for the dashed lines.

Rescaling $P(\mathrm{C})$ in this manner produces a rather uninterpretable measure and, since rescaled $P(\mathrm{C})$ appears to offer no advantages, we prefer to consider rescaled hit rate (see chapter 8 in this book).

Simulations of a Yes–No Task: How Well Does "Correction" Work?

The practical implications of the preceding analysis are encouraging in that they suggest a scheme for reducing the effects of certain nonsensory factors to levels that may be acceptable. It is not clear, however, that this scheme is practical. Specifically, the problem is whether sufficiently reliable estimates of hit rates can be obtained under the constraints of typical experimental procedures. The problem is especially severe in infant and in animal psychophysics where time and subject constraints permit only relatively few trials. To assess the effects of a limited number of trials on threshold estimates based upon the correction procedure we simulated a simple detection task.

The Simulation

A yes–no task using the method of constant stimuli was simulated. Three signal levels were used, corresponding to the 60, 90, and 99+ percentage-correct points on the PCF shown in Figure 1. One fourth of the trials were no-signal trials, and one fourth of the trials were at each of the three signal levels. These conditions were chosen with the objective of obtaining corrected threshold estimates with a minimum number of trials.

For each of the 1,000 "runs" a corrected HRF was obtained using Equation 3. The hit-rate at the highest level was used as the estimate of D; the false-alarm rate was used as the estimate of C. The two points on the corrected HRF were fitted using a probit procedure and the threshold (corresponding to a corrected hit rate of 50%) was obtained. No fits were attempted for a given run if the HRF did not monotonically increase or if the false-alarm rate was higher than the hit rate at the lowest level.

Results

Figure 8 shows the proportion of acceptable fits as a function of the number of trials at each level. As expected, the functions are monotonically increasing with increasing number of trials: An obtained function that is nonmonotonic is less likely with a larger number of trials. As the parameter p_a decreases, the proportion of fits for a given number of trials also decreases. This occurs because the raw HRFs flatten (see Figure 6), and it is therefore more likely that the raw function will be nonmonotonic and thus excluded.

The functions shown in Figure 8 were obtained with a strict criterion, specifically, that used to derive the solid functions of Figure 6. With the lax criterion used for the dashed curves of Figure 6, the proportion of "fittable" functions is considerably reduced and, up to 80 trials, never exceeds 50%. Again, this occurs because the underlying HRFs are flatter for the more lax criterion and are therefore more likely to yield an obtained HRF that is nonmonotonic.

The practical implication of Figure 8 is not encouraging. It suggests that with a realistic number of trials, a high proportion of the data from individual subjects will not yield usable threshold estimates. The situation becomes worse when the false-alarm rate increases, reflecting a more lax criterion. Possible solutions to this problem will be considered in the final section.

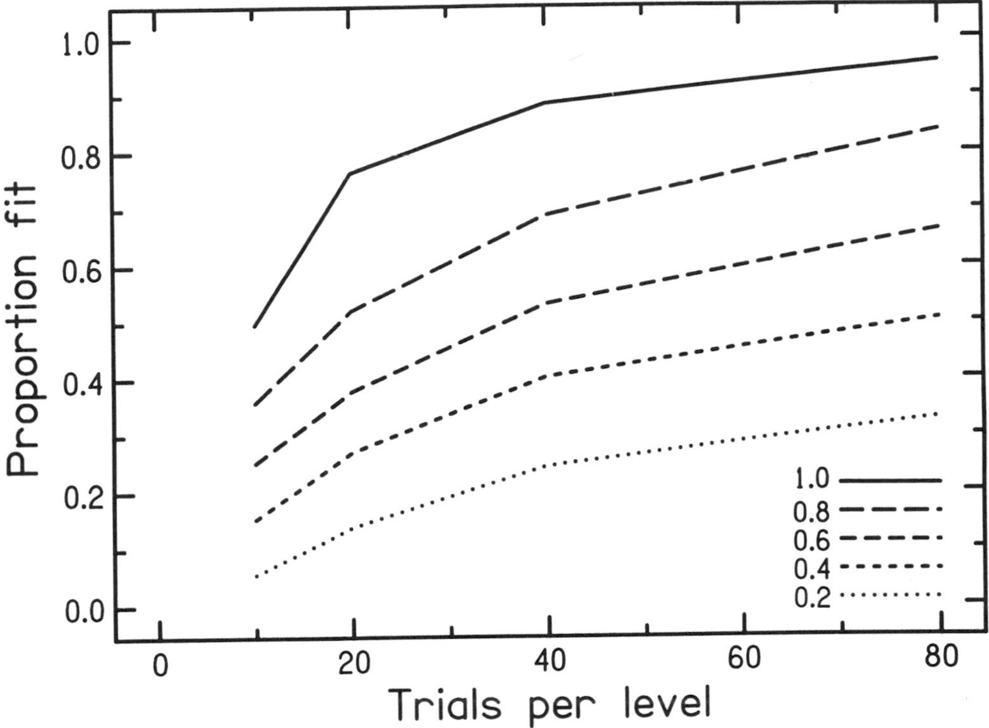

FIGURE 8 Proportion of acceptable fits to the corrected hit-rate function from the yes–no simulation. The parameter is p_a.

The situation regarding the threshold estimates from the acceptable fits is more encouraging. Figure 9 shows that for a given criterion, these threshold estimates are relatively independent of the number of trials and, especially for the strict criterion, are also independent of p_a. The thresholds for the lax criterion are about 2.5 dB lower than those for the strict criterion. This is close to that expected from the theoretical analysis (see Figure 7). Thus, the correction procedure appears to work when there is realistic variability in the data and when a fairly high proportion of the HRFs are excluded.

Figure 10 shows the standard deviation of the threshold estimates based upon acceptable fits to the HRF. Only data for the strict criterion are shown. Those for a lax criterion overlap those shown in Figure 10 but tend to be slightly larger: All the standard deviations are less than 4 dB, however. Overall, it ap-

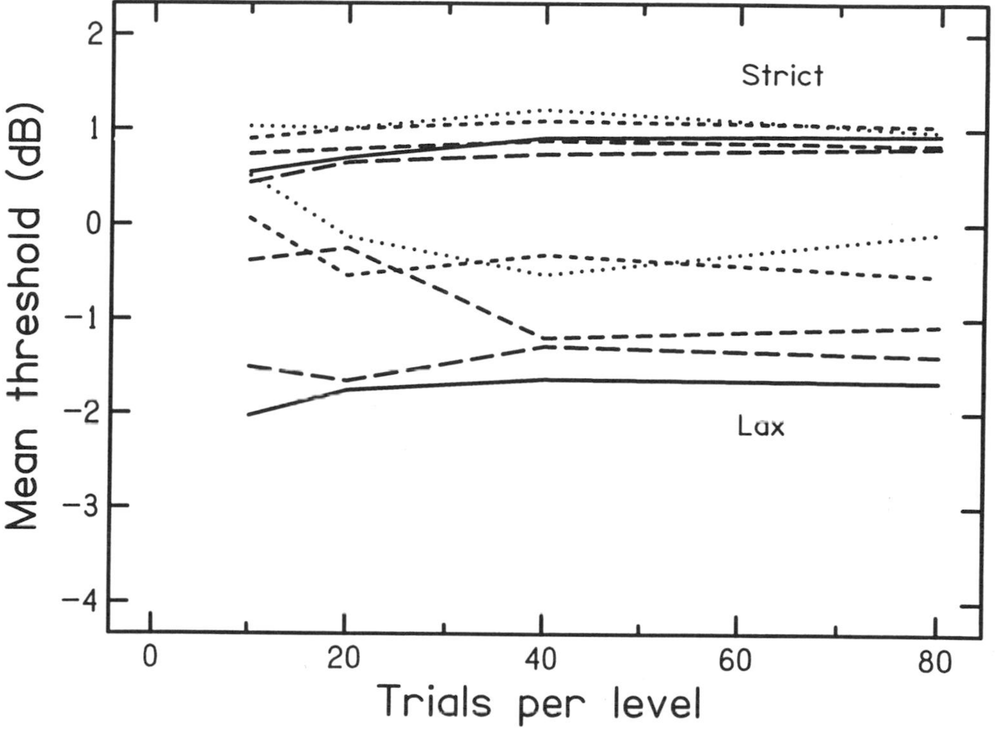

FIGURE 9 Average thresholds based on acceptable fits to the corrected hit-rate function.

pears that the variability in the threshold estimates is similar to that observed in typical psychoacoustic studies using adult observers.

Conclusions

Two conclusions are suggested by the present analysis. The first is that changes in criterion may not markedly affect threshold estimates when the criterion changes are not extreme. The second conclusion is that it may be possible to correct HRFs and thresholds for attentional effects, but at the expense of discarding data from perhaps an unacceptably high proportion of the subjects, especially if few trials are used with each subject. These conclusions must, of course, be tempered by the assumptions and limitations of this preliminary analysis. We will consider those that appear to be most important.

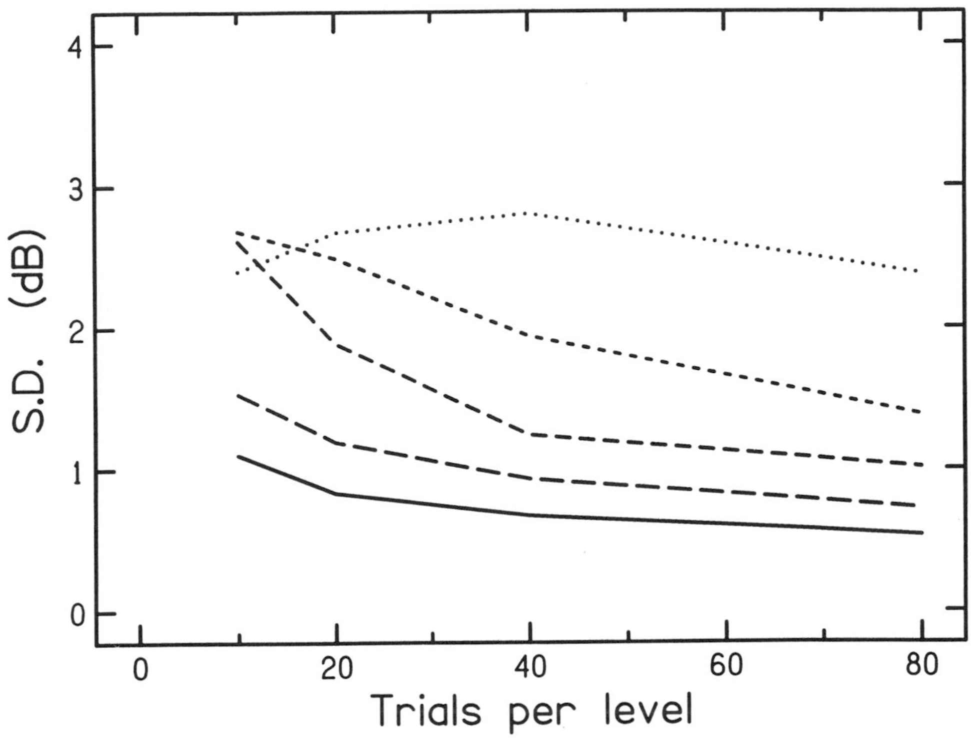

FIGURE 10 Standard deviation of the threshold estimates based on acceptable fits to the corrected hit-rate function. SD = standard deviation.

We assumed that the PCF was given by the equation used by Egan et al. (1969) with an exponent (k) of unity. If the PCF were much "flatter" than this, then the conclusion of relatively small effects of criterion changes is no longer true. Specifically, if $k = 0.25$, then a change in false-alarm rate from .05 to .40 corresponds to a change in hit rate threshold of approximately 32 dB, as compared with the 3.5 dB previously noted. It has been reported that the psychometric function (specifically, the HRF) for infants is considerably flatter than that for adults. As suggested by our analysis, this may result from inattention. If it does not, if the true psychometric function is flatter (an extremely interesting result), then even small criterion changes may wreak havoc on the threshold estimates. It would then be necessary to obtain a reliable estimate of the false-alarm rate and compute d' or a similar criterion-free measure. At this point, it seems appropriate to study extensively the psychometric function in infants (see chapter 8 in this book).

The correction for attention is based directly on a model for attention that certainly is an oversimplification. If the model is wrong, the correction is inappropriate. We have not analyzed other models for attention; those, for example, that treat attention as internal noise, or those that posit a dependence of attention on signal level. We do not wish to strenuously defend this model, but we do not think it is completely inappropriate. The model does, at least qualitatively, simulate the flattening of the HRF. Also, for the method of constant stimuli, in contrast to staircase methods, we think it is reasonable to assume that the net effect of attention is as if it were constant. Specifically, the random order of signal levels would presumably remove any systematic changes of attention with level. Similarly, if attention were to vary systematically with trial number, as seems likely, the randomization of signal levels (and no-signal trials) would likely remove this systematic dependence. Finally, it is our intuition that the model is fairly robust and that the correction of the HRF will work fairly well even in the face of substantial changes in the model. The primary goal here is not to model attention in detail; it is to arrive at a correction procedure that works reasonably well.

The most troublesome aspect of this analysis is the implication that when few trials are used, a high proportion of the HRFs will be unusable and no threshold estimate will be obtained. The situation is even worse in practice. For the simulations we chose known points on the PCF. This, of course, is not realistic. If the levels chosen are either on the upper or lower asymptote of the PCF, then the HRF will not be correctable and an even larger proportion of the functions will be unusable. Unfortunately, we do not see any clear solution to this problem other than running more trials and perhaps more levels. In the simulations there were essentially four levels, including no-signal trials. Two of these were used to estimate the upper and lower asymptotes, leaving a two-point HRF. An additional level in between these two points would greatly increase the proportion of fittable functions (see footnote 3 in McKee, Klein, & Teller, 1985), but because we did not examine three (or more) points in this preliminary analysis, we do not know how large the increase would be.

The thrust of this analysis has been geared to efficiency: To obtain a reasonably reliable and valid threshold estimate with few trials and observation intervals. Clearly, certain compromises have been made and we have made implicit judgments about the importance of various factors. We have emphasized, for example, a single-interval task with a relatively low proportion of no-signal trials. The assumption here was that one would prefer to "spend" observation intervals, or trials, for points on the HRF rather than spending them for "controlling" for criterion effects by using a two-interval, forced-choice task or a higher proportion of no-signal trials. The compromise was, again, motivated by efficiency and by the judgment that, in the grand scheme of things, the variability in threshold estimate due to criterion variability was likely to be small relative to the variability introduced by other factors, including attention. Further compromises for efficiency are possible, of course. For example, to estimate the lower asymptote, C, one might use a false-alarm rate that has been pooled over different stimulus conditions (e.g., different frequencies in measuring the audibility curve) and thereby reduce the proportion of no-signal trials for each condition. Similarly, an estimate of the upper asymptote, D, might be pooled across stimulus conditions. Group data might be used but it is our intuition that attentional differences and true differences in threshold would make such pooling very risky. Each of these compromises affects the credibility of the threshold estimates and, in our opinion, should not be undertaken without justification of their underlying assumptions.

References

Abbott, W. S. (1925). A method of computing the effectiveness of an insecticide. *Journal of Economic Entomology*, *18*, 265–267.

Berg, K. M., & Smith, M. C. (1983). Behavioral thresholds for tones during infancy. *Journal of Experimental Child Psychology*, *35*, 409–425.

Blackwell, H. R. (1963). Neural theories of simple visual discriminations. *Journal of the Optical Society of America*, *53*, 129–160.

Egan, J. P. (1975). *Signal detection theory and ROC analysis*. New York: Academic Press.

Egan, J. P., Lindner, W. A., & McFadden, D. (1969). Masking level differences and the form of the psychometric function. *Perception and Psychophysics*, *6*, 209–215.

Finney, D. J. (1971). *Probit analysis*. London: Cambridge University Press.

Green, D. M., & Swets, J. A. (1966). *Signal detection and psychophysics*. New York: Wiley.

Macmillan, N. A. (1985). What sort of psychophysics is infant psychophysics? In S. Trehub & B. Schneider (Eds.), *Auditory development in early infancy* (pp. 231–239). New York: Plenum Press.

McKee, S. P., Klein, S. A., & Teller, D. Y. (1985). Statistical properties of forced-choice psychometric functions. *Perception and Psychophysics*, *37*, 286–298.

Nozza, R. J., Miller, S. L., Rossman, R. N. F., & Bond, L. C. (1991). Reliability and validity of infant speech-sound discrimination-in-noise thresholds. *Journal of Speech and Hearing Research*, *34*, 643–650.

Nozza, R. J., Rossman, R. N. F., Bond, L. C., & Miller, S. L. (1990). Infant speech-sound discrimination in noise. *Journal of the Acoustical Society of America*, *87*, 339–350.

Olsho, L. W., Koch, E. G., Carter, E. A., Halpin, C. F., & Spetner, N. B. (1988). Pure-tone sensitivity of human infants. *Journal of the Acoustical Society of America*, *84*, 1316–1324.

Swets, J. A., Tanner, W. P., Jr., & Birdsall, T. G. (1961). Decision processes in perception. *Psychological Review*, *68*, 301–340.

Trehub, S. E., Schneider, B. A., & Endman, M. (1980). Developmental changes in infants' sensitivity to octave-band noises. *Journal of Experimental Child Psychology*, *29*, 282–293.

Trehub, S. E., Schneider, B. A., Thorpe, L. A., & Judge, P. (1991). Observational measures of auditory sensitivity in early infancy. *Developmental Psychology*, *27*, 40–49.

CHAPTER 8

Statistical Properties of 500-Trial Infant Psychometric Functions

Davida Y. Teller, Corinne Mar, and Karen L. Preston

The estimation of thresholds is a common enterprise in the psychophysical study of vision and audition, and the same is true in studies of visual and auditory development. The forced-choice preferential looking (FPL) technique (Teller, 1979; Teller, Morse, Borton, & Regal, 1974) is a method for determining visual thresholds in infant subjects. The technique combines preferential looking (Fantz, Ordy, & Udelf, 1962) with a two-alternative, forced-choice (2AFC) psychophysical format. FPL and related techniques have been used in a variety of studies of the development of visual acuity, color vision, temporal resolution, and

This work was supported by NIH research grants EY02920 to Davida Teller and EY02581 to M. Velma Dobson.

We thank Dr. Dobson and Dr. Luisa Mayer for their input throughout the course of the work. We also thank Drs. Suzanne McKee and Anthony Movshon for providing the computer programs used for probit analysis, and Dr. Michael Samek for laboratory assistance.

Corinne Mar is currently with the Department of Psychology, The Ohio State University, Columbus, Ohio, 43210.

Correspondence concerning this chapter should be addressed to Dr. Davida Y. Teller, Department of Psychology, NI-25, University of Washington, Seattle, Washington 98195.

other functions in human infants. Recent reviews of the infant vision literature can be found in Simons (in press).

To test the infant's threshold with FPL, a series of three to five stimuli that spans the range of the infant's psychometric function is chosen. Each stimulus is presented for a fixed number of trials, typically 20, leading to a total of 60 to 100 trials for each infant's psychometric function. A theoretical curve, such as a cumulative normal curve (Finney, 1971) can be fitted to the data, and interpolation performed to estimate a threshold value halfway between the upper and lower asymptotes of the fitted curve. The threshold value so derived is used to specify the *location* of the psychometric function along the stimulus axis.

Although the threshold, T, is usually the parameter of interest, the cumulative normal function also has three other parameters: the lower asymptote, L, the upper asymptote, U, and a slope or dispersion parameter, σ, the standard deviation of the cumulative normal curve. These parameters are shown schematically in Figure 1. For the 2AFC case, the lower asymptote, L, is fixed at 50%. However, the upper asymptote, U, need not be at 100%, especially for infants, and the slope parameter need not have a fixed value.

Although infants' thresholds have been estimated under many conditions, little is known about the average population values of U and σ for infant subjects, or about the variability or interrelationships of these parameters among individual infants. Since the number of stimuli and the number of trials obtained from an individual infant are usually extremely limited, it is not feasible to estimate all three parameters from each individual data set.

Thus, in fitting cumulative normal curves to infant psychometric functions, values of U and σ must be assumed, implicitly or explicitly. For example, in many probit programs, U is set to a fixed value of 100%. But the choice of a value of U may introduce systematic biasses in the estimated values of T and/or σ. An optimal choice of the value of U, based on empirical studies of infant psychometric functions, might minimize such errors.

In addition, knowledgeable estimates of σ are important in assessing the *accuracy* of estimates of T. As is usual in formulas for the standard error of estimation of a mean, the standard error of estimation of T depends directly on the value of σ (Finney, 1971). McKee, Klein, and Teller (1985) have shown that under optimal conditions, the standard error of estimation of forced-choice thresholds from probit analysis is approximately $3\sigma/\sqrt{N}$. Thus, over- or underestimates

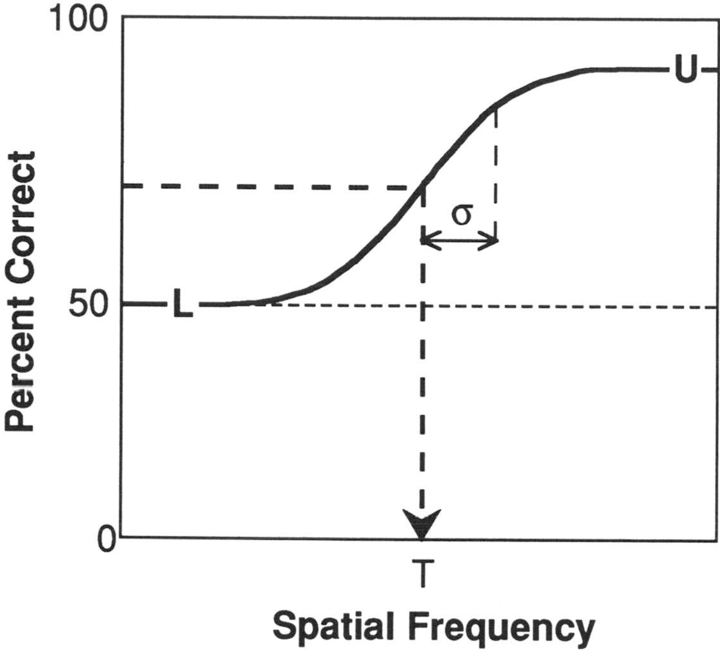

FIGURE 1 Cumulative normal curve showing the three parameters T (threshold), σ (standard deviation), and U (upper asymptote). In a two-alternative, forced-choice task, the lower asymptote, L, is fixed at 50%.

of σ will lead directly to corresponding over- or underestimates of the standard error of T.

An accurate estimate of the standard error of T is critical when one is interested in small differences among individual infants, or within the same infant over time. A major example comes from the case of clinical assessment. In clinical assessments of infant acuity, interocular acuity differences of an octave (a factor of two) can have important treatment implications for infant patients. A major goal in developing techniques of clinical acuity assessment, therefore, is to develop measures with standard errors of less than 0.5 octave, so that octave differences in acuity will approach conventional statistical significance.

The purpose of the present project was to increase our understanding of the population distributions and interactions of T, U, and σ in infant subjects. To that end, 500-trial data sets were collected on 20 2-month-old infants, 10 each by two different adult observers, in a visual acuity task. Population distributions of T, U, and σ were compiled, their intercorrelations were examined, and the effects of inaccurate estimates of U on the calculated values of T and σ were explored. In the course of the experiment, questions also arose concerning individual differences in parameter values between the two adult observers.

Obtaining the Data

Infants

Infants were recruited from the Infant Studies Subject Pool at the University of Washington. Each infant was tested for as many as 10 daily, 1-hour sessions within a 2-week period. Due to limits on individual infant testing time, the two observers tested different groups of infants, drawn from the same pool. Informed consent was obtained from parents.

Procedure

The stimuli and conditions were standard for acuity testing in our laboratory at the time the data were collected. The stimuli were a set of 10 printed black and white square-wave gratings, of nominal spatial frequencies ranging from 0.4 to 8 cycles/deg in approximately half-octave steps. The actual spatial frequencies[1] deviated slightly from these values, and are listed in Table 1. The gratings were presented on either the left or the right side of a gray screen, which matched the gratings in space-average luminance to within about 2%.

Due to apparatus limitations, the 10 different stimuli were presented in two interleaved sets: 0.5, 1, 2, 4 and 8 cycles/deg and 0.4, 0.8, 1.5, 3 and 6 cycles/deg. The initial stimulus set was chosen randomly for each infant; thereafter, on each day the set for which the fewest trials had been generated on previous days was used. The five stimuli in use were randomized in blocks of 10, and the location of the stimuli n′ randomly selected except for the constraint of equal overall numbers of appearances in the left and right positions for each stimulus.

The forced-choice preferential looking technique was used for data collection. Briefly, on each trial a stimulus was presented on either the left or the

[1] *Spatial frequency* refers to the numbers of cycles (one black and one white bar) of the grating that subtend 1 deg of visual angle; it is specified in units of cycles/deg. These units are somewhat counterintuitive, in that the *finer* the stripes of the grating, the *higher* the spatial frequency, and the *greater* the number of cycles per degree. An *octave* is a halving or doubling of spatial frequency; for example, from 1 to 2 or from 2 to 4 cycles/deg.

TABLE 1

Psychometric Functions for Visual Acuity for Twenty 2-Month-Old Infants

		Nominal Spatial Frequency[a] (cycles/deg)										T	U	σ
Observer	Infant	0.4	0.5	0.8	1	1.5	2	3	4	6	8	(cycles/deg)	(%)	(octaves)
1[b]	1	94	92	92	80	74	68	78	44	52	58	1.92	96	1.32
	2	90	92	86	80	82	62	58	66	52	48	2.00	92	1.17
	3	96	96	90	72	58	62	66	46	58	54	1.18	100	1.02
	4	88	84	84	86	70	62	64	58	56	50	2.09	88	1.17
	5	84	88	90	68	72	52	70	52	62	60	1.34	96	1.92
	6	98	98	90	94	90	74	72	46	68	44	2.68	96	0.82
	7	96	96	98	92	90	82	52	62	50	68	2.57	96	0.70
	8	90	98	90	90	82	74	70	48	68	54	2.65	94	1.09
	9	90	90	94	82	86	70	80	50	52	62	3.02	90	0.97
	10	82	86	90	72	72	60	54	58	56	60	1.65	88	0.99
2[c]	11	98	94	100	94	84	62	58	58	48	46	1.96	98	0.57
	12	98	98	100	86	66	52	48	52	52	62	1.38	98	0.39
	13	94	96	94	94	88	72	66	52	46	54	2.52	94	0.60
	14	98	96	94	96	84	82	60	56	52	52	2.56	96	0.73
	15	98	96	98	96	96	82	56	42	48	50	2.60	96	0.25
	16	100	100	100	92	90	80	68	38	38	62	2.31	100	0.73
	17	98	98	98	88	82	74	56	40	48	62	1.96	98	0.74
	18	98	100	96	100	98	92	88	66	48	52	3.95	98	0.51
	19	98	96	94	96	66	58	44	50	48	50	1.49	98	0.25
	20	94	96	96	92	88	78	48	50	52	46	2.37	94	0.39

Note. The main body of the table gives the raw data, in terms of percent correct for each spatial frequency for each infant. Best-fitting values of T, U and σ for each infant are given at the right.

[a]Actual spatial frequencies were 0.38, 0.56, 0.74, 1.1, 1.6, 2.4, 3.2, 4.8, 6.3, and 7.6 respectively.

[b]For T, $M = 2.11$, $SD = 0.61$; for U, $M = 93.6$, $SD = 4$; for σ, $M = 1.12$, $SD = 0.33$.

[c]For T, $M = 2.31$, $SD = 0.71$; for U, $M = 96.8$, $SD = 1.9$; for σ, $M = 0.51$, $SD = 0.21$.

right side of the display. A video camera was located behind a peephole at the center of the display. An adult observer, naive with respect to stimulus location, held the infant in front of the display and watched the infant's face on the video monitor. Based on the infant's looking behavior and/or head movements and postural cues, the observer judged the stimulus location on each trial. The observer's performance varied from near chance (50%) for very fine gratings (high spatial frequencies) to nearly 100% for very coarse gratings (low spatial frequencies).

Data Analysis

Each data set was fitted with a cumulative normal curve by means of probit analysis (Finney, 1971). L was set to 50% in all cases. For each of a series of fixed values of U, the curve-fitting program used an iterative procedure to determine the values of σ and T, which yielded the best simultaneous fit to the data by a minimum chi-square criterion. Fits were discarded if the procedure did not converge on values of these parameters. The values of σ, T, and U that in combination yielded the grand minimum chi-square for each infant were taken as the values of these parameters for that infant. In addition, a preliminary split-halves (first half-second half) analysis of each function was conducted, with U set to 100%.

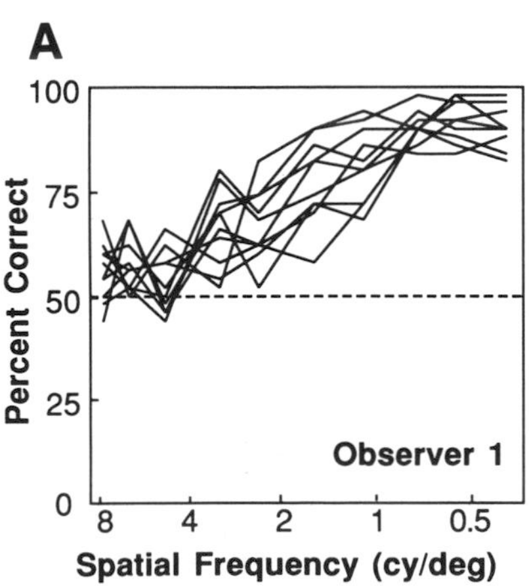

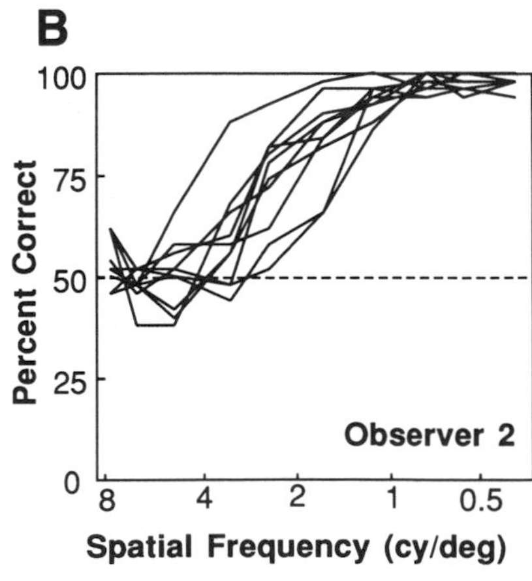

FIGURE 2 Psychometric functions for 20 infants, 10 tested by Observer 1 (Panel A) and 10 tested by Observer 2 (Panel B). The ordinate shows the spatial frequency of the grating in cycles/deg, with fine gratings (high spatial frequencies) at the left and coarse gratings (low spatial frequencies) at the right.

Results of the Experiment

The raw data for all 20 infants, along with the best estimates of T, U, and σ for each infant, and mean values for each observer, are given in Table 1.

The psychometric functions for the 20 infants are shown in Figure 2. Infants tested by Observer 1 and Observer 2 are shown in Figures 2A and 2B, respectively. Visual inspection reveals several features of the data. First, there appear to be substantial and meaningful individual differences in threshold, with individual threshold values covering a two-octave range from about 1 to about 4 cycles/deg. Second, the individual psychometric functions tend to be quite flat, spanning a range of 1 to 2 octaves or more between lower and upper asymptotes. The functions appear to be flatter for Observer 1 than for Observer 2. And third, the upper asymptotes vary from one infant to the next, especially for Observer 1, for whom U is apparently about 88% in the worst cases.

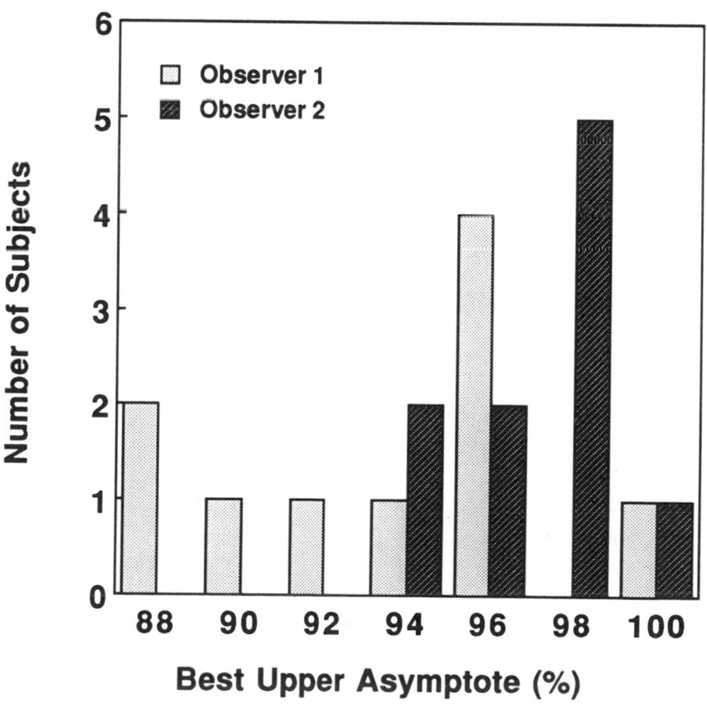

FIGURE 3 Frequency distributions of estimated upper asymptotes (U). The distributions differ for the two observers.

Frequency Distributions

Frequency distributions of the best-fitting upper asymptote values, *U*, for the 10 infants tested by each observer, are shown in Figure 3. In confirmation of the trends seen by inspection in the raw data, there are substantial differences between the two observers. The value of *U* varies from 88% to 100% for Observer 1, and from 94% to 100% for Observer 2; the averages are about 94% and 97%, respectively ($p < .05$).

Frequency distributions of the estimated standard deviations, σ, are shown in Figure 4. As in the case of *U*, the distributions of values of σ vary markedly between the two observers; in fact, the ranges of values hardly overlap. For Observer 1, the functions are relatively shallow, with σ averaging about 1 octave, while for Observer 2 the functions are steeper, with σ averaging about 0.5 octave ($p < .002$).

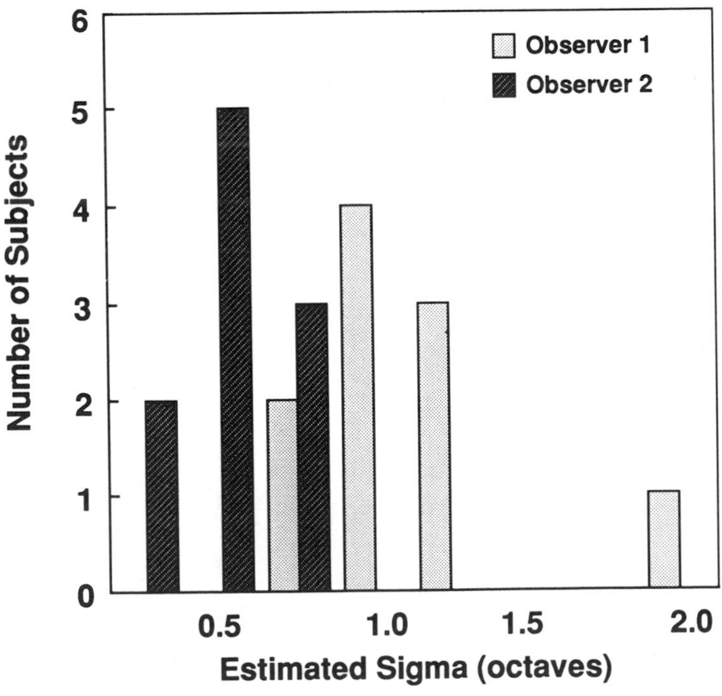

FIGURE 4 Frequency distribution of estimated standard deviations (σ). The distributions differ for the two observers.

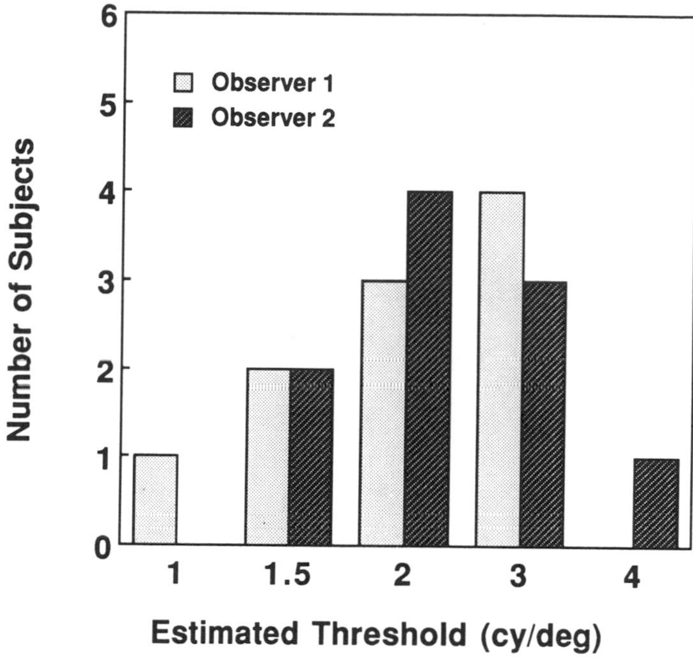

FIGURE 5 Frequency distribution of estimated thresholds (*T*). The distributions are very similar for the two observers.

Frequency distributions of the estimated threshold values, T, are shown in Figure 5. In contrast to the interobserver differences seen in the distributions of U and σ, the distributions of threshold values are similar, and the means are nearly identical at values of about 2 cycles/deg.

Correlations Among Parameters Within Infants

Within observers, all of the within-infant correlations between pairs of parameters were small, the largest being $r = 0.27$ between T and σ for Observer 1. The lack of correlation among parameters supports the supposition that these parameters vary independently. That is, an infant with a particular (high or low) threshold can have any value of σ, and any value of U; the parameter values are not interpredictable within observers.[2] In particular, it is not the case that infants with high "noise," as determined by a low value of U, also show the worst acuity.

[2]The solid symbols in Figures 6 and 7 may be visualized as correlation plots between U and T, and U and σ, respectively.

Influence of U on T

The influence of variations in the assumed value of U on the estimated value of T is shown in Figure 6. These changes are systematic: the higher the assumed value of U, the farther the estimated value of T shifts to the right along the spatial frequency axis of Figure 2; that is, the lower the estimated acuity in cycles/deg.

Intuitively, the reasons for this bias are as follows. Suppose that for a data set in Figure 2, the infant's true upper asymptote is at 90%, and data points for low spatial frequencies in fact fall near 90%. Suppose further that an upper asymptote of 100% is assumed. The curve-fitting procedure will displace the upper asymptote rightward, toward lower spatial frequencies, in order to bring the fitted curve close to the points near 90%. The fitted function will be consequently flattened, and the threshold value is likely to be shifted rightward.

How much difference do incorrect values of U make? In Figure 6, the value of U which yields the best overall fit to the data is shown with a solid symbol.

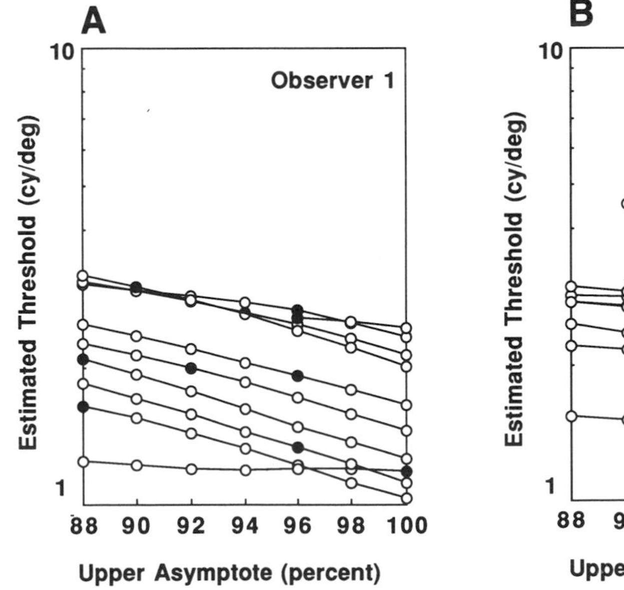

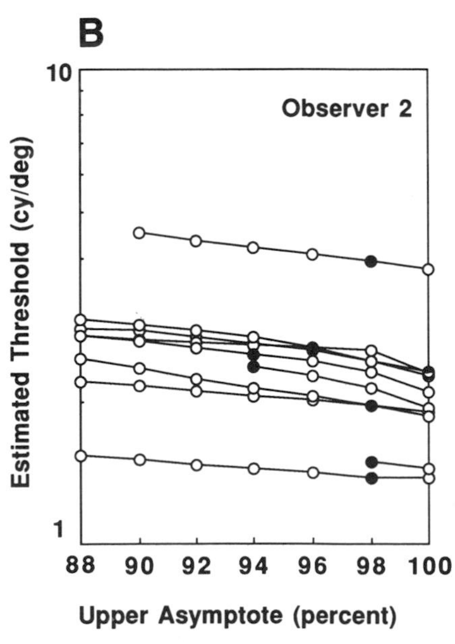

FIGURE 6 Effect of the choice of a fixed value of U on the estimated value of T. (A) shows the data from Observer 1, and (B) shows the data from Observer 2. Closed symbols mark the best-fitting values of U and T.

Compared to these values, a fixed value of U of 100% introduces an average underestimation of the threshold value of 0.35 octave for Observer 1 and 0.13 octave for Observer 2. A fixed value of 95% yields a smaller average error—0.15 octave for Observer 1 and 0.06 octave for Observer 2.

Influence of U on σ

The influence of variations in the value of U on the estimated values of σ are shown in Figure 7. The effect is again systematic: the higher the assigned value of U the larger the resulting value of σ (i.e., the shallower the fitted function). Intuitively, the argument is the same as that given for the threshold: An artificially high assumed value of U forces the upper asymptote rightward, and flattens the fitted function.

For Observer 1, the estimated value of σ changes rather uniformly over the range from 88% to 100%, with an average change of 0.85 octave. For Observer 2 the changes average 1.0 octave, and are marked with a change of U from 96% to 100%. Thus, the choice of U over this range can make a difference of a factor of 2 in estimated standard deviations, and thus in estimated standard errors of the value of T.

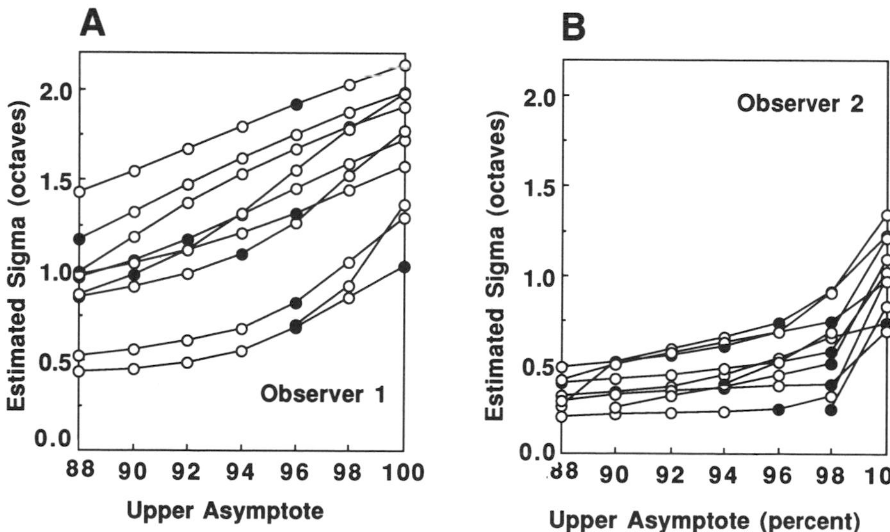

FIGURE 7 Effect of the choice of a fixed value of U on the estimated value of σ. (*A*) shows the data from Observer 1, and (*B*) shows the data from Observer 2. Closed symbols mark the best-fitting values of U and σ.

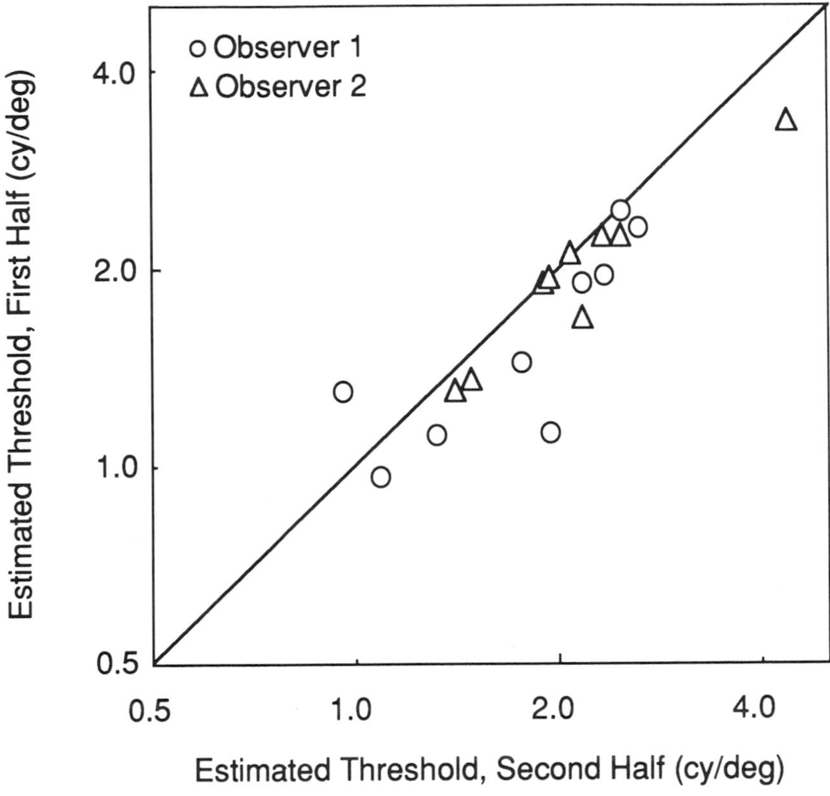

FIGURE 8 Split-half reliability of the estimated thresholds, using the first versus second halves of the data from each infant. The small improvement from the first to the second half is expected from the 1-week change in age of the infants.

The solid symbols in Figure 7 show the value of U which yielded the best overall fit to each data set. Compared to these values, setting the upper asymptote to 100% for all infants leads to an overestimation of σ by 0.5 octave for Observer 1 and 0.4 octave for Observer 2, while setting U to 95% leads to an average error of only 0.2 octave for Observer 1 and 0.1 octave for Observer 2.

Finally, Figure 8 shows a preliminary split-halves analysis of threshold values for each infant. For these fits, U was fixed at a value of 100%, and further analyses need to be done with variations of the assumed value of U. However, even with U fixed at 100%, the correlations between thresholds estimated from the first versus the second half of each data set are excellent: $r = 0.86$ for Observer 1 and 0.96 for Observer 2.

Moreover, there is a very small but systematic increase in acuity of about 0.25 cycles/deg from the first half to the second half of the data—roughly, from the first to the second week of testing. Although practice effects obviously cannot be ruled out, this improvement is almost exactly what one would expect, given the expected change of acuity from about 2 cycles/deg at 2 months to about 3 cycles/deg at 3 months (Boothe, Dobson, & Teller, 1985). This data set thus provides the first plausible example of an actual measurement of a change of acuity with a 1-week change in age, within individual infants.

Observations and Discussion

Interobserver Differences

Interobserver differences in threshold values in FPL testing have rarely been documented (cf. Teller, Lindsey, Mar, Succop, & Mahal, 1992), probably because in small data sets they are swamped by individual differences among infants and/or by measurement error. The differences between Observer 1 and Observer 2 in the distributions of threshold and slope were therefore unexpected. It is our impression that the data of Observer 1 are less typical, and those of Observer 2 more typical, for well-trained FPL observers. However, extensive testing of more observers would be required to provide evidence to support this impression.

Threshold Values

The threshold values seen in this study, ranging from about 1 to about 4 cycles/deg, with an average of about 2 cycles/deg, are entirely typical of 2-month-old infants tested with FPL and other preferential looking techniques (reviewed by Dobson & Teller, 1978). They conform almost exactly to the "rule of thumb" (Boothe et al., 1985) that the FPL acuity of infants, in cycles/deg, is numerically equal to their age in months. The correspondence of these values with the age norms for 2-month-olds tested with acuity cards (Teller, McDonald, Preston, Sebris, & Dobson, 1986; Sebris, Dobson, McDonald, & Teller, 1987) is also excellent. The use of small samples and more primitive curve-fitting techniques in earlier estimates of infant acuity therefore seems not to have produced any major bias in estimated acuity values.

In earlier studies, the population variability in observed thresholds among individual infants has been composed of true individual differences, interobserver differences, and measurement error, and no separation of these causes of variability has been possible. In contrast, in our large-sample data, measurement error is very low, and the use of only two observers reduced this source of variability as well. The high split-half correlation of acuity values (Figure 8) further supports the probable accuracy of the present acuity estimates. To our knowledge, these data thus provide the first documentation of true individual differences in FPL acuity among visually normal infants of a fixed age, and the population distributions in Figure 5 represent the best available estimates of true population variability of infant FPL acuity.

Threshold Estimation Strategies

As shown in Figure 6, inaccurate choices of the value of the upper asymptote lead to small but systematic biasses in the estimated threshold, in the direction that a fixed upper asymptote of 100% leads to an underestimation of acuity. Averaged across observers, this bias averages about 0.25 octave in our data set. The bias becomes much smaller, averaging only about 0.1 octave, when an upper asymptote of 95% is used for all infants.

Given the obvious differences between the two observers in the distribution of the upper asymptote and slope, we found it surprising that the population distributions of threshold vary so little between the two observers. Taken at face value, these data suggest that average acuity estimates are remarkably robust across interobserver variations in the upper asymptote and slope. However, we do not understand the reasons for this finding, and we feel that it should be replicated before one places much faith in it. In the meantime, since the standard error of the estimated threshold is affected by the slope, it seems wiser to avoid the use of observers with poor upper asymptotes and slopes than to count on the apparent robustness of thresholds across variations in average values of these parameters.

Standard Deviation Values

Few earlier estimates of standard deviations (or slopes) of infant psychometric functions are available. There is some prior evidence that in the acuity context, standard deviations are approximately 1 octave in infants in the 1- to 12-month age range, and 0.5 octave for children over 30 months of age (Allen, 1979; Mayer, 1980), but these values are biassed to an unknown extent by the use of small numbers of trials and probably by inflated upper asymptotes.

In our present study, the distributions of estimated standard deviations are markedly different for the two observers, with the average values being about 1 octave for Observer 1 and about 0.5 octave for Observer 2. If (as we hope and suspect) Observer 2 represents the more typical case, then the average standard deviation for 2-month-old infants is about 0.5 octave under our conditions.

McKee et al. (1985) estimated that, with the optimum deployment of trials and a minimum of 60 to 100 trials per psychometric function, the standard error of estimation of forced-choice thresholds was approximately $3\sigma/\sqrt{N}$. If so, then for observers like Observer 2, a typical 80-trial infant data set should yield an estimate of threshold with a standard error of about 0.2 octave. Such a data set should therefore be sufficient to establish the statistical significance of an interocular or intersession acuity difference as small as 0.5 octave. For Observer 1, the standard error would be about 0.4 octaves, but differences on the order of 1 octave could still be considered statistically significant.

Estimation of Standard Deviations

Unlike the negligible influence of variations in upper asymptote upon estimated thresholds, variations in upper asymptote have an important effect on estimated values of the standard deviations. This effect is in the direction that inflated upper asymptotes lead to inflated standard deviation; that is, to estimating the psychometric function to be flatter than it really is. Since estimates of the standard error of the threshold depend directly upon the slope, the use of too-high upper asymptotes with their corresponding underestimates of slope can lead to unnecessarily pessimistic assessments of the probable accuracy of threshold estimates in infant subjects (cf. Teller, 1983).

Future Analyses

In the future, it would be useful to analyse subsamples of these large data sets. A variety of studies might prove interesting, including further analyses of test–retest reliability of estimates of threshold, upper asymptote, and slope between the first and second halves of each data set. Preliminary analyses of this kind have suggested that test–retest reliability is poor for the estimated slope, suggesting either that the slope is not stable within an individual infant from week to week, or that 250 trials is not a sufficient sample size for estimation of the slope in infant subjects.

Subsamples of the stimuli could also be used to verify the findings of McKee et al. (1985) concerning the optimal placement of trials in 2AFC techniques for infant testing. In addition, it will be particularly interesting to see whether the interactions among parameters seen in the present analyses, such as the effects of inaccurate estimates of the upper asymptote, and the optimum value of the upper asymptote for the minimization of bias in estimated thresholds, will hold true for smaller subsamples of the data.

Conclusions

In conclusion, we would make three practical points. First, since the standard error of estimation of the infant's threshold varies directly with slope, avoiding the use of observers who produce low slopes is of obvious importance. The slope cannot be estimated separately for each data set when the number of trials is limited. Given the relatively high correlation between the upper asymptote and slope, across observers, we suggest that low upper asymptotes might be used as an indicator of low probable values of the slope. If so, one could monitor the percent-correct values of each observer, for the most salient stimulus used in any given experiment, and avoid the use of an observer if his or her average percent correct for this stimulus falls consistently below that of other observers.

Second, for small data sets the upper asymptote cannot be estimated separately for each infant, and it would seem wise to adopt a fixed upper asymptote value for use with all data sets. In the present data set, a fixed upper asymptote of about 95% minimizes the overall errors of estimation of both threshold and slope. In the absence of better information, we recommend this value as a fixed upper asymptote value for infants, especially in the 2-month age range.

Third, the generality of our results, across adult observers, stimuli, and ages, is unknown. It may be that other researchers will need to gather data sets like ours on an occasional basis, in order to gain some guidance about probable upper asymptotes and slopes in their particular situations.

References

Allen, J. (1979). *Visual acuity development in human infants up to 6 months of age*. Unpublished doctoral dissertation, University of Washington, Seattle, WA.

Boothe, R. G., Dobson, M. V., & Teller, D. Y. (1985). Postnatal development of vision in human and nonhuman primates. *Annals of Research in Neuroscience*, *8*, 495–545.

Dobson, M. V., & Teller, D. Y. (1978). Visual acuity in human infants: A review and comparison of behavioral and electrophysiological studies. *Vision Research*, *18*, 1469–1483.

Fantz, R. L., Ordy, J. M., & Udelf, M. S. (1962). Maturation of pattern vision in infants during the first 6 months. *Journal of Comparative Physiological Psychology*, *55*, 907–917.

Finney, D. J. (1971). *Probit analysis*. London: Cambridge University Press.

Mayer, D. L. (1980). *Operant preferential looking: A new technique provides estimates of visual acuity in infants and children*. Unpublished doctoral dissertation, University of Washington, Seattle, WA.

McKee, S. P., Klein, S. A., & Teller, D. Y. (1985). Statistical properties of forced-choice psychometric functions: Implications of probit analysis. *Perception & Psychophysics*, *37*, 286–298.

Sebris, S. L., Dobson, M. V., McDonald, M., & Teller, D. Y. (1987). Acuity cards for visual acuity assessment of infants and children in clinical settings. *Clinical Vision Sciences*, *2*, 45–48.

Simons, K. (in press). *Infant vision: Laboratory and clinical research*. New York: Oxford University Press.

Teller, D. Y. (1979). The forced-choice preferential looking procedure: A psychophysical technique for use with human infants. *Infant Behavior and Development*, *2*, 135–153.

Teller, D. Y. (1983). Measurement of visual acuity in human and monkey infants: The interface between laboratory and clinic. *Behavioral Brain Research*, *10*, 15–23.

Teller, D. Y., Lindsey, D. T., Mar, C. M., Succop, A., & Mahal, M. (1992). Infant temporal contrast sensitivity at low temporal frequencies. *Vision Research*, *32*, 1157–1162.

Teller, D. Y., McDonald, M., Preston, K., Sebris, S. L., & Dobson, M. V. (1986). Assessment of visual acuity in infants and children: The acuity card procedure. *Developmental Medicine and Child Neurology*, *28*, 779–789.

Teller, D. Y., Morse, R., Borton, R., & Regal, D. (1974). Visual acuity for vertical and diagonal gratings in human infants. *Vision Research*, *14*, 1433–1439.

CHAPTER 9

Optics, Receptors, and Spatial Vision in Human Infants

Martin S. Banks

Although the study of infant audition has become an active research area, it is fair to say that more attention has been devoted to infant vision. During the past 2 decades, a great deal has been learned about how well the eye and visual brain work when the child comes into the world and how they develop during the next few years. This chapter will review a small portion of the already massive literature on infant visual development. For more comprehensive accounts, the reader should refer to Banks and Salapatek (1983), Salapatek and Cohen (1985), or Yonas (1988).

The early stages of vision are primarily serial. Visual stimuli pass sequentially through the eye's optics, which are responsible for forming the retinal image; the photoreceptors, which sample and transduce the image into neural signals; and two to four retinal neurons which transform and transmit those signals

This research was supported by NIH Research Grant HD19927.
The author thanks David Shen for helping put the chapter together.

into the optic nerve and eventually to the central visual pathways. Considerable information is lost in these early stages of the visual process as evidenced by the close correspondence between the filtering properties of the optics and receptors and some measures of visual sensitivity (e.g., Banks, Geisler, & Bennett, 1987; Coletta, Williams, & Tiana, 1990; Pelli, 1990).

Recently, much research has been devoted to the question of how immaturities among these early stages of vision limit the spatial vision and the color vision of human neonates. It is well established that human neonates see poorly. In the first month of life, contrast sensitivity (a measure of the least luminance contrast required to detect a visual target) and visual acuity (a measure of the finest detail that can be detected) are at least an order of magnitude worse than in adulthood (Banks & Dannemiller, 1987). One would think that the anatomical and physiological causes of such striking functional deficits would have been identified, but the specific causes are still debated. Some investigators have proposed that optical and retinal immaturities are the primary constraint (Jacobs & Blakemore, 1988; Wilson, 1988), while others have emphasized immaturities in the central nervous system (Bronson, 1974; Brown, Dobson, & Maier, 1987; Salapatek, 1975; Shimojo & Held, 1987). Banks and Bennett (1988) have attempted to establish the limitations imposed by optical and receptor immaturities and to discuss how those limitations should be incorporated into our descriptions and theories of vision early in life. They concluded that many, but not all, of the spatial deficits exhibited by neonates can be explained by optical and receptor immaturities. Immaturities among postreceptoral mechanisms are responsible for the unexplained portion of the deficits. This chapter will review their analysis.

The approach Banks and Bennett (1988) used relies on ideal observer theory. By definition, the performance of an ideal observer is optimal given the physical and physiological constraints built in (Green & Swets, 1966). Ideal observers have been useful tools in vision research because their performance provides a rigorous measure of the information available at chosen processing stages (Barlow, 1958; Geisler, 1989; Pelli, 1990; Watson, Barlow, & Robson, 1983). For instance, the performance (e.g., contrast sensitivity or visual acuity) of an ideal observer with the optical and photoreceptor properties of an adult eye reveals the information available at the receptors to discriminate various spatial and chromatic stimuli. Similarly, comparing the performance of two ideal observers with different optics and receptors reveals how changes in those properties affect the information available for visual discrimination. In this sense, ideal observer analyses allow an atheoretic assessment of constraints imposed by various stages of visual processing.

Unlike more conventional neural theories that assume specific neural mechanisms at different ages (e.g., Bronson, 1974; Salapatek, 1975; Wilson, 1988), Banks and Bennett (1988) attempted to reduce assumptions to a minimum. They derived an ideal observer with the optical and photoreceptor properties of the human neonate. Those properties are now understood well enough for the young fovea to minimize the number of necessary assumptions. The performance of this ideal observer was then computed for various spatial tasks. Its performance is the best possible for a visual system with the front end of the newborn system. Comparisons of the performance of newborn and adult ideal observers revealed the information lost by optical and photoreceptor immaturities across the life span. Banks and Bennett showed that many, but not all, of the deficits human neonates exhibit in contrast sensitivity, grating acuity, and vernier acuity can be understood from information losses in the optics and photoreceptors.

Optical and Photoreceptor Development

This section reviews the literature on the development of the eye and its optics and on the development of the photoreceptors. More detail is provided in Banks and Bennett (1988).

The eye grows significantly from birth to adolescence, with most of the growth occurring in the first year. For instance, the distance from the cornea at the front of the eye to the retina at the back (the axial length) is 16–17 mm at birth, 20–21 mm at 1 year, and 23–25 mm in adolescence and adulthood (Hirano, Yamamoto, Takayama, Sugata, & Matsuo, 1979; Larsen, 1971). Shorter eyes have smaller retinal images; for example, a 1° target subtends 204 μm on the newborn's retina and 298 μm on the adult's. Thus, if newborns had the retina and visual brain of adults, one would expect their visual acuity to be about ⅔ that of adults.

Another ocular dimension relevant to visual sensitivity is the diameter of the pupil. The newborn's pupil is smaller than the adult's, but this age change probably has little effect, if any, on visual sensitivity because the eye is shorter, too. More specifically, the eye's numerical aperture (the ratio of pupil diameter divided by focal length of the eye) is nearly constant from birth to adulthood; so for a given target, the amount of light falling on the retina per degree squared should be nearly constant across age.

The ability of the eye to form a sharp retinal image is another relevant ocular factor. This ability is typically quantified by the optical transfer function. There have been no measurements of the human neonate's optical transfer function, but the quality of the retinal image almost certainly surpasses the resolution performance of the young visual system. Thus, Banks and Bennett (1988) assumed that the optical transfer function of the young eye is adultlike. This assumption is not critical because moderate changes in optical quality would not affect the main conclusions of their analysis.

If optical imperfections do not contribute significantly to the visual deficits observed in young infants, receptoral and postreceptoral processes must. The retina and central visual system exhibit immaturities at birth (for reviews, see Banks & Salapatek, 1983; Hickey & Peduzzi, 1987), but recent work has found striking morphological immaturities in the fovea, particularly among the photoreceptors.

The development of the fovea is dramatic in the first year of life, but subtle morphological changes continue until at least 4 years of age (Yuodelis & Hendrickson, 1986). To illustrate some of the more obvious immaturities, Figures 1 and 2 display Yuodelis and Hendrickson's micrographs of retinas at different ages. Figure 1 shows low-power micrographs of the fovea at birth, 4 years, and adulthood. The black lines and arrows mark the rod-free portion of the retina, the so-called *foveola*. The diameter of the rod-free zone decreases from roughly 5.4° at birth to 2.3° at maturity.

Figure 2 displays at higher magnification the human foveola at birth and adulthood. For clarity, an individual cone is outlined in each panel. The cones' outer segments are labelled OS. The inner segments are just below the outer segments. In the mature cones, the inner segment captures light, and through waveguide properties, funnels it to the outer segment where the photopigment resides. As the light travels down the outer segment, several opportunities are provided to isomerize a photopigment molecule, thereby creating a visual signal.

The micrographs of Figure 2 illustrate the striking differences between neonatal and adult cones. Neonatal inner segments are much broader and shorter, and, unlike their mature counterparts, they are not tapered from the external

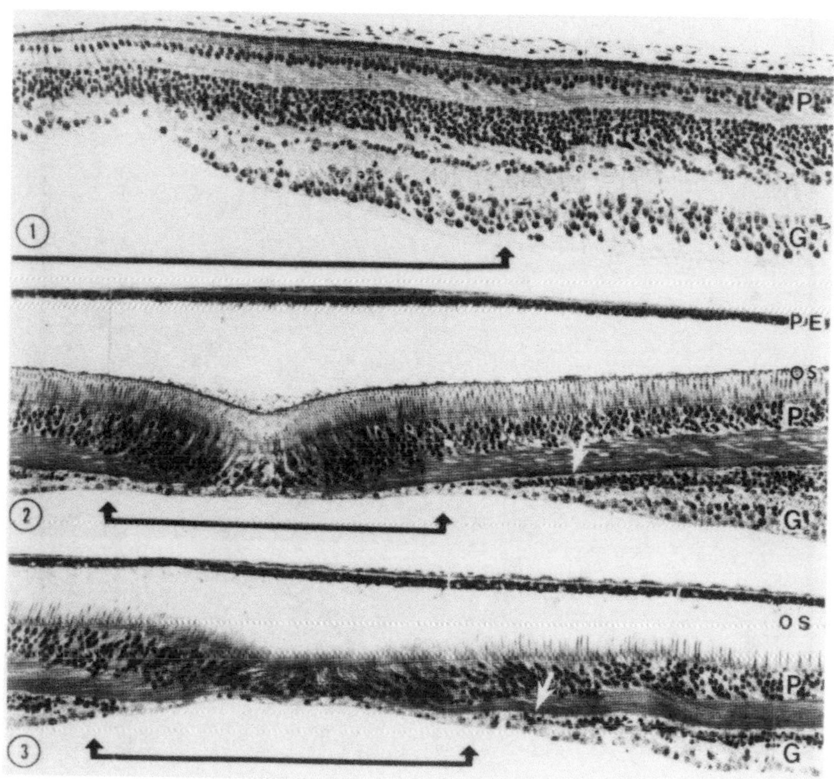

FIGURE 1 Development of the human fovea. Low-power micrographs of the developmental stages of the postnatal human fovea at birth (section 1), 45 months (section 2), and 72 years (section 3) of age. Sections are from the center of the foveola. The black lines and arrows mark the width of the rod-free foveola; at birth the foveola is so wide that only half can be shown in section 1. The retina is detached from the pigment epithelium (PE) in section 2, but a line of pigment marks the distal ends of the outer segments. The most central cone synaptic pedicles are indicated by a white arrow in sections 2 and 3. P = photoreceptor nuclei; G = ganglion cell layer; and OS = outer segments of photoreceptors. From Yuodelis and Hendrickson (1986). Copyright 1986 by Pergamon Press. Reprinted by permission.

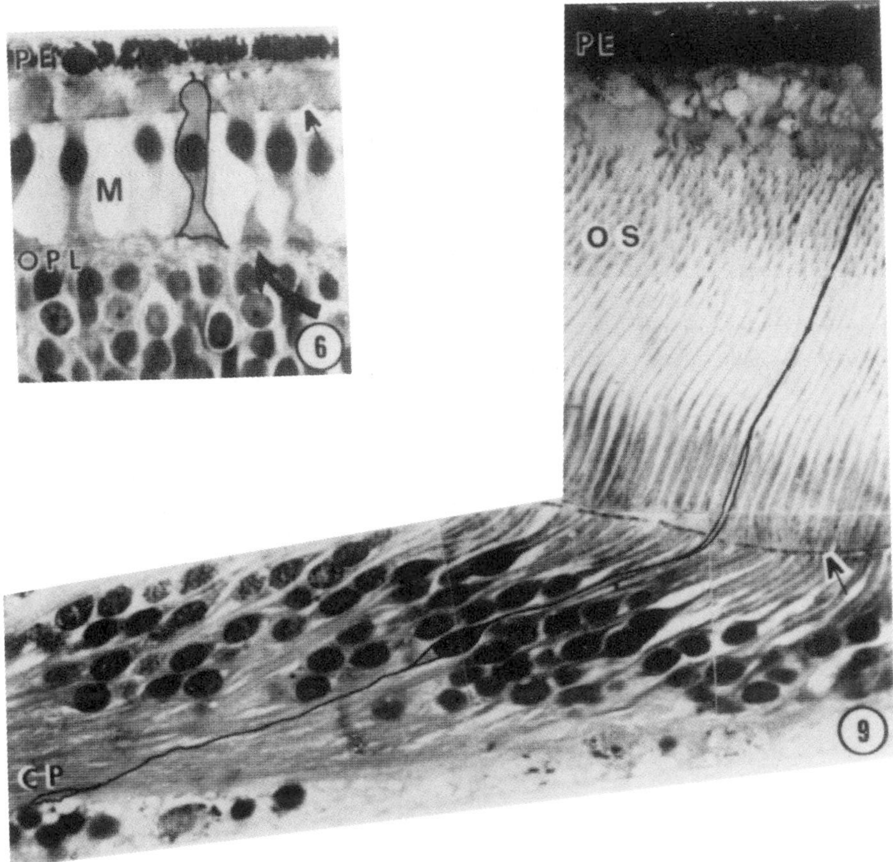

FIGURE 2 Development of human foveal cones illustrated by light micrographs. A single cone is outlined in each figure; magnification is the same in both panels. Section 6: Age is 5 days postpartum. Section 9: Age is 72 years. PE = pigment epithelium; OPL = outer plexiform layer; M = Muller glial cell processes; CP = cone synaptic pedicles; OS = outer segments. From Yuodelis and Hendrickson (1986). Copyright 1986 by Pergamon Press. Reprinted by permission.

limiting membrane to the interface with the outer segment. The outer segments are distinctly immature, too, being much shorter than their adult counterparts.

In order to estimate the efficiency of the neonate's lattice of foveal cones, Banks and Bennett (1988) calculated the ability of the newborn's cones to capture light in the inner segment, funnel it to the outer segment, and produce a visual signal. They began by estimating the effective collecting area of cones at different ages. They found that the newborn inner segment cannot funnel light to the outer segment properly: The inner segment is so short and broad that light rays approaching and reflecting off the inner segment wall at acute angles cannot reach the outer segment. If the funneling property of the inner segment does not work, the effective aperture or collecting area of newborns' cones must be the outer segment itself. Taking the smaller size of the newborn eye into account, the angular diameter of the effective collecting area is about 0.35 minutes of arc. The dimensions required to compute this value are given in Table 1. The effective aperture of adult foveal cones is, of course, the inner segment because its funneling properties are rather good. Thus, the aperture of adult cones is about 0.48 minutes.

Calculations were also made of the average spacing of cones in the newborn and adult fovea from Yuodelis and Hendrickson's (1986) data. Table 2 shows the cone–to–cone distances in minutes of arc. Cone–to–cone separation in the center of the fovea is about 2.3 minutes, 1.7 minutes, and 0.58 minutes in neonates, 15-month-olds, and adults, respectively. It is very important to note that these lattice dimensions impose a limit on the highest spatial frequency that can be resolved without distortion or aliasing (Williams, 1985). This highest resolvable spatial frequency is called the *Nyquist limit*. From these cone spacing estimates, Nyquist limits of 15, 27, and 60 cycles/deg were calculated for newborns, 15-month-olds, and adults, respectively. Adult grating acuity is similar to the Nyquist sampling limit of the foveal cone lattice (Green, 1970; Williams, 1985), so one naturally asks whether a similar relationship is observed in newborns. The answer is evident from a comparison of Table 2 and Figure 5. Although newborn Nyquist limits are much lower than adults, they are not nearly as low as the highest grating acuity observed early in life. Thus, in human newborns, the Nyquist sampling limit of the foveal cone lattice far exceeds the observed visual resolution, implying that coarse sampling by widely spaced receptors is not the sole cause of low acuity in newborns.

Banks and Bennett (1988) used the information listed in Table 1 to construct receptor lattices for newborns and adults. They found that the percentage of the retinal area covered by receptor apertures was much lower in neonates than in adults. The effective collecting areas cover 65% and 2% of the retinal patches for the adult and newborn foveas, respectively. Consequently, the vast majority of incident photons are not collected within newborn cone apertures and are consequently not useful for vision.

TABLE 1
Ideal-Observer Parameters

Factor	Source	Neonate Foveal Slope	Neonate	Central Fovea of a 15-Month-Old Infant	Adult
Pupil diameter	Banks & Salapatek, 1983	2.2 mm	2.2 mm	2.7 mm	3.3 mm
Axial length	Larsen, 1971; Stenstrom, 1946	16.6 mm	16.6 mm	20.4 mm	24.0 mm
Posterior nodal distance	Axial length ratios	11.7 mm	11.7 mm	14.4 mm	16.7 mm
Receptor aperture	Yuodelis & Hendrickson, 1986; Miller & Bernard, 1983	0.35 arcmin	0.35 arcmin	0.67 arcmin	0.48 arcmin
Receptor spacing	Yuodelis & Hendrickson, 1986	1.66 arcmin	2.30 arcmin	1.27 arcmin	0.58 arcmin

Note. From Banks and Bennett (1988). Copyright 1988 by the Optical Society of America. Reprinted by permission.

TABLE 2
Nyquist Limits

Source of Measurement	*D* (arcmin)	Nyquist Limit (cycles/deg)
Neonate central fovea	2.30	15.1
Neonate foveal slope	1.66	20.9
15-month central fovea	1.27	27.2
Adult central fovea	0.58	59.7

Note. Assuming a regular hexagonal lattice, the Nyquist limit in cycles per degree is $60/(\sqrt{3}D)$, where D is the center-to-center distance (arcmin). From Banks and Bennett (1988). Copyright 1988 by the Optical Society of America. Reprinted by permission.

The next factor considered is how efficiently the outer segment—where the photopigment resides—absorbs photons and produces the isomerization that triggers the visual process. As can be seen in Figure 2, the lengths of newborn and adult outer segments differ substantially. In the central fovea, for instance, the ratio of adult to newborn outer segment length is about 16:1. Intuitively, longer outer segments should provide more opportunities for a photon to produce an isomerization. Banks and Bennett calculated the proportion of photons incident on the outer segment that produce an isomerization. The 16:1 difference calculated between adult and newborn outer segment lengths produces about a 10:1 difference in the number of isomerizations for a given number of incident photons. These calculations imply that once photons are delivered to outer segments, newborn cones are much less efficient than mature cones in producing isomerizations.

One can see from these calculations that the cone lattice of the newborn fovea is quite inefficient in delivering photons to the photopigment-laden outer segments. Moreover, because the path length of the outer segment is short, its efficiency is low, too. Taking into account the age-related changes in the factors listed in Table 1, Banks and Bennett estimated that the adult foveal cone lattice absorbs 350 more quanta than the newborn foveal lattice. Stated another way, if identical patches of light are presented to newborn and adult eyes, roughly 350 photons are effectively absorbed in adult foveal cones for every photon absorbed in newborn cones.

Ideal observers were built for the adult fovea and newborn fovea. As mentioned earlier, ideal observers employ an optimal decision rule to discriminate stimuli on the basis of different effective photon catches among photoreceptors.

Thus, they allow one to assess, without assumptions about subsequent neural mechanisms, the contributions of optical and receptoral properties to the detection and discrimination of spatial and chromatic stimuli. Likewise, the performance of the neonatal ideal observer relative to the adult is a measure of the information lost by immature optics and photoreceptors.

Contrast Sensitivity

The contrast sensitivity function (CSF) represents the visual system's sensitivity to sinusoidal gratings of various spatial frequencies. The CSF is a reasonably general index of visual sensitivity because any two-dimensional pattern can be represented by its spatial frequency content (Banks & Salapatek, 1981; Cornsweet, 1970). Thus, an understanding of how optical and receptoral immaturities limit contrast sensitivity should offer insight into how they limit spatial vision in general.

Before discussing infant contrast sensitivity, consideration is given to how optics and photoreceptor efficiency affect contrast sensitivity in adults. Banks, Geisler, and Bennett (1987) and Crowell and Banks (1991) used the ideal observer detailed in Table 1 to calculate the best contrast sensitivity the human fovea could possibly have given the quantal fluctuations in the stimulus (photon noise), the optics of the eye, and the size, spacing, and efficiency of the foveal cones. They also included considerations of a postreceptoral factor: the functional summation area for gratings of different spatial frequencies (Howell & Hess, 1978). (Summation experiments suggest that the intermediate- to high-frequency detecting mechanisms summate information over a constant number of grating bars or cycles.)

Figure 3 displays the CSF of the ideal observer for sine wave gratings of a constant number of cycles. Different functions illustrate the contributions of various preneural factors. The function labelled "quantal fluctuations" represents the performance of an ideal machine with no optical defocus and arbitrarily small and tightly packed photoreceptors. This function has a slope of -1, which is to say that contrast sensitivity is inversely proportional to patch width. The inverse proportionality is a manifestation of the square-root law behavior of ideal machines (Banks et al., 1987; Barlow, 1958; Rose, 1942). The function labelled "aperture and quantal fluctuations" represents performance when the photoreceptors

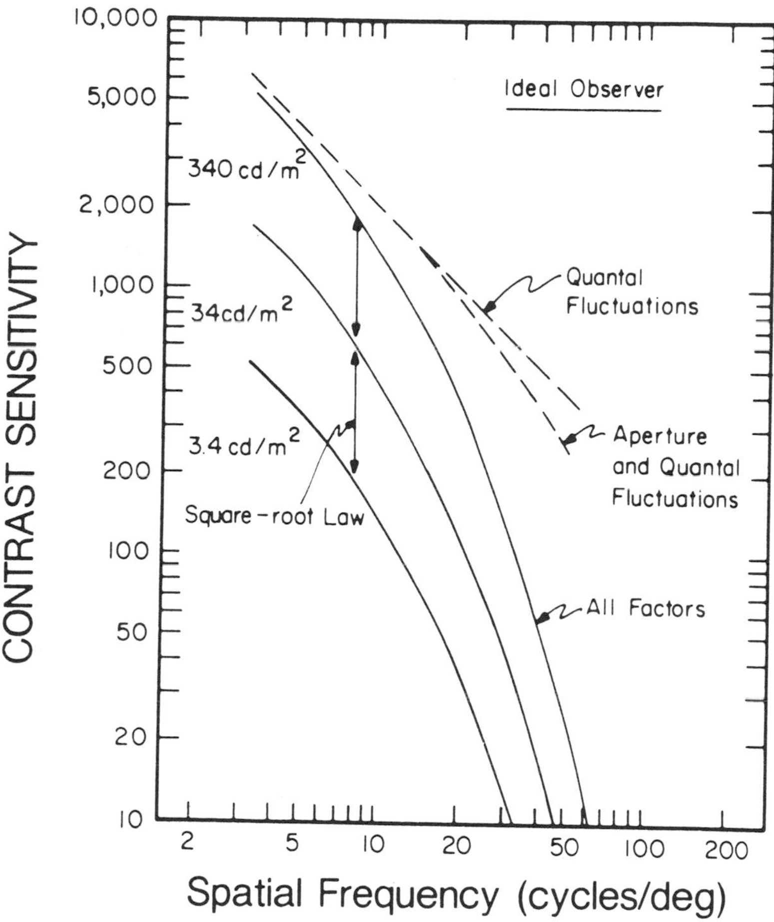

FIGURE 3 CSFs of an ideal observer incorporating different properties of the human adult fovea. Contrast sensitivity is plotted against the spatial frequency of fixed-cycle sine wave gratings. The highest dashed curve shows the contrast sensitivity of an ideal machine limited by quantal noise, ocular media transmittance, and photoreceptor quantum efficiency. The slope of −1 is dependent on the use of sine wave gratings of a constant number of cycles. Space-average luminance is 340 cd/m^2. The lower dashed curve shows the contrast sensitivity with the receptor aperture effect added in. Finally, the highest solid curve shows the sensitivity with the optical transfer function added. The other solid curves represent the contrast sensitivities for 34 and 3.4 cd/m^2. From Banks, Geisler, and Bennett (1987). Copyright 1987 by Pergamon Press. Reprinted by permission.

are given the dimensions of the adult foveal cones; comparing it to the function above it reveals the contribution of the finite aperture of foveal cones (which has the effect of attenuating high spatial frequencies slightly). The solid lines represent performance with all preneural factors included; the difference between this function and the one above it represents the contribution of optical defocus (Campbell & Gubisch, 1966). The other solid lines represent the contrast sensitivities for luminances of 340, 34, and 3.4 cd/m^2. As expected for ideal machines, these functions follow square-root law: Reducing luminance by a log unit produces a half log unit reduction in contrast sensitivity.

Figure 4 shows the performance of real adult observers when they are shown the same targets presented to the ideal observer. The data points are contrast sensitivities from 5 to 40 cycles/deg for two adult observers. As is normally observed, contrast sensitivity is greater for high luminances. As expected, the contrast sensitivity values for the real adult observers are substantially lower than those of the ideal observer. The solid lines are the three ideal functions of Figure 3, shifted vertically as a unit to fit the real observer's data. The ideal functions fit the experimental data reasonably well, which shows that the shapes of the ideal and real CSFs are similar. The similarity of shapes demonstrates that the high-frequency rolloff of the human adult's foveal CSF, for gratings with a fixed number of cycles, can be explained by the operation of optical and receptoral factors alone. This observation implies in turn that neural efficiency (by which I mean the efficiency with which information at the outputs of the receptors is transmitted through the rest of the visual system) is constant from 5 to 40 cycles/deg for adult foveal vision. Moreover, the luminance dependance of intermediate- and high-frequency sensitivity is similar in real and ideal adult observers, which means that adults exhibit square-root behavior just like ideal observers do.

These two observations—that the spatial-frequency dependence and luminance dependence of human adult contrast sensitivity are similar to those exhibited by an ideal observer placed at the receptors—are important in the analysis of contrast sensitivity development: They legitimize comparisons of ideal and real observer performance at different ages.

Figure 5 displays neonatal and adult CSFs. Contrast sensitivity is obviously quite low in newborns. Newborns' peak sensitivities, whether measured by forced-choice preferential looking (FPL; Atkinson, Braddick, & Moar, 1977; Banks & Sa-

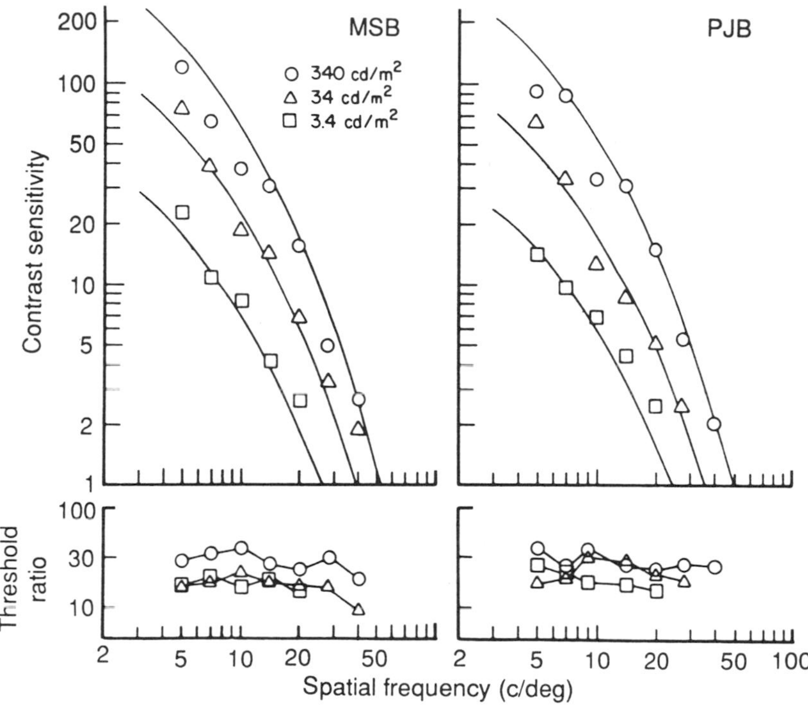

FIGURE 4 CSFs of human adult and ideal observers. The upper panels plot contrast sensitivity for two human observers for three luminances. The solid lines are the CSFs of the ideal observer, which are shifted downward by 1.33 log units for MSB and 1.43 log units for PJB. The lower panels plot threshold ratios as a function of spatial frequency. The ratios are the human observers' contrast thresholds divided by the ideal observer's thresholds. From Banks, Geisler, and Bennett (1987). Copyright 1987 by Pergamon Press. Reprinted by permission.

lapatek, 1978) or by visual evoked potential (VEP; Norcia, Tyler, & Allen, 1986; Pirchio, Spinelli, Fiorentini, & Maffei, 1978), are substantially lower than those of adults. One can also see that visual acuity in neonates is very limited, being roughly 25 times worse than that of normal adults (Dobson & Teller, 1978; Norcia & Tyler, 1985).

To examine the extent to which the development of contrast sensitivity can be explained by optical and receptoral maturation, CSFs of the neonatal ideal and adult observers were computed for gratings of a fixed number of cycles. The space-average luminance was 50 cd/m^2. The ideal CSFs are shown in Figure 6. As

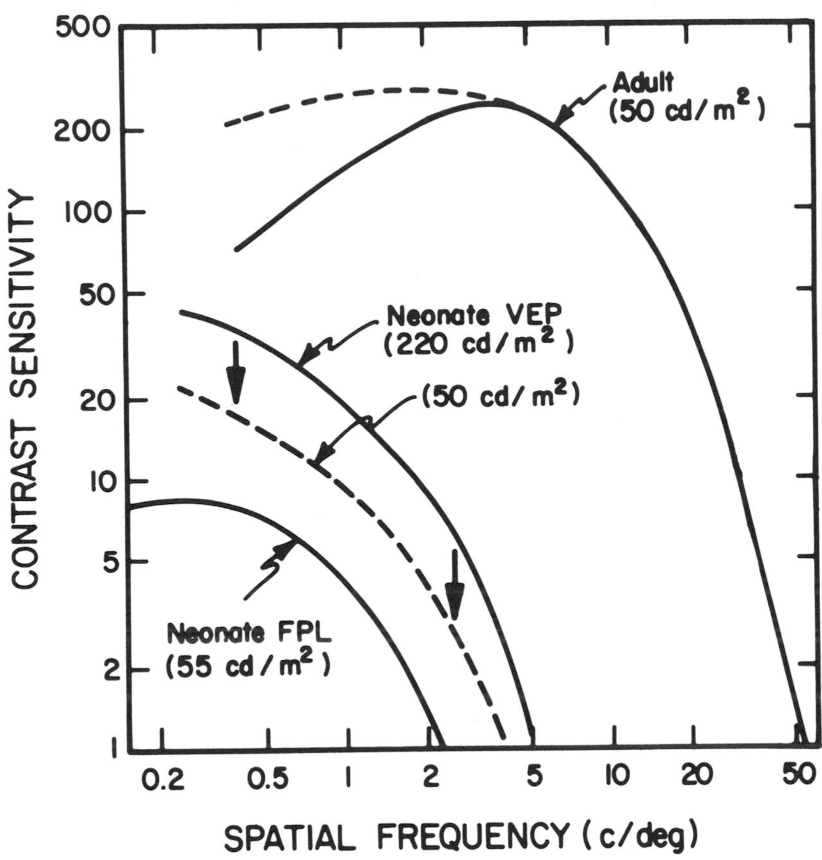

FIGURE 5 Empirically determined adult and neonate CSFs. The curve labeled Neonate FPL is from Banks and Salapatek (1978) and was collected at 55 cd/m^2. The curve labeled Neonate VEP is from Norcia (personal communication, 1988). The VEP data were collected at a space-average luminance of 220 cd/m^2 and the function was shifted downward by 0.32 log units to indicate its expected location at 50 cd/m^2. The curve labeled Adult represents data from Campbell and Robson (1968) that were collected at 50 cd/m^2. From Banks and Bennett (1988). Copyright 1988 by the Optical Society of America. Adapted by permission.

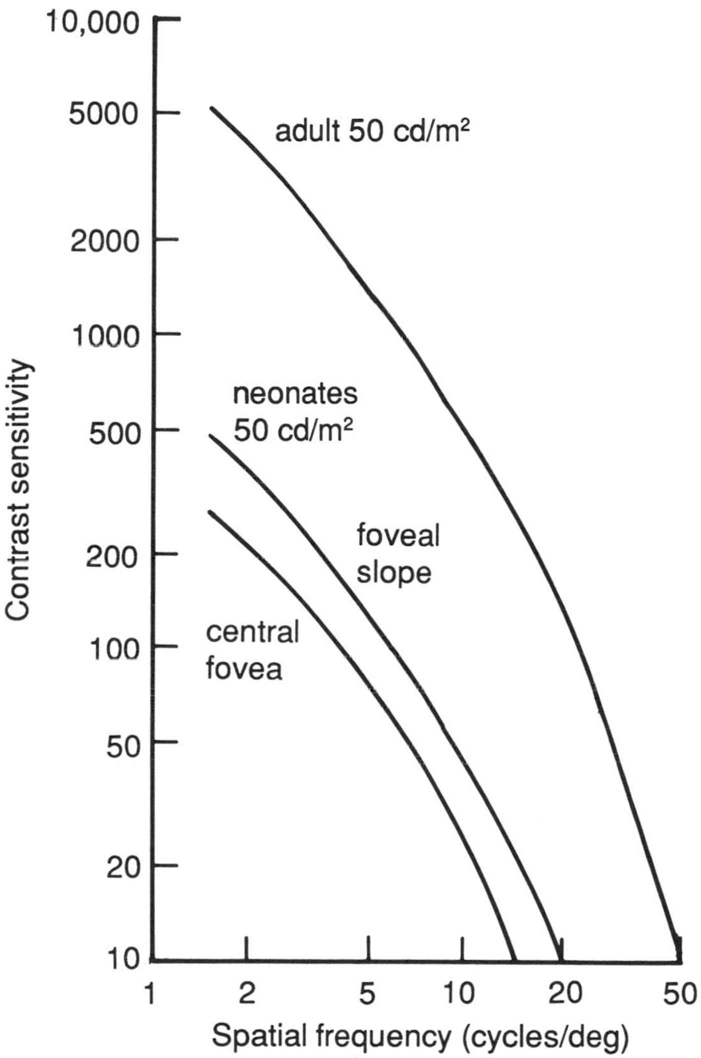

FIGURE 6 CSFs for ideal observers incorporating the preneural factors of the adult, neonatal central foveas, and the neonatal foveal slope. The stimuli were grating patches of a constant number of cycles. Space-average luminance is 50 cd/m^2. The differences between adult and neonatal sensitivities are due primarily to the reduced quantum capture of the neonate's cone lattice. From Banks and Bennett (1988). Copyright 1988 by the Optical Society of America. Reprinted by permission.

in Figure 3, these functions reflect performance limitations imposed by quantal fluctuations in the stimulus, ocular media transmittance, optical transfer, and the aperture spacing, efficiency, and spacing of photoreceptors. Notice that the ideal sensitivity is higher at the margin of the newborn's foveola than in the central 250 μm because of the greater efficiency of foveal slope cones.

Most noteworthy are the differences between the contrast sensitivities of the adult and neonatal ideal observers. They are substantial. For example, the ratio between adult sensitivity and neonatal central foveal sensitivity at 5 cycles/deg is about 21:1 (1.32 log units). The major cause of decreased sensitivity in the newborn is the reduced photon capture of its cone lattice.

Of course, neither adults nor newborns are ideal observers. So one naturally asks whether these predicted differences in sensitivity can explain the differences observed between real adult and real newborn performance.

If the visual systems of newborns and adults were identical except for the observed differences in eye size, and in cone aperture, efficiency, and spacing, one would expect the neonatal CSF to simply be a vertically shifted version of the adult CSF. To examine this possibility, empirically determined adult and newborn CSFs were compared. Figure 7 displays an adult CSF at 50 cd/m^2 along with neonatal CSFs obtained at similar luminances with FPL and VEP. The vertical arrows indicate the amount of shifting one would expect if the visual systems of adults and newborns were identical except for the optical and receptoral factors listed in Table 1. The vertical shifts correspond to information lost by small eye size and inefficient photon capture and photoisomerization. As mentioned previously, the fact that ideal and real adult contrast sensitivities are affected in similar ways by changes in spatial frequency and luminance makes plausible the implicit assumption behind vertical shifting. In keeping with this, the adult function was not shifted at frequencies below 3 cycles/deg because Banks et al. (1987) and Crowell and Banks (1991) were unable to show that differences in contrast sensitivity below 3 cycles/deg can be explained by the factors considered. This shifting accounted for a substantial fraction of the observed newborn–adult disparity, but not all of it. Evidently additional factors contribute to the newborn contrast sensitivity deficit.

The disparity between the real newborn's CSF and the shifted adult function is called the *postreceptoral gap*. It is illustrated in Figure 8. Banks and Bennett's (1988) analysis suggests that the postreceptoral loss is roughly 7-fold (0.85

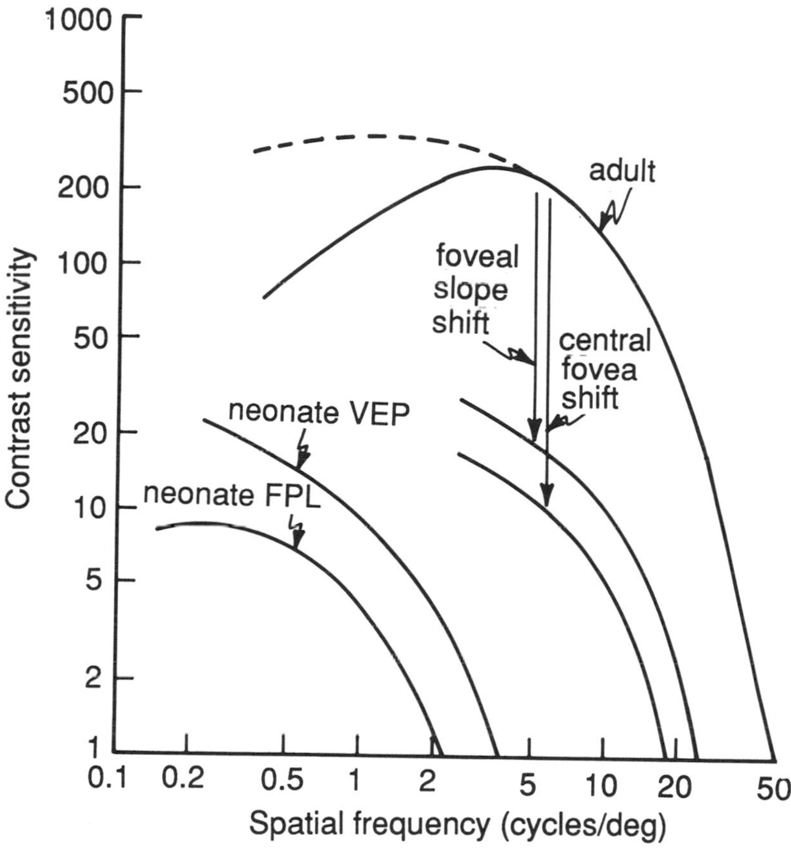

FIGURE 7 Empirically determined adult and neonatal CSFs and predictions of neonate contrast sensitivity based on ideal observer analysis. The curves labeled Adult, Neonate FPL, and Neonate VEP are the same as those in Figure 5. The vertical arrows represent the ratios of the ideal neonate sensitivity to the ideal adult sensitivity at each spatial frequency. The reductions in contrast sensitivity indicated by the arrows represent the effects of smaller image magnification, coarser spatial sampling by the cone lattice, and less efficient photoreception in the neonate. The curves at the bottom of the arrows are the CSFs that one would expect if adult and neonatal visual systems were identical except for the preneural factors listed in Tables 1 and 2. From Banks and Bennett (1988). Copyright 1988 by the Optical Society of America. Reprinted by permission.

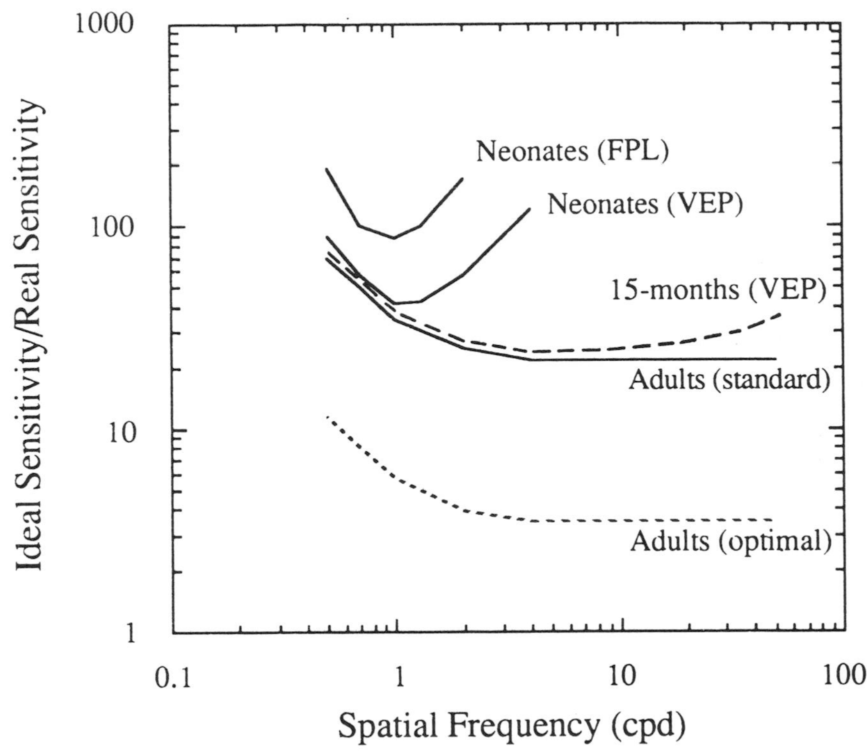

FIGURE 8 Visual efficiency at different ages. The ratio of ideal contrast sensitivity divided by real contrast sensitivity is plotted as a function of spatial frequencies for the central fovea of neonates and adults. The function labeled Adult (standard) is calculated from the data of Banks, Geisler, and Bennett (1987). The function labeled Adult (optimal) is calculated from the data of Crowell and Banks (1988). The neonatal functions were calculated from the central fovea ideal sensitivities and the FPL data of Banks and Salapatek (1978) and the VEP data of Norcia (personal communication, 1988). From Banks and Bennett (1988). Copyright 1988 by the Optical Society of America. Adapted by permission.

log units) at 3 cycles/deg and 22-fold (1.34 log units) at 5 cycles/deg. An important question is: What factors not considered in their analysis determine the magnitude and shape of the postreceptoral gap? There are, of course, numerous candidates; including intrinsic neural noise (such as random addition of action potentials at central sites), inefficient neural sampling (such as lack of appropriate cortical receptive fields for detecting sine wave gratings), poor motivation to respond, and so forth.

A caveat is warranted before concluding this section. Despite the fact that the fovea subtends a large area at birth, newborns may use extrafoveal loci in contrast sensitivity experiments. There are no quantitative data on the morphological development of extrafoveal cones, so it is possible that the extrafoveal cones are actually more efficient than foveal cones at birth (Abramov et al., 1982). If this were the case, the disparity between predicted and observed contrast sensitivity (the postreceptoral gap) would be greater than that indicated in Figures 7 and 8. There is some evidence, however, that suggests, but by no means proves, that newborns fixate visual targets foveally. Hainline and Harris (1988), Slater and Findlay (1975), and Salapatek and Kessen (1966) all showed that neonates use a consistent retinal locus when fixating a high-contrast target. They could not, however, prove that this locus is the fovea because of uncertainties about the location of the visual axis with respect to the optic axis. Other evidence relevant to the issue of peripheral and foveal viewing concerns the relative sensitivity of foveal and peripheral vision in neonates; some of this evidence is from macaques and some from humans. Retinal and central nervous development in macaques and humans is similar, except that macaques are somewhat more advanced at birth and mature more rapidly (Boothe, Williams, Kiorpes, & Bito, 1980; Hendrickson & Kupfer, 1976; Kiely, Crewther, Nathan, Brennan, & Efron, 1987). Blakemore and Vital-Durand (1980) measured the visual resolution of lateral geniculate cells supplied by different retinal regions. In newborn macaques, the acuity of foveal cells was similar but higher than the acuity of peripheral cells. Thus, in macaque infants anyway, the highest resolution is likely to be observed with central vision. The same appears to be true for human infants. Lewis, Maurer, and Kay (1978) found that newborns could detect a narrower light bar against a dark background when it was presented in central vision rather than in the periphery. More recently, Allen, Norcia, and Tyler (1989) showed that VEP acuity is higher in central than in peripheral vision in infants as young as 2 months. These observations suggest that the newborn contrast sensitivity and acuity estimates are manifestations of central rather than peripheral processing, but more direct experimental evidence is needed to show that central fixation is the same as foveal fixation in such young infants.

In conclusion, within the assumptions of the aforementioned analysis, much but not all of the contrast sensitivity and acuity deficits observed early in life can be accounted for by small eye size and by photoreceptor immaturities in and around the fovea. The major constraint is the poor photon catching and isomerization of the newborn's foveal cone lattice. The unexplained portion of the sensitivity deficit—the postreceptoral gap—must reflect immaturities among postreceptoral retinal circuits and central visual pathways.

Implications

Ideal observer analyses were used to estimate the information available at the photoreceptors for the discrimination of spatial stimuli. The information is much reduced in the human neonate compared to the adult mainly because of immaturities among neonates' photoreceptors. This reduction in information available for discrimination sets an upper bound on the visual performance human neonates are capable of, given their optics and photoreceptors. Real newborns can do no better than the neonatal ideal observer. The discrimination information lost by inefficient photoreception accounts for a substantial fraction of the gap between adult and infant contrast sensitivity and grating acuity. Nonetheless, the magnitude of the information gain with age is insufficient by itself to account for the entire developmental gap in these tasks. In the following section, consideration is given to various hypotheses about the sources of the postreceptoral loss and to the sorts of visual tasks for which this analysis is likely or unlikely to yield useful insights.

Contributors to Postreceptoral Loss

The performance of the neonatal ideal observer was much better than that of human neonates in all of the tasks considered. This is hardly surprising given that the human adult performance does not equal ideal performance in these same tasks. More interestingly, the gap between real and ideal neonate values is significantly larger than that between real and ideal adult values (see Figures 7 and 8). This means that neonates, although significantly limited by optical and receptoral deficiencies, use the information that is available at the photoreceptors less efficiently than adults do. What postreceptoral factors contribute to this additional developmental deficit? Some of the obvious candidates are considered here.

Before considering mechanistic explanations of postreceptor loss, I should mention a methodological explanation: Perhaps the sensitivity of the young visual system is actually better than believed, so the postreceptoral loss is properly ascribed to motivational deficiency. There is no good theory of how motivation should affect visual performance, so unfortunately it is difficult to know where to look for its effects. For the sake of argument though, suppose that behavioral estimates of visual thresholds are uniformly higher than the true sensory thresholds. This would imply that the postreceptoral gap is smaller than Banks and Bennett's (1988) estimates. Behavioral procedures, like FPL, rely on an infant's willingness to perform the appropriate looking behavior. It is well known that infants tend to preferentially fixate on patterned rather than unpatterned stimuli, but their looking preference is entirely voluntary and certainly not mandated whenever they detect a target. The VEP technique used in infant vision studies only requires that the infant look in the direction of the target for fairly brief periods. For these reasons, it has been assumed that the FPL measurements are more subjective to motivational deficits. VEP measurements commonly reveal greater sensitivities than behavioral measurements. For instance, grating acuity measured by VEP is typically an octave higher (Dobson & Teller, 1978). If this argument is accepted, it should be noted that VEP estimates of neonatal contrast sensitivity and grating acuity still fall well short of the values predicted from the front-end losses as plotted in Figure 7. That is to say, whether one relies on FPL or VEP measurements of visual sensitivity, one cannot explain all of the difference between neonatal and adult performance from front-end losses alone.

There are a number of possible explanations involving inefficient neural processing that might explain age changes in the postreceptoral loss. Real observers' deviations from ideal performance are characterized by two general factors: the level of internal noise and the efficiency with which the observer utilizes available stimulus information. These two factors have been called *intrinsic noise* and *sampling efficiency,* respectively (Legge, Kersten, & Burgess, 1987). Here the possibility is discussed that one or both of these causes of less-than-ideal performance contribute to the postreceptoral loss observed in neonates.

Intrinsic noise refers to sources of random error within the visual system. There are numerous sources of noise within the visual system that could degrade visual performance. Let me discuss one plausible example, because it might be particularly important in developing systems. A consistent and striking physiological observation is that cells in the visual cortex of kittens respond sluggishly compared to adult cells (Bonds, 1979; Derrington & Fuchs, 1984; Hubel & Wiesel, 1963). Their response latency, fatigability, and peak firing rate are much lower than in mature neurons. The firing rates of retinal ganglion cells, in contrast, do not differ markedly across age (Hamasaki & Flynn, 1977). Peak firing rates also decrease at successive sites in the geniculostriate pathway of adult cats, but the effect is more dramatic in kittens. Thus, it appears that peak firing rate drops dramatically in the ascending visual pathway of kittens. The human visual cortex appears to be quite immature early in life, too (Atkinson & Braddick, 1981; Braddick & Atkinson, 1987; Naegele & Held, 1982), so the same drop in firing rate may occur in human neonates. Reduced firing rates from retina to cortex, if caused by random or nearly random dropping of spikes from one cell to the next, would decrease the total number of spikes in an unpredictable way. If the spike trains are Poisson distributed (an approximation to the binomial distribution) or nearly so, a drop in the mean number of spikes reduces the signal-to-noise ratio. It is equivalent to adding noise and, therefore, is best thought of as a source of intrinsic noise. Thus, successive reductions in firing rate may well be a significant source of information loss in the young visual system.

Poor sampling efficiency may also contribute significantly to the postreceptoral loss. The optimal strategy in detecting a visual stimulus is one which extracts the greatest signal information possible while keeping the effects of external or internal noise to minimum. When the parameters of the signal are known, the optimal strategy is implemented, for all intents and purposes, by a weighting function that matches the profile of the expected signal (for a rigorous treatment, see Geisler, 1989). This is probably accomplished in the visual system by monitoring the activity of neurons whose receptive fields nearly match the profile of the expected signal. The newborn visual system might exhibit poorer sampling efficiency than the adult for a couple of reasons. First, because of the immaturity of the visual cortex, neurons with receptive fields that match experimental stimuli (sine wave gratings, for example) may be rare or nonexistent. Second, and perhaps most importantly, in behavioral experiments, the situation is surely quite different for a neonate compared to an adult. The adult can be coached to anticipate the spatial configuration and temporal characteristics of the signal to be detected. Thus, an adult observer can choose more wisely which neurons to monitor the activity of. Newborns, on the other hand, cannot be coached in such a fashion. The experimenter has to rely on the general orienting response of the child to salient or novel targets. The child presumably has to monitor the activity of a very large number of neurons any of which could indicate the appearance of a salient or novel event. The consequence is a reduction in sampling efficiency.

Banks, Stephens, and Hartmann (1985) provided some data relevant to measuring intrinsic noise and sampling inefficiency in young infants. This experiment, however, was conducted for another purpose so there are too few measurements to draw any firm conclusions. Nonetheless, it is interesting to consider their findings. Banks et al. presented sine wave gratings with and without a noise masker to 6-week-olds, 12-week-olds, and adults. They found that adults exhibited a significantly larger masking effect than did 6- or 12-week-olds. That is to say, the presence of the noise elevated threshold much more in adults than in infants. This implies that the 6- and 12-week-olds have more intrinsic noise than adults do; stated another way, the equivalent noise in infants appears to be higher than in adults. It also appears from their data that infants' sampling efficiency is poorer, too.

As stated earlier, the spatial visual deficits infants exhibit are due to both front-end and postreceptoral immaturities. The postreceptoral immaturities—whose effects are evidenced by the postreceptoral gap shown in Figure 8—may well be caused by both elevated intrinsic noise and by low sampling efficiency.

Conclusions

This chapter has reviewed evidence that the spatial vision of human neonates is very poor compared to adults. One useful indicant of this difference is the spatial contrast sensitivity function. Neonates' CSFs are shifted to lower spatial frequencies and lower sensitivities, which means that they require higher contrasts and coarser patterns to see. Much, but by no means all, of the gap between neonatal and adult CSFs can be explained by an analysis of the information lost by immature optics and (particularly) photoreceptors. To understand the cause of the unexplained portion of the gap, we will need more information about how retinal neurons and central visual pathways mature during the first few years.

We are in a better position to understand how "front-end" mechanisms affect age-related changes in vision than in audition right now because we know more about how morphological changes in optics and receptors ought to affect visual sensitivity than we know about how such changes in the outer, inner, and middle ear ought to affect hearing. One hopes, however, that advances in the analysis of front-end mechanisms in hearing will soon change this situation.

References

Abramov, I., Gordon, J., Hendrickson, A., Hainline, L., Dobson, V., & LaBossiere, E. (1982). The retina of the newborn human infant. *Science, 217*, 265–267.

Allen, D., Norcia, A. M., & Tyler, C. W. (1989). Development of grating acuity and contrast sensitivity in the central and peripheral visual field of the human infant. *Investigative Ophthalmology and Visual Science, 30* (Suppl.), 311.

Atkinson, J., & Braddick, O. (1981). Development of optokinetic nystagmus in infants: An indicator of cortical binocularity? In D. F. Fisher, R. A. Monty, & J. W. Sanders (Eds.), *Cognition and visual perception* (pp. 17–39). Hillsdale, NJ: Erlbaum.

Atkinson, J., Braddick, O., & Moar, K. (1977). Development of contrast sensitivity over the first three months of life in the human infant. *Vision Research, 17*, 1037–1044.

Banks, M. S., & Bennett, P. J. (1988). Optical and photoreceptor immaturities limit the spatial and chromatic vision of human neonates. *Journal of the Optical Society of America, 5*, 2059–2079.

Banks, M. S., & Dannemiller, J. L. (1987). Infant visual psychophysics. In P. Salapatek &. L. B. Cohen (Eds.), *Handbook of infant perception* (pp. 115–184). New York: Academic Press.

Banks, M. S., Geisler, W. S., & Bennett, P. J. (1987). The physical limits of grating visibility. *Vision Research, 27*, 1915–1924.

Banks, M. S., & Salapatek, P. (1978). Acuity and contrast sensitivity in 1-, 2-, and 3-month-old human infants. *Investigative Ophthalmology and Visual Science, 17*, 361–365.

Banks, M. S., & Salapatek, P. (1981). Infant pattern vision: A new approach based on the contrast sensitivity function. *Journal of Experimental Child Psychology, 31*, 1–45.

Banks, M. S., & Salapatek, P. (1983). Infant visual perception. In M. M. Haith &. J. J. Campos (Eds.), *Handbook of child psychology* (pp. 113–224). New York: Wiley.

Banks, M. S., Stephens, B. R., & Hartmann, E. E. (1985). The development of basic mechanisms of pattern vision: Spatial frequency channels. *Journal of Experimental Child Psychology, 40*, 501–527.

Barlow, H. B. (1958). Temporal and spatial summation in human vision at different background intensities. *Journal of Physiology, 141*, 337–350.

Blakemore, C., & Vital-Durand, F. (1980). Development of the neural basis of visual acuity in monkeys. Speculation on the origin of deprivation amblyopia. *Transactions of the Ophthalmological Society of the United Kingdom, 99*, 363–368.

Bonds, A. B. (1979). Development of orientation tuning in the visual cortex of kittens. In R. Freeman (Ed.), *Developmental neurobiology of vision* (pp. 61–77). New York: Plenum.

Boothe, R. G., Williams, R. A., Kiorpes, L., & Teller, D. Y. (1980). Development of contrast sensitivity in infant *Maccaca nemestrina* monkeys. *Science, 208*, 1290–1292.

Braddick, O., & Atkinson, J. (1987). Sensory selectivity, attentional control, and cross-channel integration in early visual development. In A. Yonas (Ed.), *Perceptual development in infancy: The Minnesota Symposium on Child Psychology* (pp. 105–143). Hillsdale, NJ: Erlbaum.

Bronson, G. W. (1974). The postnatal growth of visual capacity. *Child Development, 45*, 874–890.

Brown, A. M., Dobson, V., & Maier, J. (1987). Visual acuity of human infants at scotopic, mesopic and photopic luminances. *Vision Research, 27*, 1845–1858.

Campbell, F. W., & Gubish, R. W. (1966). Optical quality of the human eye. *Journal of Physiology*, *186*, 558–578.

Campbell, F. W., & Robson, J. G. (1968). Application of Fourier analysis to the visibility of gratings. *Journal of Physiology*, *197*, 551–566.

Colleta, N. J., Williams, D. R., & Tiana, C. L. M. (1990). Consequences of spatial sampling for human motion perception. *Vision Research*, *30*, 1631–1648.

Cornsweet, T. (1970). *Visual perception*. Orlando: Harcourt Brace Jovanovich.

Crowell, J. A., & Banks, M. S. (in revision). The efficiency of foveal vision. *Journal of the Optical Society of America*.

Derrington, A. M., & Fuchs, A. F. (1981). The development of spatial-frequency selectivity in kitten striate cortex. *Journal of Physiology*, *316*, 1–10.

Dobson, V., & Teller, D. Y. (1987). Visual acuity in human infants: A review and comparison of behavioral and electrophysiological techniques. *Vision Research*, *18*, 1469–1483.

Geisler, W. S. (1989). Sequential ideal-observer analysis of visual discriminations. *Psychological Review*, *96*, 267–314.

Green, D. G. (1970). Regional variations in the visual acuity for interference fringes on the retina. *Journal of Physiology*, *207*, 351–356.

Green, D. M., & Swets, J. A. (1966). *Signal detection theory and psychophysics*. New York: Robert E. Krieger.

Hainline, L., & Harris, C. (1988). Does foveal development influence the consistency of infants' point of visual regard? *Infant Behavior and Development*, *11*, 129.

Hamaski, D. I., & Flynn, J. T. (1977). Physiological properties of retinal ganglion cells of 3-week-old kittens. *Vision Research*, *17*, 275–284.

Hendrickson, A., & Kupfer, C. (1976). The histogenesis of the fovea in the macaque monkey. *Investigative Ophthalmology*, *15*, 746–756.

Hickey, T. L., & Peduzzi, J. D. (1987). Structure and development of the visual system. In P. Salapatek & L. B. Cohen (Eds.), *Handbook of infant perception: From sensation to perception* (pp. 1–32). New York: Academic Press.

Hirano, S., Yamamoto, Y., Takayama, H., Sugata, Y., & Matsuo, K. (1979). Ultrasonic observations of eyes in premature babies. Part 6. Growth curves of ocular axial length and its components. *Acta Society Ophthalmologica, Japan*, *83*, 1679–1693.

Howell, E. R., & Hess, R. F. (1978). The functional area for summation to threshold for sinusoidal gratings. *Vision Research*, *18*, 369–374.

Hubel, D. H., & Wiesel, T. N. (1963). Receptive fields of cells in striate cortex of very young, visually inexperienced kittens. *Journal of Neurophysiology*, *26*, 994–1002.

Jacobs, D. S., & Blakemore, C. (1988). Factors limiting the postnatal development of visual acuity in the monkey. *Vision Research*, *28*, 947–958.

Kiely, P. M., Crewther, S. G., Nathan, J., Brennan, N. A., Efron, N., & Madigan, M. (1987). A comparison of ocular development of the cynomolgus monkey and man. *Clinical Visual Science*, *3*, 269–280.

Larsen, J. S. (1971). The sagittal growth of the eye. IV. Ultrasonic measurement of the axial length of the eye from birth to puberty. *Acta Ophthalmologica*, *49*, 873–886.

Legge, G., Kersten, D., & Burgess, A. E. (1987). Contrast discrimination in noise. *Journal of the Optical Society of America*, *4*, 391–404.

Lewis, T. L., Maurer, D., & Kay, D. (1978). Newborns' central vision: Whole or hole? *Journal of Experimental Child Psychology*, *26*, 193–203.

Miller, W. H., & Bernard, G. D. (1983) Averaging over the foveal receptor aperture curtails aliasing. *Vision Research*, *23*, 1365–1370.

Naegele, J. R., & Held, R. (1982). The postnatal development of monocular optokinetic nystagmus in infants. *Vision Research*, *22*, 341–346.

Norcia, A. M., & Tyler, C. W. (1985). Spatial frequency sweep VEP: Visual acuity during the first year of life. *Vision Research*, *25*, 1399–1408.

Norcia, A. M., Tyler, C. W., & Allen, D. (1986). Electrophysiological assessment of contrast sensitivity in human infants. *American Journal of Optometry and Physiological Optics*, *63*, 12–15.

Pelli, D. (1990). Quantum efficiency of vision. In C. Blakemore (Ed.), *Vision: Coding and efficiency* (pp. 98–117). Cambridge, England: Cambridge University Press.

Pirchio, M., Spinelli, D., Fiorentini, A., & Maffei, L. (1978). Infant contrast sensitivity evaluated by evoked potentials. *Brain Research*, *141*, 179–184.

Rose, A. (1942). The relative sensitivities of television pick-up tubes, photographic film, and the human eye. *Proceedings of the Institute of Radio-Engineers*, *30*, 293–300.

Salapatek, P., & Kessen, W. (1966). Visual scanning of triangles by the human newborn. *Journal of Experimental Child Psychology*, *3*, 155–167.

Salapatek, P. (1975). Pattern perception in early infancy. In P. Salapatek & L. B. Cohen (Eds.), *Infant perception: From sensation to cognition* (pp. 133–234). New York: Academic Press.

Salapatek, P. & Cohen, L. B. (1985) *Handbook of infant perception*. New York: Academic Press.

Shimojo, S., & Held, R. (1987). Vernier acuity is less than grating acuity in 2- and 3-month-olds. *Vision Research*, *27*, 77–86.

Slater, A. M., & Findlay, J. M (1975). Binocular fixation in the newborn baby. *Journal of Experimental Child Psychology*, *20*, 248–273.

Stenstrom, S. (1946). Investigation of the variation and correlation of the optical elements of human eyes. *American Journal of Optometry*, *25*, 5.

Watson, A. B., Barlow, H. B., & Robson, J. G. (1983). What does the eye see best? *Nature*, *31*, 419–422.

Williams, D. R. (1985). Aliasing in human foveal vision. *Vision Research*, *25* (2), 195–206.

Wilson, H. R. (1988). Development of spatiotemporal mechanisms in infant vision. *Vision Research*, *28*, 611–628.

Yonas, A. (1988) Perceptual development in infancy. *The Minnesota Symposium on Child Psychology*. Hillsdale, NJ: Erlbaum.

Yuodelis, C., & Hendrickson, A. (1986). A qualitative and quantitative analysis of the human fovea during development. *Vision Research*, *26*, 847–876.

PART THREE

Developmental Psychoacoustics in the Context of Hearing Science

CHAPTER 10

The Refinement of Central Auditory Form and Function During Development

Dan H. Sanes

Our success in demonstrating a causal relationship between central neuronal structure or function and auditory perception in adult animals has been limited (Suga, 1988; Young & Rubel, 1983). The most compelling strategies—to stimulate, reversibly inactivate, or record from neural tissue in awake, behaving animals—are available only with highly trained animals (Jay & Sparks, 1984; Moiseff & Konishi, 1981; Penfield & Rasmussen, 1950; Riquimaroux, Gaioni, & Suga, 1991; Takahashi, Moiseff, & Konishi, 1984). Of course, this challenge is magnified during development when nonspecific behavioral factors (e.g., level of arousal) and the fragility of the nervous system (e.g., rapid fatigue) introduce experimental constraints. However, the study of immature *brains*, and the *behaviors* that

Portions of this work were supported in part by the Mendik Research Fund, a Whitehead Fellowship, and NIH grant DC00540. Dan Sanes is a Sloan Foundation Fellow.

Correspondence concerning this chapter should be sent to D. Sanes at his present address: Center for Neural Science, 4 Washington Place, New York University, New York, NY 10003.

they manufacture should prove informative in that it is one of the only ways to "obtain" a major transformation in both.

In cases where central auditory development does appear to explain the emergence of perceptual abilities, one must carefully eliminate the maturation of cochlear mechanics and electrophysiology as the proximal basis. In order to circumvent the cochlea, my strategy will be to describe developmental changes that are known to occur in the central auditory system. Both functional and morphological studies using animal models suggest a critical role for central auditory maturation. Possible perceptual consequences of these ontogenetic events within the central nervous system are discussed herein, but it should be recognized that they have not been directly demonstrated in any system.

The simple psychophysical properties for which cochlear or central explanations are sought include: absolute threshold, dynamic range, intensity discrimination, frequency resolution, frequency discrimination, and sound localization. There are at least three general neuronal properties that may reasonably be associated with such perceptual attributes. First, it appears that acoustically evoked activity must ascend bilaterally through the central auditory pathways to have its full impact on behavior (Neff, Diamond, & Casseday, 1975). Therefore, the *quantity* of sound-evoked neural activity should give us some indication of competence. Second, one would assume that gradations in neural activity patterns would accompany the discernable gradations in sound stimuli. Neuronal attributes such as the number of afferent inputs per neuron, convergence, and the *specificity* of these afferent connections are likely to impact the response characteristics of the postsynaptic cell. Third, the temporal characteristics of sound-evoked activity play a crucial role during synaptic integration, or the process by which a single auditory neuron synthesizes a response from the great deal of afferent activity impinging on it. A simple example of this is a neuronal mechanism called temporal summation: If two excitatory synaptic potentials are elicited at the same time, then their effect at the postsynaptic cell is additive. In this regard, the maturation of *temporal properties* such as response latency, phase-locking, and fatigue may also inform us about the central limitations for processing an acoustic signal in young animals.

The following sections describe the measurement of these three general neuronal characteristics during the course of development in several mammals. The results of these studies generally establish that the central auditory system initially operates under somewhat severe constraints. To the extent that sensitive measures of auditory perception can be obtained during this time period, one may begin to understand the behavioral relevance of these neural properties.

Functional Limitations of Central Auditory Synapses

A group of binaural neurons located in the mammalian brain stem, the lateral superior olive (LSO), provide a favorable location to study the development of central auditory function for two reasons (Figure 1). First, as schematized in Figure 1B, these neurons encode a relatively simple percept, the location of an azimuthal sound source using interaural sound level differences (Boudreau & Tsuchitani, 1968; Caird & Klinke, 1983; Harnischfeger, Neuweiler, & Schlegel, 1985; Sanes & Rubel, 1988). Second, LSO neurons receive two relatively discrete sets of afferent contacts. They are excited when sound stimuli are presented to the ipsilateral ear, and are inhibited when sound stimuli are presented to the contralateral ear (Figure 1A). Both the excitatory and the inhibitory afferents are topographically arranged along the frequency axis (Boudreau & Tsuchitani, 1970; Sanes & Rubel, 1988).

In order to address some of the underlying cellular mechanisms of sound localization during development, we have begun to extract the part of the central auditory system that first performs binaural computations, the superior olivary complex, for in vitro analyses (Sanes, 1990). The brain is rapidly removed from a deeply anesthetized gerbil, and a 400–500 μm section through the brain stem is produced. Sections through the central auditory system are kept alive in an oxygenated artificial cerebrospinal fluid for 3–5 hours, depending on the age of the animal. This preparation allows the investigator superior access and mechanical stability compared to an in vivo preparation. Using this brain slice preparation, we are able to record intracellularly from single LSO neurons while electrically stimulating the ipsilateral excitatory pathway and/or the contralateral inhibitory pathways that provide the majority of synaptic input to these cells.

In postnatal 18-to-25-day-old gerbils, approximately 1 week after the onset of hearing, the synaptic potentials are of fairly short duration. For example, the hyperpolarizing inhibitory synaptic events last for 3–8 ms, while the synaptically evoked action potentials last for less than 1 ms (Sanes, 1990). Figure 2A illustrates characteristic synaptic responses from a 19-day-old animal when electric

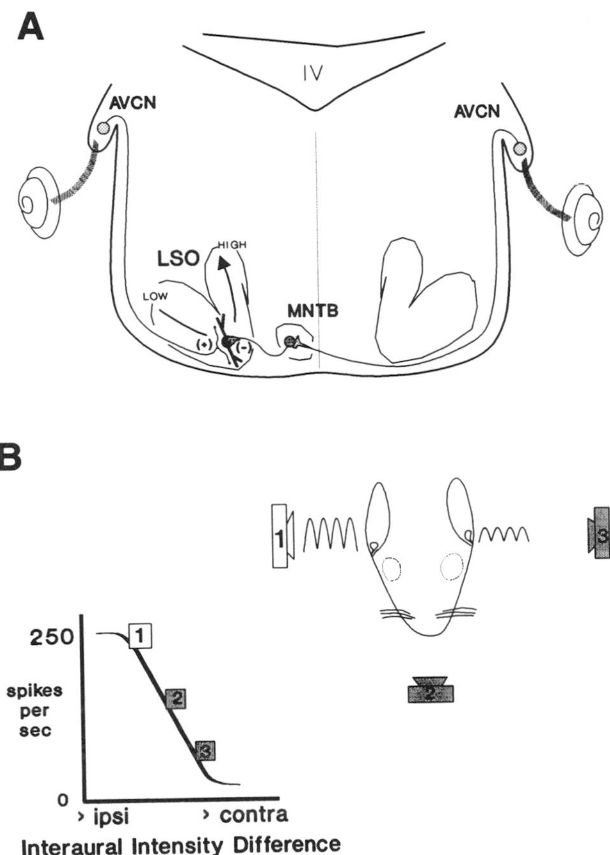

FIGURE 1 The superior olive and its role in binaural processing. (*A*) A schematic through the brain stem at the level of the cochlear nuclei and superior olive. Neurons in the lateral superior olive (LSO) receive a prominent excitatory projection from the ipsilateral cochlear nucleus. The contralateral ear evokes an inhibitory response because the glycinergic neurons of the medial nucleus of the trapezoid body (MNTB) are interposed in the pathway. Note that both sets of afferents project topographically along the frequency axis (arrow) of the LSO. Although evidence exists for other minor projections to the LSO, depending on the species, the illustrated afferents account for the vast majority of input. (*B*) A schematic illustrating the response of a single LSO neuron to changes in sound-source location. As interaural intensity difference is altered with the speaker's location, due to shadowing of sound by the head, the neuron shows a graded change in discharge rate. For example, when the speaker is located at position 1, ipsilateral to the LSO neuron (see *A*), the neuron receives maximum excitatory input, minimum inhibitory input, and is maximally activated.

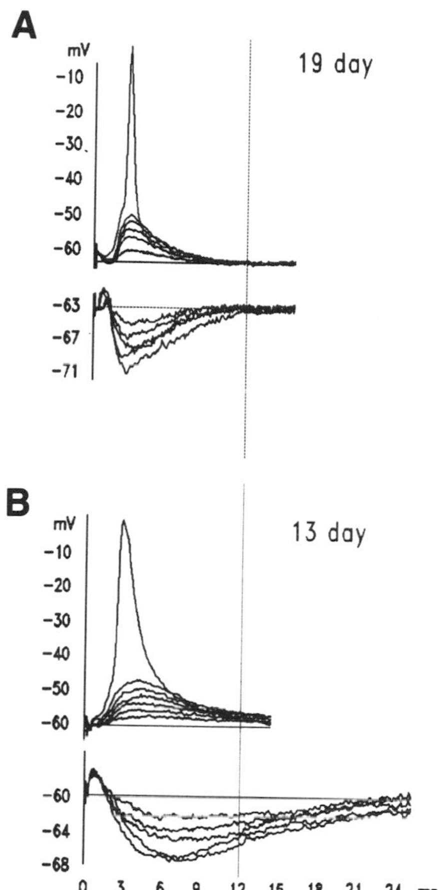

FIGURE 2 Synaptic potentials from intracellular recordings at 19 postnatal days (*A*), and 13 postnatal days (*B*), using the brain slice preparation. The duration of both the excitatory (positive-going) and inhibitory (negative-going) potentials is much longer in the 13-day-old animal. For ease of comparison, the dotted line indicates the time at which all inhibitory potentials have returned to baseline in the 19-day neuron. Note that the gain is greater for inhibitory potentials at both ages.

stimulus pulses were delivered to either the ipsilateral or contralateral pathways. The amplitude increments are related to stimulus strength and presumably the number of afferent connections that have been recruited by the stimulus pulse. When the synaptic responses obtained in a 13-day-old animal, about the time of hearing onset, were directly compared, it was clear that they were of longer duration (Figure 2B). In fact, recordings from LSO neurons prior to external ear canal opening revealed a functional state that can be an order of magnitude longer in the time domain. Synaptic responses recorded from 3-to-4-day-old animals demonstrated that the potentials can last for up to 100 ms.

The consequence of such long-lasting synaptic potentials is better demonstrated when one compares the response to a rapid train of electric stimulus pulses delivered to either the ipsilateral or contralateral pathways. Whereas the synaptic responses are relatively discrete entities in more mature animals (Figure 3A), there is a complex pattern of temporal summation of events, and fatigue or habituation in the neurons from neonatal animals. For example, in the neuron from a 7-day animal, the first stimulus to the excitatory pathway produces an action potential, the next three stimuli produce a summation of excitatory potentials, and the final three stimuli lead to a decrement in response (Figure 3B). Alternatively, the recording at 3 days demonstrates a summation of the first five stimulus-evoked potentials to produce an action potential (Figure 3C). Therefore, the longevity of a single potential constrains the amount of information that is able to be processed during any given stimulus period, thus limiting the dynamic range of the neuron. Furthermore, these prolonged potentials lend a measure of unpredictability as to when an action potential will occur.

In some sense, the time domain of these synaptic events—the ability to produce discrete responses—could be characterized as the clock speed of this simple circuit. In order for the central nervous system to operate properly in the time domain, an inhibitory postsynaptic potential should only be effective at blocking an action potential for a discrete amount of time, as shown in Figure 4. Although the inhibitory event lasted for 6 ms, it was able to prevent the ipsilaterally evoked action potential for only about 1.5 ms. We are currently quantifying the effective duration of inhibition in neonatal animals.

The alterations in postsynaptic potential size and duration were not unexpected. In fact, a decrease in the duration of postsynaptic potentials has been documented in a wide variety of central neuronal systems (Gardette, Debono, Dupont, & Crepel, 1985; Naka, 1964; Purpura, Shofer, & Scarff, 1965; Schwob, Haberly, & Price, 1984; Wilson & Leon, 1986). In addition, we have previously shown that the transmitter receptor molecule mediating neural inhibition in the LSO, the glycine receptor, undergoes a dynamic change in distribution during postnatal development (Sanes & Wooten, 1987).

Since an increase in stimulus duration often leads to improved perceptual resolution (Hafter, Dye, & Gilkey, 1979; Tobias & Zerlin, 1959), these extremely

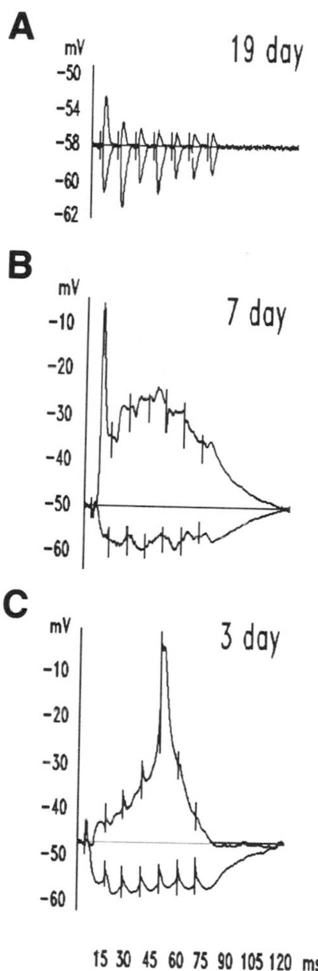

FIGURE 3 Synaptic potentials evoked by a 100-Hz train of electrical stimuli at 19 (*A*), 7 (*B*), and 3 (*C*) postnatal days using the brain slice preparation. Whereas each stimulus evokes a discrete excitatory or inhibitory potential at 19 days, the long-lasting synaptic potentials summate at 3 and 7 days.

long-lasting synaptic potentials may affect many aspects of auditory perception, including gap detection and voice onset time discrimination tasks. This is not to say that infants cannot perform these tasks. Rather, we expect resolution to be poor if synaptic events are prolonged in the time domain, much as was shown for single neuron interaural intensity difference (IID) functions in young gerbils and cats (see next section).

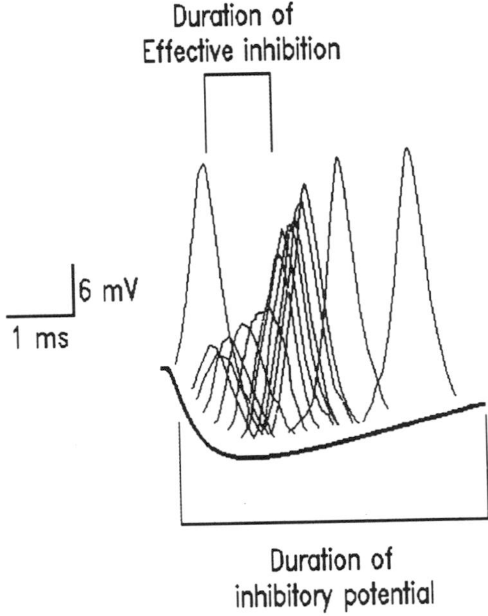

FIGURE 4 An inhibitory synaptic potential, and the ipsilaterally evoked excitatory potentials at increasing latency. The action potential was not blocked by the inhibitory potential if it occurred at a very short latency, but was blocked for about 1.5 ms (duration of effective inhibition) at slightly greater latencies. After this point, the inhibitory potential was unable to block the ipsilaterally evoked action potential, even though it had not yet returned to baseline.

Temporal Processing in the Immature Central Auditory System

The functional characteristics of single synaptic potentials in neonatal and mature animals, discussed earlier, illustrated two fundamental constraints in processing information: temporal resolution and dynamic range. Temporal properties have long been a focus of neurophysiological study, particularly in terms of the stimulus response latency, the ability to synchronize, or phase-lock, to an acoustic signal, and the fatigue with repeated presentations.

The response latency to a sound stimulus decreases with age at all levels of the neuraxis (Moore, 1983; Mysliveek, 1983). The contribution of central modifications to this process is readily apparent when one compares the decrease in latency at the level of the cochlea and cortex in the cat (Ellingson & Wilcott, 1960; Romand, 1971). The decrease in latency occurs simultaneously in the periphery and centrally, and reaches the mature state at approximately 30 postnatal days. However, from 15 to 30 postnatal days, the decrease in response latency is only 0.4 ms at the level of the cochlea (Romand, 1971), but nearly 13 ms at the level of the cortex (Ellingson & Wilcott, 1960). Quantitative assessment of auditory evoked potentials demonstrated much the same feature in the mouse and the cat (Mikaelian & Ruben, 1965; Sanes & Constantine-Paton, 1985; Shnerson & Pujol, 1982; Walsh, McGee, & Javel, 1986).

Most of the parametric data on response latency is obtained by detecting the peak amplitude of a sound-evoked compound potential, presumably reflecting the synchronous discharge of many neuronal elements. Moore and Irvine (1979) have pointed out that the utility of a compound potential in detecting threshold may ultimately depend on the temporal characteristics of the response (i.e., the ability of many neurons to discharge in synchrony). For example, the threshold values obtained when recording from single neurons in the auditory midbrain reveal that a stable state is reached by 30 postnatal days, whereas the thresholds determined with the compound potentials continue to decline, suggesting a continued improvement in discharge synchrony. This caveat likely applies to the use of compound potentials as an estimator of response latency as well. The disparities between measures obtained with extremely sensitive assays of neural function (e.g., intracellular recording), and those obtained on large populations of neurons (i.e., evoked compound potential), highlight an additional difficulty in relating brain to behavior.

The ability of single auditory neurons to synchronize their discharge to a particular phase of the stimulus waveform is generally thought to play a crucial role in the discrimination of low-frequency sounds and interaural time differences. A direct comparison of phase-locking at the level of the auditory nerve and the anteroventral cochlear nucleus in the cat reveals a contribution to maturation centripetal to the cochlea (Brugge, Javel, & Kitzes, 1978; Kettner, Feng, & Brugge, 1985). Since this represents the first synaptic transformation within the central auditory system, one would expect a further corruption of temporal information as one ascends the auditory pathway. In fact, infants and immature animals generally exhibit a protracted period of improved discrimination with low-frequency sounds and an impressive variability of response (see chapter 2 in this volume). The variability of the behavioral response may be partially related to the absolute failure of neurons in young animals to respond to repeated stimuli, even at low repetition rates (Fitzakerly, McGee, & Walsh, 1991).

Whereas measures of latency and phase-locking tell us about temporal acuity, a more significant problem lies in the modest evoked response amplitudes found in young animals, the neuron's dynamic range (Brugge et al., 1978; Romand, 1983; Sanes & Rubel, 1988; Woolf & Ryan, 1985). For example, the mean maximum discharge rate in the LSO of 13-to-14-day-old gerbils is about 80 discharges/s but increases to 350 discharges/s in adult animals (Sanes & Rubel, 1988). Even though LSO neurons from 13-to-14-day-old gerbils encode smaller changes in stimulus level, they still end up devoting fewer action potentials to a given change in sound level. In other words, they have a poorer resolution. Unless neonatal animals are able to employ normalized activity levels (e.g., to assign perceptual significance to a discharge rate of 50% of maximum, whether this corresponded to 10 discharges/s or 200 discharges/s), they must necessarily make decisions based upon less neural information.

The modest evoked activity levels may be further eroded in that sensory and neural elements are especially prone to adaptation or fatigue during development (Mysliveek, 1983; Saunders, Coles, & Gates, 1973). Once again, it is clear that there is a process of fatigue or habituation in the developing central auditory system that is independent of the cochlea. The decrement of evoked response amplitudes during the presentation of repetitive clicks was examined quantitatively at the levels of the eighth nerve, cochlear nucleus, and auditory midbrain in mice of increasing postnatal age (Sanes & Constantine-Paton, 1985). The response amplitudes in 13-to-16-day-old mice were severely attenuated with click repetition rates above 1/s, and this was more pronounced in the auditory midbrain. Furthermore, the improved stimulus following that was seen with increasing age was slower developing at the level of the auditory midbrain, even at click repetition rates as low as 2/s.

Taken together, the modest evoked activity levels and the rapid decrease in response to repetitive auditory stimuli in young animals suggest that (a) young animals must listen for a longer period of time to acquire the same information, in neural terms, as an adult and (b) the most efficacious stimuli for young animals must contain periods of silence to allow for neural recovery. These suggestions are consistent with the behavioral attributes of human infants (Clarkson, Clifton, Swain, & Perris, 1989).

Neuron Form and Frequency Selectivity: Afferent Arborizations

In addition to the immature electrophysiological characteristics at central auditory synapses, the question arises as to whether afferent connections are in the proper location, a feature commonly referred to as synaptic specificity. We have been able to use the brain slice preparation to stain single inhibitory afferents from the medial nucleus of the trapezoid body (MNTB) and follow the development of arbor specificity along the tonotopic axis of the LSO (Figure 1A). A computer-directed morphometry system has allowed us to reconstruct complete afferent arborizations and measure salient features of their anatomy (Sanes & Siverls, 1991).

A comparison between single arborizations from 2-, 13-, and 19-day-old animals is shown in Figure 5. In general, the projections from neonatal animals are accurate and occupy a fairly discrete region of the tonotopic axis within the LSO (Figure 5A). However, from 7 to 13 postnatal days, a subpopulation of arbors displays a rather broad spread along the tonotopic axis (Figure 5B).

In order to quantify the specificity of these arborizations along the tonotopic axis, we measured the distance that the presynaptic boutons (i.e., enlargements of the arbor thought to be the site of synaptic transmission), shown as dot patterns in Figure 5B and C, spread across the frequency axis. This distance decreases 25%, from 123 μm in animals at 12–13 postnatal days to 93 μm in animals at 18–25 postnatal days. Since LSO is increasing in size during the same period (Sanes, Merickel, & Rubel, 1989; Sanes & Siverls, 1991), the retracting MNTB arbors also occupy a much smaller fraction of postsynaptic space as development progresses.

We may speculate that the less refined arbors affect those auditory percepts involving frequency selectivity. The responses of single LSO neurons to tonal stimuli during development do exhibit a degree of refinement that cannot be solely explained by the maturation of the cochlea (Sanes & Rubel, 1988). For example, single neurons may respond to two discrete frequency ranges in 13- to 16-day animals, whereas only a single frequency range is found in neurons from adult animals (Figure 6). One may also record from single neurons having both

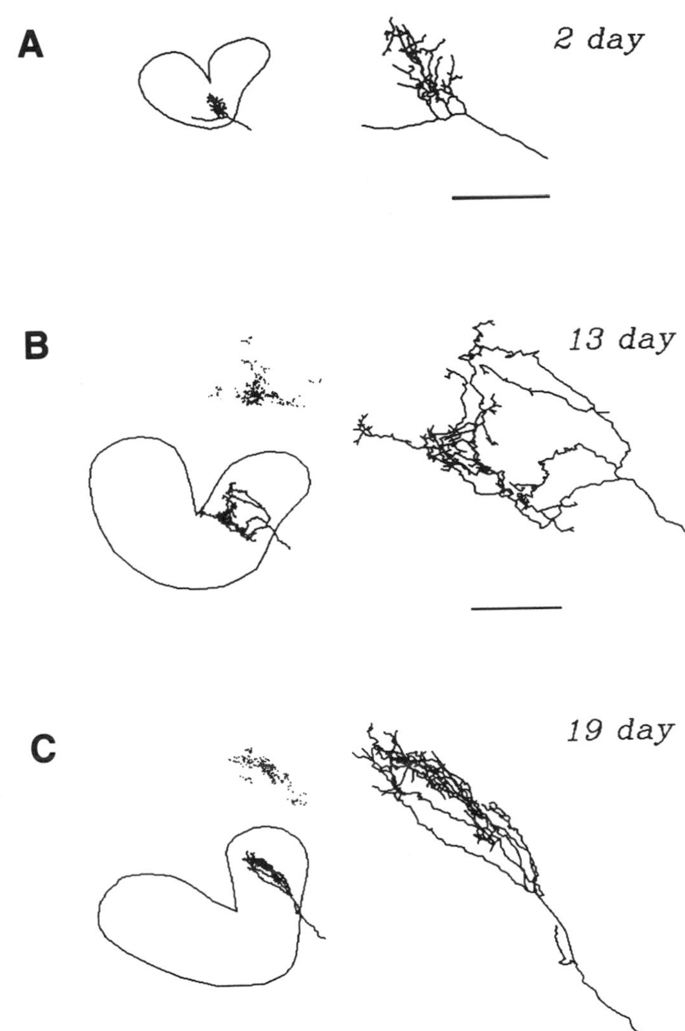

FIGURE 5 Examples of single MNTB axonal arborizations within the LSO at (*A*) 2, (*B*) 13, and (*C*) 19 postnatal days. In each case, the position of the arborization within the LSO is shown to the left, and the complete reconstructed arbor is shown to the right. In (*B*) and (*C*) the dot pattern above the nucleus outline is the terminal bouton (presumed presynaptic release sites) pattern for the arbor. Whereas the initial projections are quite punctate (*A*), a sizable percentage of fibers adopt a more diffuse arborization pattern prior to the time of hearing onset (*B*). The inappropriate arborization patterns appear to reach a more mature morphology over the 3rd postnatal week (*C*). Bars = 100 μm. From Sanes and Siverls (1991). Copyright 1991 by John Wiley & Sons.

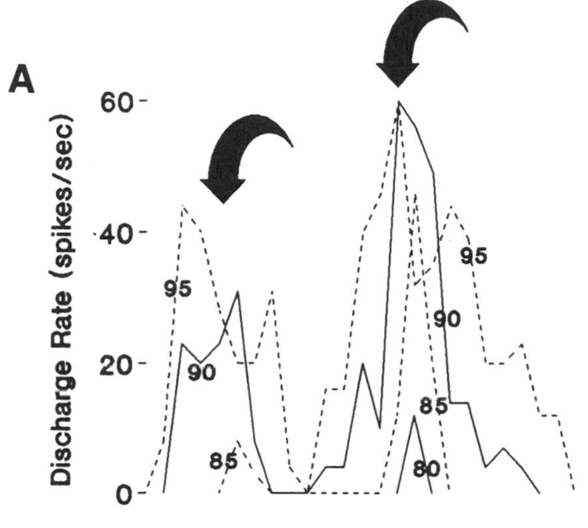

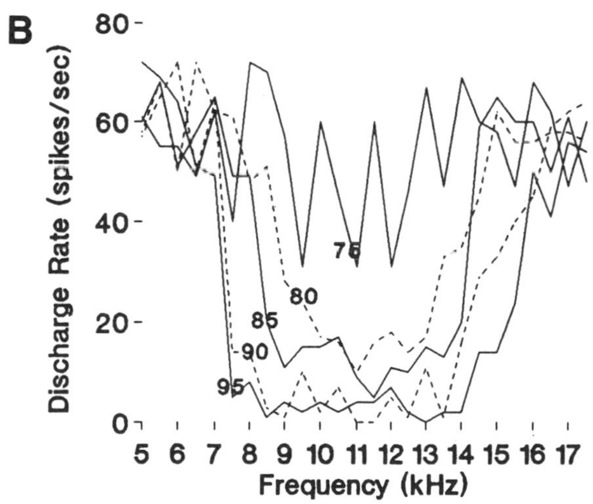

FIGURE 6 Excitatory (*A*) and inhibitory (*B*) frequency response areas from a single neuron in the LSO of a 15-day-old gerbil. Note that the neuron responds to two discrete frequency regions when sound stimuli are presented to the ipsilateral excitatory ear (arrows). The inhibitory response area from the same neuron shows only a single broad response area. The intensity of stimulation is shown in dB SPL for each isointensity curve. From Sanes and Rubel (1988). Copyright 1988 by Society for Neuroscience. Adapted by permission.

normal and exceptionally broad tuning in the same immature animal (Sanes & Rubel, 1988). Therefore, it is unlikely that the cochlea is solely responsible for immature frequency selectivity following the onset of response to airborne sound.

There have been two studies on the specificity of afferents within the developing chick auditory brain stem. In the first, Jackson and Parks (1982) were able to demonstrate that single neurons in the avian cochlear nucleus went through a period of synapse elimination from embryonic day 13 to embryonic days 17–18. Whereas neurons were originally innervated by about four afferents, this decreased to about 2.2 over the following 5 days. Therefore, there is a period when central neuronal connections are refined after the chick has begun to respond to airborne sound (Jackson & Rubel, 1978; Saunders et al., 1973). This period of dynamic change in the connections between neurons may not be an obligatory process. Young and Rubel (1986) have shown that the projection from the avian cochlear nucleus to the dorsal dendrites of *n. laminaris* does not show signs of refinement along the frequency axis, whereas the projection to the ventral dendrites does alter its projection.

Neuron Form and Frequency Selectivity: Dendritic Arborizations

Although the arrangement of single afferent arborizations tells us something about the maturity of synaptic connections, one must also consider the form of a postsynaptic structure, the dendritic arborization. There are several examples of dendrite modification in the central auditory system, each one suggesting a possible functional consequence (Glaser, Van derLoos, & Gissler, 1979; McMullen, Goldberger, & Glaser, 1988; Meininger & Baudrimont, 1981; Morest, 1969; Rogowski & Feng, 1981; Smith, 1981). We have previously shown that the morphology of LSO neurons varies, in a predictable way, along the tonotopic axis (Sanes, Goldstein, Ostad, & Hillman, 1990). Low-frequency dendrites spread a greater distance across the frequency axis, and with greater variability, than high-frequency dendrites (see asterisks in Figure 7A). Surprisingly, the octave bandwidths of single low-frequency neurons, at 50–60 dB above their threshold, are also much larger than those of high-frequency neurons (see asterisks in Figure 7B). In short, the morphometric finding bears an interesting resemblance to the functional property.

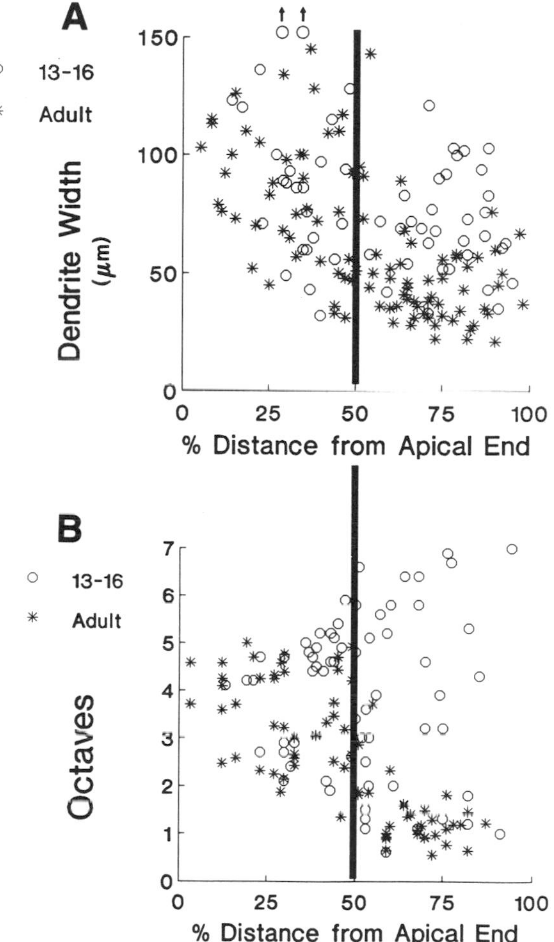

FIGURE 7 A comparison of LSO dendritic width along the frequency axis (*A*), and frequency selectivity (*B*), at 13–16 postnatal days (open circle) and in the adult gerbil (asterisk). The frequency axis has been converted to % distance from the apical–most projection region to correct for changes in the cochlear tonotopic map during development (Harris & Dallos, 1984; Sanes et al., 1989). (*A*): The dendritic width for both age groups is virtually identical from 0–50% of the distance from the apical–most projection region (to the left of the solid vertical line). However, above 50% the dendritic width is generally greater for 13-to-16-day-old animals. (*B*): The octave bands for both age groups largely overlap from 0–50% of the distance from the apical–most projection region (to the left of the solid vertical line), but are much greater for 13-to-16-day-old animals above 50%. From Sanes, Song, and Tyson (in press). Copyright 1992 by Elsevier. Reprinted by permission.

Since there is some reason to believe that the morphology of these central auditory neurons plays at least a partial role in the generation of frequency selectivity, we have now examined this correlation between neuronal geometry and frequency selectivity during the period of postnatal maturation. Figure 8 shows computer reconstructions of two neurons at 14 and at 21 postnatal days, with the high-frequency neuron showing a much more constrained dendritic arborization along the tonotopic axis at 21 days.

A quantitative analysis of dendritic spread along the frequency axis revealed that dendritic arbors do become more refined along the frequency axis, but only in the high-frequency projection region of the LSO (Sanes, Song, & Tyson, in press). The spread of dendrites across the frequency axis for neurons in adult animals and all animals between 13 and 16 postnatal days is shown in Figure 7A. Whereas there does not appear to be any change in this parameter for low-frequency neurons (i.e., less than 50% of the distance from the apical–most projection region), there is a significant decrease in this value for high-frequency neurons. The dendritic spread of high-frequency neurons decreases by 44% during the 3rd postnatal week. Therefore, neurons in one part of the LSO, the high-frequency region, change their geometry significantly, whereas the others do not.

If dendritic form is related to the range of frequencies to which a neuron will respond, then we predict that high-frequency neurons, but not low-frequency neurons, should have broader octave bandwidths following the onset of hearing. A comparison of the octave bandwidths of neurons in 13-to-16-day-old animals to those of adults indicated that this is the case. The octave bandwidth of single low-frequency neurons is similar to that of adults, but those from high-frequency neurons are significantly larger (Figure 7B). For both morphological and physiological criteria, there was a change towards greater specificity in the high-frequency neuronal population.

The failure of low-frequency neurons to change their dendritic form and frequency selectivity during this postnatal period is not necessarily an indication that behavioral capabilities are fully matured. As discussed earlier, the discrimination of low-frequency sounds relies heavily on temporal coding, and this may improve independently of the effective frequency range of a neuron. However, the refinement of dendrite morphology and frequency selectivity in high-frequency neurons does suggest behavioral consequences.

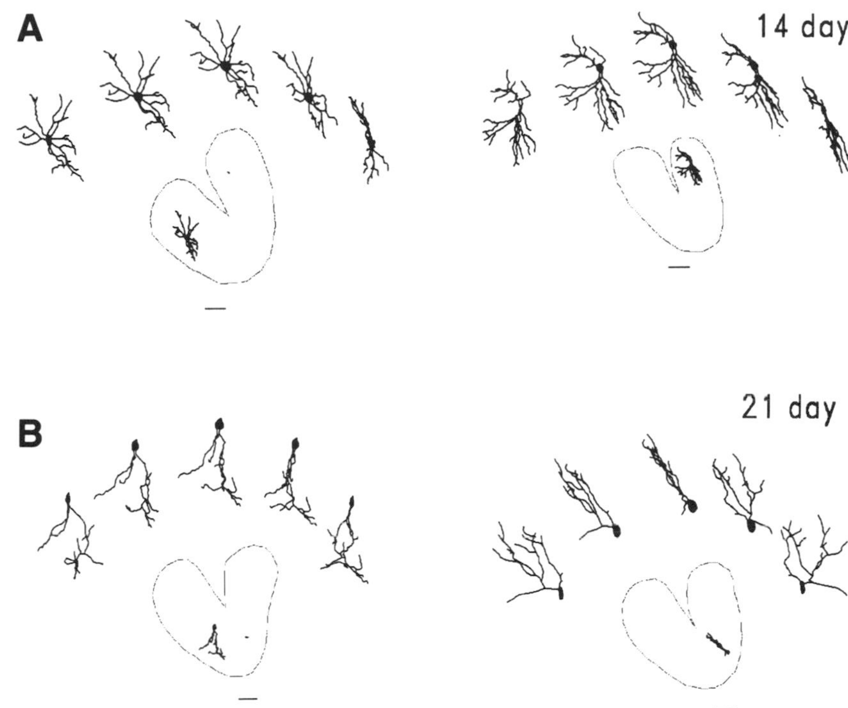

FIGURE 8 Computer reconstructions of LSO dendrites from postnatal day 14 (*A*) and day 21 (*B*) gerbils. The position of each neuron is shown along the frequency axis of the LSO, and the neuron is rotated at 30° intervals (from −60° to +60°) about the Y axis (sagittal plane). There is a marked refinement of dendrite spread along the frequency axis for high-frequency neurons (right), but not low-frequency neurons (left). Note that there are fewer branch points in the neurons from 21-day-old animals. Bars = 100 μm. From Sanes, Song, and Tyson (in press). Copyright 1992 by Elsevier. Reprinted by permission.

The Development of Binaural Processing

Behavioral analyses have demonstrated that adult gerbils have a minimal audible angle of 14–27°, and are able to localize both high- and low-frequency sounds (Heffner & Heffner, 1988). Although it is clear that young rodents use binaural cues to localize a sound source soon after their ear canal opens (Kelly, Judge, & Fraser, 1987; Kelly & Potash, 1986; Potash & Kelly, 1980), the resolution and temporal constraints have not been examined.

The response of single LSO neurons to IIDs has been studied immediately following ear canal opening and in the adult gerbil (Sanes & Rubel, 1988). As shown in Figure 9, the resolution of single neurons is very poor in young animals, primarily because the discharge rate is so low. In addition, some neurons appear to have a very irregular response as IID is altered. This functional immaturity is more apparent in single neurons recorded from the kitten inferior colliculus (Moore & Irvine, 1981). Single neurons display irregular changes in discharge rate as IID is altered, and these responses are quite variable.

A more elegant central neuronal response to sound location is found within the maps of auditory space that have been described in the midbrain of several mammals (King & Hutchings, 1987; Middlebrooks & Knudsen, 1984; Palmer & King, 1982; Wong, 1984). A recent study on the emergence of single neuron auditory receptive fields in the guinea pig demonstrates that the orderly progression of responses to auditory space is not apparent until postnatal day 32, even though hearing begins in utero (Withington-Wray, Binns, & Keating, 1990). Before

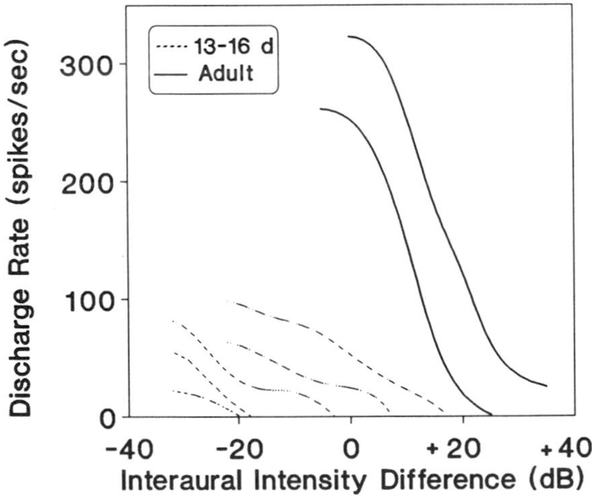

FIGURE 9 Single LSO neuron interaural intensity difference functions from 13-to-16-day-old and adult gerbils (see Figure 1B for explanation of interaural intensity difference functions). Note that neurons from young animals display a very poor dynamic range and that some have an irregular change in discharge rate as intensity difference is altered. From Sanes and Rubel (1988). Copyright 1988 by Society of Neuroscience. Reprinted by permission.

this age, individual neurons respond diffusely to stimuli located in the contralateral hemifield. Presumably, the integration of several monaural and binaural cues is required to attain adultlike spatial sensitivity, and the developmental process operates over an extended period of time. It has previously been suggested that an extended period of maturation might facilitate the central modifications necessary to accommodate alterations of interaural cues attendant to head growth (Knudsen, Esterly, & Knudsen, 1984).

Conclusions

I have attempted to point out specific differences between the central auditory system of young and mature animals and to relate these differences to computational abilities, namely binaural coding and frequency selectivity. No doubt, some of the ontogenetic changes observed in the animal models may be peculiar to one system or another. Taken as a whole, however, they provide ample evidence that the central auditory system is as dynamically regulated as the peripheral auditory system during development.

While I attached a fair amount of speculation to the developmental data under review, I have carefully avoided drawing direct parallels between any single parametric value obtained in nonhuman species and the psychophysical abilities of baby humans. In order to make valid correlations, the functional and structural features of the developing human auditory system must be determined separately. However, I am optimistic that the animal studies serve to identify the neural mechanisms that will be found to underlie the maturation of human auditory behavior.

References

Boudreau, J. C., & Tsuchitani, C. (1968). Binaural interaction in the cat superior olive s-segment. *Journal of Neurophysiology*, *31*, 442–454.

Boudreau, J. C., & Tsuchitani, C. (1970). Cat superior olive s-segment cell discharge to tonal stimulation. In W. D. Neff (Ed.), *Contributions to sensory physiology: Vol. 4* (pp. 143–213). New York: Academic Press.

Brugge, J. F., Javel, E., & Kitzes, L. M. (1978). Signs of functional maturation of peripheral auditory system in discharge patterns of neurons in anteroventral cochlear nucleus of kitten. *Journal of Neurophysiology*, *41*, 1557–1579.

Caird, D., & Klinke, R. (1983). Processing of binaural stimuli by cat superior olivary complex neurons. *Experimental Brain Research*, *52*, 385–399.

Clarkson, M. G., Clifton, R. K., Swain, I. U., & Perris, E. E. (1989). Stimulus duration and repetition rate influence newborns' head orientation toward sound. *Developmental Psychobiology*, *22*, 683–705.

Ellingson, R. J., & Wilcott, R. C. (1960). Development of evoked responses in visual and auditory cortices of kittens. *Journal of Neurophysiology*, *23*, 363–375.

Fitzakerly, J. L., McGee, J., & Walsh, E. J. (1991). Variability in discharge rate of cochlear nucleus neurons during development. *Abstracts Society for Neuroscience*, *17*, 304.

Gardett, R., Debono, M., Dupont, J.-L., & Crepel, F. (1985). Electrophysiological studies on the postnatal development of intracerebellar nuclei neurons in rat cerebellar slices maintained in vitro. I. Postsynaptic potentials. *Developmental Brain Research*, *19*, 47–55.

Glaser, E. M., Van der Loos, H., & Gissler, M. (1979). Tangential orientation and spatial order in dendrites of cat auditory cortex: A computer microscope study of golgi-impregnated material. *Experimental Brain Research*, *36*, 411–431.

Hafter, E. R., Dye, R. H., & Gilkey, R. H. (1979). Lateralization of tonal signals which have neither onsets nor offsets. *Journal of the Acoustical Society of America*, *65*, 471–477.

Harnischfeger, G., Neuweiler, G., & Schlegel, P. (1985). Interaural time and intensity coding in superior olivary complex and inferior colliculus of the echo locating bat *Molossus ater*. *Journal of Neurophysiology*, *53*, 89–109.

Harris, D., & Dallos, P. (1984). Ontogenetic changes in frequency mapping in a mammalian cochlea. *Science*, *225*, 741–743.

Heffner, R. S., & Heffner, H. E. (1988). Sound localization and use of binaural cues by the gerbil (*Meriones unguiculatus*). *Behavioral Neuroscience*, *102*, 422–428.

Jackson, H., & Parks, T. N. (1982). Functional synapse elimination in the developing avian cochlear nucleus with simultaneous reduction in cochlear nerve axon branching. *Journal of Neuroscience*, *2*, 1736–1743.

Jackson, H., & Rubel, E. W. (1978). Ontogeny of behavioral responsiveness to sound in the chick embryo as indicated by electrical recordings of motility. *Journal of Comparative Physiology and Psychology*, *92*, 682–696.

Jay, M. F., & Sparks, D. L. (1984). Auditory receptive fields in primate superior colliculus shift with changes in eye position. *Nature*, *309*, 345–347.

Kelly, J. B., Judge, P. W., & Fraser, I. H. (1987). Development of the auditory orientation response in the albino rat (*Rattus norvegicus*). *Journal of Comparative Psychology*, *101*, 60–66.

Kelly, J. B., & Potash, M. (1986). Directional responses to sounds in young gerbils (*Meriones unguiculatus*). *Journal of Comparative Psychology*, *100*, 37–45.

Kettner, R. E., Feng, J.-Z., & Brugge, J. F. (1985). Postnatal development of the phase-locked response to low frequency tones of auditory nerve fibers in the cat. *Journal of Neuroscience*, *5*, 275–283.

King, A. J., & Hutchings, M. E. (1987). Spatial response properties of acoustically responsive neurons in the superior colliculus of the ferret: A map of auditory space. *Journal of Neurophysiology*, *57*, 596–624.

Knudsen, E. I., Esterly, S. D., & Knudsen, P. F. (1984). Monaural occlusion alters sound localization during a sensitive period in the barn owl. *Journal of Neuroscience*, *4*, 1001–1011.

McMullen, N. T., Goldberger, B., & Glaser, E. M. (1988). Postnatal development of lamina III/IV nonpyramidal neurons in rabbit auditory cortex: Quantitative and spatial analyses of golgi-impregnated material. *Journal of Comparative Neurology*, *278*, 139–155.

Meininger, V., & Baudrimont, M. (1981). Postnatal modifications of the dendritic tree of cells in the inferior colliculus of the cat. A quantitative golgi analysis. *Journal of Comparative Neurology*, *200*, 339–355.

Middlebrooks, J. C., & Knudsen, E. I. (1984). A neural code for auditory space in the cat's superior colliculus. *Journal of Neuroscience*, *4*, 2621–2634.

Mikaelian, D., & Ruben, R. J. (1965). Correlation of physiological observations with behavioral responses and with cochlear anatomy. *Acta Otolarynologica*, *59*, 451–461.

Moiseff, A., & Konishi, M. (1981). Neuronal and behavioral sensitivity to binaural time differences in the owl. *Journal of Neuroscience*, *1*, 40–48.

Moore, D. R. (1983). Development of inferior colliculus and binaural audition. In R. Romand (Ed.), *Development of auditory and vestibular systems* (pp. 121–166). New York: Academic Press.

Moore, D. R., & Irvine, D. R. F. (1979). The development of some peripheral and central auditory responses in the neonatal cat. *Brain Research*, *163*, 49–59.

Moore, D. R., & Irvine, D. R. F. (1981). Development of responses to acoustic interaural intensity differences in the cat inferior colliculus. *Experimental Brain Research*, *41*, 301–309.

Morest, D. K. (1969). The differentiation of cerebral dendrites: A study of the post-migratory neuroblast in the medial nucleus of the trapezoid body. *Zeitschrift für Anatomie und Entwicklungsgeschichte*, *128*, 271–289.

Mysliveek, J. (1983). Development of the auditory evoked responses in the auditory cortex in mammals. In R. Romand (Ed.), *Development of auditory and vestibular systems* (pp. 167–209). New York: Academic Press.

Naka, K.-I. (1964). Electrophysiology of the fetal spinal cord. I. Action potentials of the motoneuron. *Journal of General Physiology*, *47*, 1003–1022.

Neff, W. D., Diamond, I. T., & Casseday, J. H. (1975). Behavioral studies of auditory discrimination. In W. D. Keidel & W. D. Neff (Eds.), *Handbook of sensory physiology: Vol. 5/2* (pp. 307–400). Berlin, Germany: Springer.

Palmer, A. R., & King, A. J. (1982). The representation of auditory space in the mammalian superior colliculus. *Nature*, *299*, 248–249.

Penfield, W., & Rasmussen, T. (1950). *The cerebral cortex of man. A clinical study of the localization of function*. New York: Macmillan.

Potash, M., & Kelly, J. (1980). Development of directional responses to sounds in the rat (*Rattus norvegicus*). *Journal of Comparative & Physiological Psychology*, *94*, 864–877.

Purpura, D. P., Shofer, R. J., & Scarff, T. (1965). Properties of synaptic activities and spike potentials of neurons in immature neocortex. *Journal of Neurophysiology*, *28*, 925–942.

Riquimaroux, H., Gaioni, S. J., & Suga, N. (1991). Cortical computational maps control auditory perception. *Science, 251*, 565–568.

Rogowski, B. A., & Feng, A. (1981). Normal postnatal development of medial superior olivary neurons in the albino rat: A Golgi and Nissl study. *Journal of Comparative Neurology*, *196*, 85–97.

Romand, R. (1971). Maturation des potentiels cochléaires dans la période postnatale chez le chat et chez le cobaye [Maturation of cochlear potentials during the postnatal period in the cat and in the guinea pig]. *Journal of Physiology*, *63*, 763–782.

Romand, R. (1983). Development of the cochlea. In R. Romand (Ed.), *Development of auditory and vestibular systems* (pp. 47–88). New York: Academic Press.

Sanes, D. H. (1990). An in vitro analysis of sound localization mechanisms in the gerbil lateral superior olive. *Journal of Neuroscience*, *10*, 3494–3506.

Sanes, D. H., & Constantine-Paton, M. (1985). The development of stimulus following in the cochlear nerve and inferior colliculus of the mouse. *Developmental Brain Research*, *22*, 255–267.

Sanes, D. H., Goldstein, N. A., Ostad, M., & Hillman, D. E. (1990). Dendritic morphology of central auditory neurons correlates with their tonotopic position. *Journal of Comparative Neurology*, *294*, 443–454.

Sanes, D. H., Merickel, M., & Rubel, E. W. (1989). Evidence for an alteration of the tonotopic map in the gerbil cochlea during development. *Journal of Comparative Neurology*, *279*, 436–444.

Sanes, D. H., & Rubel, E. W. (1988). The ontogeny of inhibition and excitation in the gerbil lateral superior olive. *Journal of Neuroscience*, *8*, 682–700.

Sanes, D. H., & Siverls, V. (1991). The development and specificity of inhibitory terminal arborizations in the central nervous system. *Journal of Neurobiology*, *22*, 837–854.

Sanes, D. H., Song, J., & Tyson, J. (in press). Refinement of dendritic arbors along the tonotopic axis of the gerbil lateral superior olive. *Developmental Brain Research*.

Sanes, D. H., & Wooten, G. F. (1987). Development of glycine receptor distribution in the lateral superior olive of the gerbil. *Journal of Neuroscience*, *7*, 3803–3811.

Saunders, J. C., Coles, R. B., & Gates, G. R. (1973). The development of auditory evoked responses in the cochlea and cochlear nuclei of the chick. *Brain Research*, *63*, 59–74.

Schwob, J. E., Haberly, L. B., & Price, J. L. (1984). The development of physiological responses of the piriform cortex in rats to stimulation of the lateral olfactory tract. *Journal of Comparative Neurology*, *223*, 223–237.

Shnerson, A., & Pujol, R. (1982). Age related changes in the C57BL/6J mouse cochlea. I. Physiological findings. *Developmental Brain Research*, *2*, 65–75.

Smith, Z. D. J. (1981). Organization and development of brain stem auditory nuclei of the chicken: Dendritic development in *n. laminaris*. *Journal of Comparative Neurology*, *203*, 309–333.

Suga, N. (1988). Auditory neuroethology and speech processing: complex-sound processing by combination-sensitive neurons. In G. M. Edelman, W. E. Gall, & W. M. Cowan (Eds.), *Auditory function. neurobiological bases of hearing* (pp. 679–720). New York: Wiley.

Takahashi, T., Moiseff, A., & Konishi, M. (1984). Time and intensity cues are processed independently in the auditory system of the owl. *Journal of Neuroscience*, *4*, 1781–1786.

Tobias, J. V., & Zerlin, S. (1959). Localization thresholds as a function of stimulus duration. *Journal of the Acoustical Society of America*, *31*, 1591–1594.

Walsh, E. J., McGee, J., & Javel, E. (1986). Development of auditory evoked potentials in the cat. II. Wave latencies. *Journal of the Acoustical Society of America*, *79*, 725–744.

Wilson, D. A., & Leon, M. (1986). Early appearance of inhibition in the neonatal rat olfactory bulb. *Developmental Brain Research*, *26*, 289–292.

Withington-Wray, D. J., Binns, K. E., & Keating, M. J. (1990). The developmental emergence of a map of auditory space in the superior colliculus of the guinea pig. *Developmental Brain Research*, *51*, 225–236.

Wong, D. (1984). Spatial tuning of auditory neurones in the superior colliculus of the echolocating bat, *Myotis lucifugus*. *Hearing Research*, *16*, 261–270.

Woolf, N. K., & Ryan, A. F. (1985). Ontogeny of neural discharge patterns in the ventral cochlear nucleus of the mongolian gerbil. *Developmental Brain Research*, *17*, 131–147.

Young, S. R., & Rubel, E. W. (1983). Frequency specific projections of individual neurons in chick brain stem auditory nuclei. *Journal of Neuroscience*, *3*, 1373–1378.

Young, S. R., & Rubel, E. W. (1986). Embryogenesis of arborization pattern and topography of individual axons in *n. laminaris* of the chicken brain stem. *Journal of Comparative Neurology*, *254*, 425–459.

CHAPTER 11

Developmental Considerations in Binaural Hearing Experiments

Constantine Trahiotis

Both classic and more recent contributions to our understanding of binaural hearing appear to be relevant and potentially important for the study of developmental psychoacoustics. The literature dealing with topics directly or indirectly related to binaural hearing is truly enormous and highly complex. Fortunately, several excellent, topically oriented review chapters have recently been written by key investigators, and the reader is referred to an excellent book edited by Yost and Gourevitch and entitled *Directional Hearing* (1987) and to two very detailed and comprehensive reviews concerning binaural phenomena and models of binaural processes that were written by Durlach and Colburn and by Colburn and Durlach for the fourth volume of Carterette and Friedman's *Handbook of Perception* (1978). Instead of summarizing, or otherwise presenting information available in those sources, I have selected several issues and notions that

Preparation of this manuscript was supported by a grant from the National Institutes of Health (DC00234).

I thank Doug Bradway, who prepared the manuscript, for his patience, perseverance, and almost constant good humor.

might be useful to those who study newborns and infants. The discussion will be principally restricted to studies concerning behavior and will only touch on the wealth of anatomical and physiological knowledge in this area. The reader is referred to Clifton's chapter (chapter 5) in this volume for a summary of recent binaural studies of infants.

Our discussion will assume that the *binaural* processing of information occurs via comparisons between the physical stimuli impinging on each ear (i.e., *monaural* channels). Such comparisons are mediated by, or dependent upon, neural interactions within the *central* auditory nervous system in several places, including the superior olivary complex, the inferior colliculus, the medial geniculate body, and the auditory cortex. The neural interactions that occur within cells in each of those nuclei are typically defined, studied, and described in terms of the centripetal (or afferent) flow of information from ear to brain. An all-inclusive definition of binaural hearing could also include peripheral and central interactions that are influenced by, or depend upon, *centrifugal* effects, some possibly mediated by the crossed, efferent, olivo-cochlear bundle. Although it would be highly interesting to speculate about such effects and their potential contribution or import for auditory development, such speculations are omitted from this discussion. Perhaps a similar chapter written a decade or so from now will include a detailed account of these sorts of mechanisms and interactions. We may even find that what we include here as the classical binaural system actually involves such centrifugal effects.

For the present, we will retain the more restrictive, classical, definition of *binaural*. This will make the discussion more straightforward and much easier to relate to the primary and secondary literature. We will be concerned with the listener's ability to utilize *fused perceptual images* formed from information presented to each ear in detection, discrimination, lateralization, and localization tasks. Fusion, in turn, depends upon the essentially simultaneous occurrence of activity within each ear and, especially, within *common frequency channels* emanating from each ear. In other words, we will be concerned with comparisons between the two ears only when those comparisons occur between highly similar (if not identical) spectral regions. These comparisons, at the behavioral level, can be thought of as between "critical bands" of the same center frequency (Nuetzel & Hafter, 1981). Of course, physiologically they could also be thought of as comparisons between peripheral nerve fibers of very similar characteristic frequency. In that manner, fusion would ultimately depend upon mechanical events and transduction processes that occur within specific regions of the cochlea.

That is why all comprehensive modern models of binaural information processing (e.g., Blauert & Cobben, 1978; Lindemann, 1986; Stern & Colburn, 1978; Stern, Zeiberg, & Trahiotis, 1988) implicitly and quite often explicitly incorporate the bandpass filtering, rectification and low-pass filtering of frequency-specific monaural channels as input to binaural mechanisms. This approach makes clear that the understanding of binaural hearing depends heavily on our understanding of at least the peripheral aspects of monaural hearing. It also means, however, that most modern theoretical formulations deal only indirectly with the physical stimuli arriving at each ear. They really focus on, or implicitly assume, a general description of the transformations that occur to physical stimuli within the cochlea and eighth nerve. Any departures from the normal adult ear at maturity, be they due to abnormal development, acoustic trauma, or drugs, potentially can have implications or repercussions for binaural interactions and mechanisms because "normal" central interactions could be altered, diminished or precluded. Colburn and Trahiotis (1991) have reviewed recent studies concerning the effect of acoustic trauma on binaural hearing.

Methodological Factors Affecting Measures of Binaural Hearing

Several factors that could affect the design and interpretation of experiments in developmental psychoacoustics arise from the methods used to gather behavioral data. As in most areas of psychoacoustic research, those who study binaural hearing have used several variations of only a few psychophysical tasks. Other chapters in this volume (e.g., chapters 4, 7, and 8) contain discussions of behavioral procedures, especially adaptive tracking tasks. Trahiotis, Bernstein, Buell, and Spektor (1990) document the recent increase in use of adaptive procedures in binaural experiments and discuss several factors that determine and limit their appropriateness. The point to be made here is that the details concerning the actual psychophysical procedures used may affect greatly the measurement used to infer the sensitivity of the listener and, perhaps more important, the types of cues that the listener has available to solve the task.

For example, let us suppose that we perform a seemingly simple experiment that requires a listener to detect an interaural delay of the stimulus in the right ear in either a single interval, yes/no task or in a two-alternative, temporal forced-choice task. Suppose the "other choice" or foil presented on the nonsignal trials (or in the nonsignal interval) is a diotic stimulus (i.e., identical waveforms at each ear). What are the actual cues available or used by the subjects? At face value, the listener might be discriminating between two classes of acoustic images: one in the middle of the head (produced by the diotic stimulus), and the other *lateralized* more toward the leading ear. Let's call this a "center/left judgment." Is it necessary, however, that the listener actually use the *position* of the acoustic image to solve this task? Not really. The listener could, instead, make judgments based on the *variability* of the distribution of interaural differences of time and/or intensity for each of the two classes of input. Changing the task to a truly symmetric, left/right, forced-choice task (perhaps by replacing the diotic stimulus with one delayed to the opposite ear) would force the listener to use positional information and completely remove the interaural distribution of differences or the variability of interaural stimuli as a potential cue (Dye, 1990).

Merely choosing a simple yes/no single interval task instead of a two-alternative, temporal forced-choice task can affect greatly the listener's ability to detect cues binaurally in what are termed binaural masking level difference (MLD) paradigms. As reported by several investigators (e.g., Gilkey, Simpson, & Weisenberger, 1990; McFadden, 1966; Robinson & Trahiotis, 1972; Yost, 1985), listeners can be very much less sensitive when detecting the presence of out-of-phase targets if those targets are relatively brief (less than 150 ms or so) and presented against a burst of masking noise of similar duration. Sensitivity can be improved in at least three ways: (a) lengthening the duration of both the signal and the masker; (b) turning on the noise masker earlier and earlier before the signal is turned on (i.e., providing a noise fringe); and (c) changing to a two-alternative, temporal forced-choice procedure.

As discussed by McFadden (1966), an important element of people's ability to utilize binaural cues to detect tonal signals against a background of noise appears to be "memory" for the intracranial position of the potential acoustic images. What appears to be especially important is memory for the center of the head produced by the diotic masking noise that is typically used in such experiments. That is, in such tasks, the *nonsignal* interval is almost always diotic broadband noise and is heard in the middle of the head by the listener. It appears that having the masking noise available either (a) *before* the signal by turning the noise on earlier and earlier (in a single interval task); or (b) by having the diotic noise available in the *nonsignal* interval (in the two-alternative, temporal forced-choice task) provides enough memorial information to produce a 6–8 dB difference in threshold. This rather large difference could easily occur across two experiments, perhaps one utilizing infants and the other adults. The data could be misinterpreted in terms of developmental differences because the same procedure was not used for both groups. Alternatively, it could be the case that the same procedure was used for both groups and the measured sensitivity would be different than those reported in the literature. In either case, the experimenter would have difficulty interpreting the data without noting the special and subtle nature of the issues that are involved.

Although many of us are impressed with 6-dB effects, an even more dramatic example of how information in nonsignal intervals (i.e., cues) can affect performance in binaural experiments is discussed by Smith (1976) and Bernstein and Trahiotis (1982). Hafter and Carrier (1972) and Ruotolo, Stern, and Colburn (1979) had each noted that listeners require an enormous amount of practice (upwards of 25,000 trials) in order to learn to discriminate between stimuli composed of small values of interaural time and intensity differences presented in special combinations so that the two cues were in opposition between ears. Babkoff, Sutton, and Barris (1973) in a quite similar experiment found that their listeners were unable to respond better than by chance. Hafter and Carrier used a "cued" yes/no task that could have provided some information about the middle of the head. Their first stimulus, or cue, was a 500-Hz diotic tone. Bernstein and Trahiotis (1982) provided two cues: one before and one after the two observation intervals that compose a two-alternative, temporal forced-choice task. By simply changing the two-alternative, temporal forced-choice task into what we now call a two-cue, two-interval, temporal forced-choice task, we discovered that listeners were able to discriminate between stimuli like those used by Hafter and Carrier and Ruotolo et al. within the first 150 trials or so! The actual analysis of the types of information provided by the two cues within and across trials and between intervals and how that information could be used in the task is somewhat complicated and beyond the scope of this discussion. However, for our purposes it should be stressed that subtle details concerning the psychophysical tasks can have serious consequences in studies concerning binaural hearing.

I would urge those who study developmental aspects of binaural hearing to consider the recent efforts of Colburn and his colleagues (Koehnke, Colburn, & Durlach, 1986). They have embarked on a large program of binaural research designed to identify and to assess deleterious effects produced by noise and other insults to the auditory system. Particularly germane is their use of a battery of tests. The tests are designed to reveal defects by using a wide variety of theoretically important stimuli. Those stimuli are carefully chosen to tap important abilities while simultaneously providing information that may permit a better theoretical understanding of the mechanisms involved.

Stimulus Effects and Recent Models of Binaural Hearing

The distinction between judgments based on the intracranial position of acoustic images and judgments based on the underlying variability of interaural cues (or on some other property of acoustic images, such as their shape) is useful to remember when evaluating the literature concerning the use of interaural differences of time conveyed by complex, high-frequency stimuli such as two-tone complexes, sinusoidally amplitude-modulated tones, and bands of noise. A large number of excellent investigations have shown that listeners can detect interaural delays that are conveyed by the ongoing envelope of such stimuli (e.g., David, Guttman, & Van Bergeijk, 1959; Henning, 1974, 1980; Klumpp & Eady, 1956; Leakey, Sayers, & Cherry, 1958; McFadden & Pasanen, 1976; Nuetzel & Hafter, 1976, 1981). In fact, sensitivity to interaural time delays at high frequencies can rival that measured with low-frequency stimuli.

Those findings are quite important and could lead one to predict that interaural time delays would be equally potent in terms of mediating lateral movement independent of the spectral region that carries the information. It turns out, however, that measures of *lateral displacement* produced by interaural delays conveyed by the envelope of high-frequency complex signals are very much smaller than those produced by delays conveyed by the fine structure of low-frequency signals (Bernstein & Trahiotis, 1985a, 1985b; Blauert, 1983; Trahiotis &

Bernstein, 1986). It would appear to be important and interesting to use both discrimination and lateralization tasks with infants.

The divergence in outcome that can occur when one compares data gathered from discrimination experiments to data obtained from tasks requiring measures of lateral position can be truly remarkable. Recently, Buell, Trahiotis, and Bernstein (1991) measured extents of laterality produced by delays occurring within the gating (onset and/or offset) or ongoing portions of pure tones. The relative potency of the type of delay was assessed by presenting the delays singly or in combination (where the types of delay were consistent or in opposition). Rise/decay time, duration and frequency of the tonal targets were also varied. The major finding was that ongoing delays were much more potent than were gating delays in determining extent of laterality. Gating delays were effective only when the interaural phase of the ongoing portion of the tone provided more or less ambiguous information about which ear was really leading.

The effects in the Buell et al. (1991) study were very robust, and similar lateralizations occurred for all durations between 15 μs and 200 μs. These data contrast greatly with the conclusion one could draw from two earlier experiments that utilized similar stimuli in a task that required that the listener only indicate which ear was actually leading (Abel & Kunov, 1983; Kunov & Abel, 1981). It is important to note that both types of experiments provide valid information about the binaural system's use of interaural differences of time. What varies greatly are the conclusions drawn from the data and the generality of those conclusions.

Buell et al. (1991) interpreted their experiments in terms of the binaural processing of off-frequency information or "spectral splatter" produced by gating tonal signals on and off. They argued that their listener's judgments of lateral position could be affected by gating delays via information present in the very low spectral regions. They went on to link their results to much earlier data and arguments provided by Yost, Wightman, and Green (1971) and McFadden and Pasanen (1976), who clearly outlined how nominally high-frequency transients or clicks can provide low-frequency energy that forms the basis of the subject's judgments. Both of those articles deserve careful scrutiny because they contain important discussions concerning how the auditory system can be provided a variety of cues in experiments dealing with repeated transients, clicks, and also with stimuli that are gated on and off with rise/decay times (typically on the order of 4–10 ms or so) that produced spectral splatter.

Perhaps the most impressive use of remote, low-frequency information in a binaural task was provided several years ago by Bernstein and Trahiotis (1982). We were astonished to find that listeners were detecting the presence of an interaural time delay conveyed by a nominally narrow band of noise presented with a center frequency of 4 kHz on the basis of very small amounts of energy present in the low-frequency skirts of the stimulus. In other words, sensitivity to interaural delay was actually determined by the listeners' utilization of interaural differences of time conveyed by energy around 500 Hz to 800 Hz or so. This occurred even though that particular spectral region was presented at a level that was 50–55 dB or so below the level of the 4 kHz pass band! Would infants "lock on" to such cues? We don't know. But we do know (Gray & Rubel, 1985; Rubel & Ryals, 1983) that spectrally related changes in sensitivity to sound do occur early in development, and such changes could make information in remote spectral regions salient enough to be the primary determiner of behavior.

Two contexts in which sensitivity to interaural delay and extent of laterality can be affected greatly by neighboring spectral information have recently been reported. First, Zurek (1985) and Trahiotis and Bernstein (1990) have shown that sensitivity to interaural delays of high-frequency, narrow-band noises can be severely degraded by the presence of other, flanking, diotic noise. To be sure, the properties of the flanking noise, including whether it is continuous or gated on and off with the information-bearing band of noise, are important. Another important factor is whether the flanking bands are interaurally uncorrelated or correlated. The important aspect of these results is that one cannot correctly predict interaural sensitivity to a particular spectral region without also knowing something about temporally and spectrally adjacent acoustic information.

Second, Stern et al. (1988), Trahiotis and Stern (1989) and Stern and Trahiotis (1992) have recently demonstrated that extents of laterality (and even the side of the head where listeners hear interaurally delayed noises) may depend heavily on the bandwidth of the noises, and equally importantly, upon features of the cross-correlations of the stimuli. Their theoretical analysis was done by considering a very complex model that incorporates a neural cross-correlation of the information in the stimuli that is realized by a matrix of so-called coincidence detector neurons as first postulated by Jeffress (1948). Of course, such elements are incorporated in every modern model of binaural hearing. The principal features of the patterns of cross-correlation that are relevant appear to be what are called the *centrality* and the *straightness* of their trajectories as a function of frequency. Centrality refers to how small the interaural delay (a delay of zero signals sounds perceived at midline). Straightness refers to how consistent the delay is over a range of frequency. One can account for the behavioral data by postulating a central integration of information utilizing neural channels that are stimulated by similar external delays but are tuned to slightly different frequencies. Recently, it has been found that there are cells in the midbrains of owls (Takahashi & Konishi, 1986) and rabbits (Stanford, 1989) that appear to respond to complex stimuli by performing the integration that is proposed (and appear to be necessary to account for the behavioral data). The general idea is that the colliculus contains a second level of relatively broadband coincidence detection units. Those cells receive inputs from several narrow band coincidence detection units emanating from the superior olivary complex. Both the behavioral and physiological studies are quite recent. Presently we do not have information regarding any developmental affects that bear on such processing of information, but the phenomena appear to be ripe for study.

It should also be mentioned that there are many recent developments concerning the digital construction, presentation, and measurement of complex signals that have the potential of furthering knowledge in developmental psychoacoustics. It is now possible to construct bands of noise while delaying, interaurally, one or more aspects of waveforms (i.e., the ongoing envelope, the carrier, and the phase modulation) singly or in combination. Amenta, Trahiotis, Bernstein, and Nuetzel (1987) have presented a thorough discussion of how this can be done and have illustrated how the stimuli can be used in binaural psychophysical experiments. Several other important aspects of complex signals can be manipulated to produce a plethora of desired waveforms that may prove interesting and important for developmental research (e.g., Bernstein, 1991; Hartmann & Pumplin, 1988; Hsueh & Hamernik, 1990; Pumplin, 1985). These advances should help make detailed tests of hypotheses concerning the nature of the cues utilized by the maturing auditory system.

In summary, it appears that there are many examples drawn from the literature concerning binaural hearing that offer potential avenues for exploration in studies of developmental psychoacoustics. Perhaps what would be most useful would be the cooperative efforts of investigators trained in a number of different areas who could pool their talents. Such collaboration would foster sophisticated and interesting physiological and behavioral experiments that would surely shed light on how developmental processes influence hearing.

References

Abel, S. M., & Kunov, H. (1983). Lateralization based on interaural phase differences: Effects of frequency, amplitude, duration, and shape of rise/decay. *Journal of the Acoustical Society of America*, *73*, 955–960.

Amenta, C. A., III, Trahiotis, C., Bernstein, L. R., & Nuetzel, J. M. (1987). Some physical and psychological effects produced by selective delays of the envelope of narrow bands of noise. *Hearing Research*, *29*, 147–161.

Babkoff, H., Sutton, S., & Barris, M. (1973). Binaural interaction of transients: Interaural time and intensity asymmetry. *Journal of the Acoustical Society of America*, *53*, 1028–1036.

Bernstein, L. R. (1991). Measurement and specification of the envelope correlation between two narrow bands of noise. *Hearing Research*, *52*, 189–194.

Bernstein, L. R., & Trahiotis, C. (1982). Detection of interaural delay in high frequency noise. *Journal of the Acoustical Society of America*, *71*, 147–152.

Bernstein, L. R., & Trahiotis, C. (1985a). Lateralization of low-frequency, complex waveforms: The use of envelope-based temporal disparities. *Journal of the Acoustical Society of America*, *77*, 1868–1880.

Bernstein, L. R., & Trahiotis, C. (1985b). Lateralization of sinusoidally amplitude-modulated tones: Effects of spectral locus and temporal variation. *Journal of the Acoustical Society of America*, *78*, 514–523.

Blauert, J. (1983). *Spatial hearing*. Cambridge, MA: MIT Press.

Blauert, J., & Cobben, W. (1978). Some consideration of binaural cross correlation analysis. *Acustica*, *39*, 96–103.

Buell, T. N., Trahiotis, C., & Bernstein, L. R. (1991). Lateralization of low-frequency tones: Relative potency of gating and ongoing interaural delay. *Journal of the Acoustical Society of America*, *90*, 3077–3085.

Colburn, H. S., & Durlach, N. I. (1978). Models of binaural interaction. In E. C. Carterette & M. P. Friedman (Eds.), *Handbook of perception: Vol. IV. Hearing* (pp. 467–518). New York: Academic Press.

Colburn, H. S., & Trahiotis, C. (1991). Effects of noise on binaural hearing. In A. Dancer, D. Henderson, R. Salvi, & R. Hamernik (Eds.), *Noise induced hearing loss* (pp. 293–302). New York: Mosby Yearbook.

David, E. E., Jr., Guttman, N., & van Bergeijk, W. A. (1959). Binaural interaction of high-frequency complex stimuli. *Journal of the Acoustical Society of America*, *31*, 774–782.

Durlach, N. I., & Colburn, H. S. (1978). Binaural phenomena. In E. C. Carterette & M. P. Friedman (Eds.), *Handbook of perception: Vol. IV. Hearing* (pp. 365–466). New York: Academic Press.

Dye, R. H. (1990). The combination of interaural information across frequencies: Lateralization on the basis of interaural differences of time. *Journal of the Acoustical Society of America*, *88*, 2159–2170.

Gilkey, R. H., Simpson, B. D., & Weisenberger, J. M. (1990). Masker fringe and binaural detection. *Journal of the Acoustical Society of America*, *88*, 1323–1332.

Gray, L., & Rubel, E. W (1985). Development of absolute thresholds in chickens. *Journal of the Acoustical Society of America*, *77*, 1162–1172.

Hafter, E. R., & Carrier, S. C. (1972). Binaural interaction in low-frequency stimuli: The inability to trade time and intensity completely. *Journal of the Acoustical Society of America*, *51*, 1852–1862.

Hartmann, W. M., & Pumplin, J. (1988). Noise power fluctuations and the masking of sine signals. *Journal of the Acoustical Society of America*, *83*, 2277–2289.

Henning, G. B. (1974). Detectability of interaural delay in high-frequency complex waveforms. *Journal of the Acoustical Society of America*, *55*, 84–90.

Henning, G. B. (1980). Some observations on the lateralization of complex waveforms. *Journal of the Acoustical Society of America*, *68*, 446–453.

Hsueh, K. D., & Hamernik, R. P. (1990). A generalized approach to random noise synthesis: Theory and computer simulation. *Journal of the Acoustical Society of America*, *87*, 1207–1217.

Jeffress, L. A. (1948). A place theory of sound localization. *Journal of Comparative & Physiological Psychology*, *41*, 35–39.

Klumpp, R. G., & Eady, H. R. (1956). Some measurements of interaural time difference thresholds. *Journal of the Acoustical Society of America*, *28*, 859–860.

Koehnke, J., Colburn, H. S., & Durlach, N. I. (1986). Performance in several binaural-interaction experiments. *Journal of the Acoustical Society of America*, *79*, 1558–1562.

Kunov, H., & Abel, S. M. (1981). Effects of rise/decay time on the lateralization of interaurally delayed 1-kHz tones. *Journal of the Acoustical Society of America*, *69*, 769–773.

Leakey, D. M., Sayers, B. McA., & Cherry, C. (1958). Binaural fusion of low- and high-frequency sounds. *Journal of the Acoustical Society of America*, *30*, 222.

Lindemann, W. (1986). Extension of a binaural cross-correlation model by contralateral inhibition. II. The law of the first wavefront. *Journal of the Acoustical Society of America*, *80*, 1623–1630.

McFadden, D. M. (1966). Masking-level differences with continuous and with burst masking noise. *Journal of the Acoustical Society of America*, *40*, 1414–1419.

McFadden, D., & Pasanen, E. G. (1976). Lateralization at high frequencies based on interaural time differences. *Journal of the Acoustical Society of America*, *59*, 634–639.

Nuetzel, J. M., & Hafter, E. R. (1976). Lateralization of complex waveforms: Effects of fine-structure, amplitude, and duration. *Journal of the Acoustical Society of America*, *60*, 1339–1346.

Nuetzel, J. M., & Hafter, E. R. (1981). Discrimination of interaural delays in complex waveforms: Spectral effects. *Journal of the Acoustical Society of America*, *69*, 1112–1118.

Pumplin, J. (1985). Low-noise noise. *Journal of the Acoustical Society of America*, *78*, 100–104.

Robinson, D. E., & Trahiotis, C. (1972). Effects of signal duration and masker duration on detectability of pulsed diotic and dichotic tonal signals. *Perception & Psychophysics*, *12*, 333–334.

Rubel, E. W, & Ryals, B. M. (1983). Development of the place principal: Acoustic trauma. *Science, 219*, 512–514.

Ruotolo, B. R., Stern, R. M., & Colburn, H. S. (1979). Discrimination of symmetric time-intensity traded binaural stimuli. *Journal of the Acoustical Society of America, 66*, 1733–1737.

Smith, L. E. (1976). *The effects of time and intensity on the lateralization of sounds*. Unpublished master's thesis, University of Illinois, Urbana.

Stanford, T. R. (1989). *A comparison of the interaural time sensitivity of neurons in the inferior colliculus and thalamus of the unanesthetized rabbit*. Unpublished doctoral dissertation, University of Connecticut, Farmington.

Stern, R. M., & Colburn, H. S. (1978). Theory of binaural interaction based on auditory-nerve data. IV. A model for subjective lateral position. *Journal of the Acoustical Society of America, 64*, 127–140.

Stern, R. M., & Trahiotis, C. (1992). The role of consistency of interaural timing over frequency in binaural lateralization. In Y. Cazals, L. Demany, & K. Horner (Eds.), *Auditory physiology and perception* (pp. 547–554). Riverside, NJ: Pergamon Press.

Stern, R. M., Zeiberg, A. S., & Trahiotis, C. (1988). Lateralization of complex binaural stimuli: A weighted image model. *Journal of the Acoustical Society of America, 84*, 156–165.

Takahashi, T. A., & Konishi, M. (1986). Selectivity for interaural time differences in the owl's midbrain. *Journal of Neuroscience, 6*, 3413–3422.

Trahiotis, C., & Bernstein, L. R. (1986). Lateralization of bands of noise and sinusoidally amplitude-modulated tones: Effects of spectral locus and bandwidth. *Journal of the Acoustical Society of America, 79*, 1950–1957.

Trahiotis, C., & Bernstein, L. R. (1990). Detectability of interaural delays over select spectral regions: Effects of flanking noise. *Journal of the Acoustical Society of America, 87*, 810–813.

Trahiotis, C., Bernstein, L. R., Buell, T. N., & Spektor, Z. (1990). On the use of adaptive procedures in binaural experiments. *Journal of the Acoustical Society of America, 87*, 1359–1361.

Trahiotis, C., & Stern, R. M. (1989). Lateralization of bands of noise: Effects of bandwidth and differences of interaural time and phase. *Journal of the Acoustical Society of America, 86*, 1285–1293.

Yost, W. A. (1985). Prior stimulation and the masking-level difference. *Journal of the Acoustical Society of America, 78*, 901–907.

Yost, W. A., & Gourevitch, G. (Eds.). (1987). *Directional hearing*. New York: Springer.

Yost, W. A., Wightman, F. L., & Green, D. M. (1971). Lateralization of filtered clicks. *Journal of the Acoustical Society of America, 50*, 1526–1530.

Zurek, P. M. (1985). Spectral dominance in sensitivity to interaural delay for broadband stimuli. *Journal of the Acoustical Society of America, 78*, S18.

CHAPTER 12

Psychoacoustics and Speech Perception: Internal Standards, Perceptual Anchors, and Prototypes

Patricia K. Kuhl

Historically, psychoacousticians and speech scientists have adopted different approaches to the study of auditory perception. Psychoacousticians focus on the basic sensory mechanism that underlies hearing. They use signals, such as tones, clicks, and noises that do not convey meaning, to assess the ear's resolving power. A psychoacoustician's goal is to define the absolute limits of the ability to hear, and to relate those findings to the underlying physiology. Factors such as learning, memory, and attention can thwart this goal, and psychoacousticians strive to eliminate such factors from their experiments (chapters 1 and 9 in this volume).

Speech scientists focus on a complex signal that conveys meaning—spoken language. The speech scientist's goal is to discover not only how listeners trans-

This research was supported by grants to Patricia K. Kuhl from the National Institutes of Health (DC 00520).

The author thanks D. Padden and E. Stevens for animal testing and statistical analyses, and Andrew Meltzoff and Ed Burns for helpful comments on an earlier draft of the paper.

Correspondence concerning this chapter should be sent to Patricia K. Kuhl, Department of Speech and Hearing Sciences, WJ-10, University of Washington, Seattle, WA 98195.

duce the physical information contained in speech into a neural code, but how the neural code is attached to meaning. Moreover, studies have shown that perception of even the most basic units of speech—the consonants and vowels that make up words—relies on the integration of information from sources outside of audition, such as the visual speech information conveyed as we watch a talker speak. Finally, factors that are not of primary interest to a psychoacoustician—those induced by learning, memory, and attention—are of primary interest to speech scientists. Speech is a signal that we have listened to all our lives. Listening experience profoundly alters the perception of speech, and a fundamental goal of the discipline is to develop theories that account for the effects of learning on speech perception.

Given these differences, what is to be gained by taking a traditional psychoacoustic approach to the study of speech perception—that is, what do speech scientists learn by examining the listener's resolving power for speech sounds? And similarly, what can the study of speech teach psychoacousticians about basic hearing mechanisms?

Researchers from both camps have historically replied: "Precious little." Research in the 1950s and 1960s in psychoacoustics and speech perception could not have been more different. At that time, psychoacousticians were steeped in a new view of signal processing, signal detection theory (Green & Swets, 1966), while speech scientists were involved in the discovery of a new phenomenon, categorical perception (Liberman, Harris, Hoffman, & Griffith, 1957). Psychoacousticians were engaged in mathematical models that lawfully described how to separate a listener's absolute sensitivity from response bias, while speech scientists were describing categorical perception, which appeared to defy a number of psychophysical laws. It did so in two ways. Findings from categorical perception experiments suggested that the discrimination of speech signals was limited by the degree to which the signals were identified as different, defying G. A. Miller's (1956) classic principle that listeners can discriminate far more stimuli than they can identify. Moreover, the phenomenon suggested that listeners' discrimination of speech stimuli was characterized by a peak in performance in the midrange of a physical continuum where none was expected, a result that defied a classic psychoacoustic principle, Weber's law. These departures from traditional findings in sensation and perception did nothing to enhance speech scientists' credibility in the eyes of psychoacousticians.

Separation between the two groups was further exacerbated by formulation of the "motor theory," which was developed by the Haskins group to explain categorical perception (Liberman, Cooper, Shankweiler, & Studdert-Kennedy, 1967). According to motor theory, speech perception relied on special processing by mechanisms that had evolved in humans for speech; speech perception was mediated with reference to the articulatory acts that produced it (Liberman et al., 1967). On this view, purely auditory processing did not play a critical role in explaining the perceptual phenomena that characterized speech. Auditory processing transduced the signal, but did so in a linear, straightforward way. Speech perception was considered beyond the domain of general sensory, perceptual, and cognitive processing. It constituted the canonical case of a specialized "module" (Fodor, 1983), a self-contained perceptual processor dedicated solely to speech sounds.

In short, psychoacousticians and speech researchers had little to say to one another in the 1950s and 1960s. Each considered the other's approach unlikely to provide key data that would address their particular phenomena and theories.

The Psychoacoustics of Speech

In the 1970s this situation changed. Three new approaches were developed to examine the role of psychoacoustics in explaining speech phenomena. All three produced data suggesting that auditory perception played a significant role in speech perception and served as a turning point for theory.

During this period, speech scientists themselves began to examine psychoacoustic explanations for speech phenomena. They were motivated to test whether categorical perception could be explained by general auditory mechanisms rather than ones that were specialized for speech (Cutting & Rosner, 1974[1]; Kuhl & J. D. Miller, 1975; J. D. Miller, Wier, Pastore, Kelly, & Dooling, 1976; Pastore et al., 1977; Pisoni, 1977). The approaches taken by speech researchers did not involve direct tests of the psychoacoustics of speech. In other words, they did not involve the manipulation of task factors to get at the auditory system's resolving

[1]Cutting and Rosner's (1974) results have not been replicated because the actual rise-times for the stimuli used in the Cutting and Rosner study were different from those that were specified in the report. Rosen and Howell (1987) provide an excellent review of the work on the perception of rise-time in speech and nonspeech stimuli.

power for speech sounds. Rather, speech scientists' goal was to test the claim that speech perception *required* specially evolved mechanisms that were unique to speech and unique to human beings.

One approach was to study the perception of nonspeech auditory signals that mimicked the critical properties of speech signals without being perceived as speech (Cutting & Rosner, 1974; J. D. Miller et al., 1976; Pisoni, 1977; see also Pastore et al., 1977, for the use of a nonspeech visual signal). The logic was that if nonspeech signals produced categorical perception, then the mechanisms responsible for categorical perception were general in nature rather than specialized. The results showed that categorical perception was reliably obtained with nonspeech signals (see Repp, 1984, for review). The data demonstrated that the categorical perception effect was not unique to speech, countering the claim made by the motor theory of speech perception.

The second approach was one I adopted (Kuhl, 1981; Kuhl & J. D. Miller, 1975, 1978; Kuhl & Padden, 1982, 1983). My goal was to study categorical perception in a nonhuman animal. The rationale was that if the categorical perception of speech signals was due to specialized mechanisms that had evolved for speech, then an animal who had no access to phonetic processing should not demonstrate the effect. Alternatively, if categorical perception did not necessitate specialized mechanisms, but rather general auditory mechanisms were sufficient, then an animal whose basic auditory abilities were similar to those of humans would replicate the effect. The results of a series of experiments revealed that animals did indeed exhibit the categorical perception phenomenon. I proposed that categorical perception of consonants did not necessitate specialized processing and might instead be attributed to the existence of "natural psychophysical boundaries," ones inherent in the auditory processing of these signals (Kuhl, 1979a, 1986b, 1988; Kuhl & J. D. Miller, 1975; see Kuhl, 1987 for summary).

Both of these approaches produced results that moved theory forward (Ades, 1977; Pastore et al., 1977; K. N. Stevens, 1981). Both sets of results supported the conclusion that *general auditory* factors, as opposed to *specialized phonetic* factors, could explain the categorical perception effect. The nonspeech results showed that the categorical perception effect was not unique to speech. The animal results demonstrated that the categorical perception effect was not unique to humans. Taken together, these findings suggested, for the first time, that categorical perception effects might be rooted in basic sensory mechanisms.[2] This ran directly counter to the prevailing theories of the Haskins group, who had initially discovered the intriguing phenomenon.

In the late 1970s a third factor increased interest in the psychoacoustics of speech perception. Psychoacousticians themselves began to study and theorize about the phenomenon of categorical perception (Macmillan, Kaplan, & Creelman, 1977). These authors were interested in redefining categorical perception in signal detection terms and in testing the claim that discrimination and identification tasks produced the same estimates of resolving power. They were also interested in testing the claim that resulted from the studies of nonspeech and animals, namely, that the peak typically observed in discrimination tasks in tests of categorical perception was due to a "natural psychophysical boundary" (Kuhl & J. D. Miller, 1975).[3] Macmillan et al. advocated study of the auditory system's *resolving power* for speech signals using signal detection theory (Green & Swets, 1966) and the theory of intensity resolution proposed by Durlach and Braida (1969).

Macmillan et al. (1977) reviewed various techniques for assessing identification and discrimination and demonstrated that certain designs came closer to identifying the absolute limits of auditory processing. They noted that the experimental techniques typically used to study categorical perception in experiments on speech were not optimal for assessing whether resolving power in discrimination and identification tasks was the same, nor whether absolute sensitivity increased at the boundaries between phonetic categories. The recommendation was that identification be assessed using more than the usual two-response-alternative

[2]After these findings were published, interactions between speech researchers taking a psychoacoustic approach and those taking a motor theory approach continued to follow this course. Motor theorists produced new findings, such as those showing that changes in the rate of speech shifted the identification and discrimination functions of stimuli such as [ba] and [wa], and attributed these findings to specialized mechanisms that took rate of articulation information into account (J. L. Miller & Liberman, 1979). However, this interpretation was countered by investigators who showed that the effects of rate could be replicated with nonspeech sounds (Diehl & Walsh, 1989; Pisoni, Carrell, & Gans, 1983), and data showing that monkeys listening to the same [ba] and [wa] speech sounds replicated the effects observed in people (E. B. Stevens, Kuhl, & Padden, 1988).

[3]Note that psychoacousticians and speech researchers were invested in slightly different aspects of the claims that resulted from the nonspeech and animal studies. Speech researchers were invested in the fundamental claim allowed by those studies—namely, that categorical perception could be attributed to *auditory* rather than *phonetic* processing. This claim countered the motor theory. Psychoacousticians, on the other hand, were invested in the claim that the phenomenon was attributable to a basic sensory limitation.

approach and that discrimination be assessed using a "fixed" discrimination format, in which the two stimuli to be discriminated remained the same throughout a block of trials, rather than a "roving" discrimination format, in which the two stimuli to be discriminated varied from trial to trial. The latter form typifies speech perception experiments but is not optimal for eliminating nonsensory effects (Macmillan et al., 1977).

Later, Macmillan, Goldberg, and Braida (1988) undertook the recommended experiments. Their data showed that the signal detection definition of categorical perception, where resolution as measured in identification equals resolution in fixed discrimination (Macmillan et al., 1977), was never fully achieved but that consonants came closer than tones varying in intensity (or vowels) in achieving that goal. More important, the Macmillan et al. (1988) psychoacoustic experiments on speech revealed that the perception of consonants from continua varying in voicing or place of articulation were indeed characterized by increases in basic sensitivity at the locations of phonetic boundaries.[4]

Thus, the results of three very different approaches to the psychoacoustics of speech—tests involving nonspeech signals, tests on animals, and tests employing psychoacoustic methods—supported the same conclusion. The peak in discrimination observed for consonant stimuli in tests of categorical perception appeared to have an auditory basis. The exact cause of the increases in sensitivity at phonetic boundaries could not be specified, but it was assumed that they were sensory in nature.

From a theoretical point of view, the importance of the discovery of "natural boundaries" was twofold (Kuhl, 1987, 1988; Kuhl & J. D. Miller, 1978): First, from the standpoint of developmental theory, the results suggested that infants' demonstration of enhanced discriminability at the boundaries of phonetic categories could be attributed to general psychoacoustic mechanisms that were present at birth, rather than an innate speech module, and this was an important turning point in developmental speech perception theory (Eimas, J. L. Miller, & Jusczyk, 1987; Kuhl, 1987; Kuhl & J. D. Miller, 1978). And second, the results had an impact on conjectures regarding the evolution of human communication

[4]This was not shown to be true for vowels. The vowel stimuli tested by Macmillan et al. (1988) did not show an increase in basic sensitivity at the location of the phonetic boundary. Thus, categorical-like perception results are not always associated with natural boundaries.

systems. The results supported the view that at least some of the speech units used to distinguish meaning in communication systems were chosen because they were located on either side of natural boundaries; this was optimal for communication (Kuhl & J. D. Miller, 1978; Lieberman, 1991; K. N. Stevens, 1981).

An Unresolved Question

These attempts to address the psychoacoustics of speech perception did not, however, address a critical question: What is the role of learning in speech perception? A large body of literature has convincingly demonstrated that adult listeners whose native languages differ behave very differently in speech perception experiments (Abramson & Lisker, 1970; Miyawaki et al., 1975; Strange & Dittmann, 1984; Werker & Logan, 1985). The notable case is that of Japanese adults, whose difficulty in discriminating the English segments /r/ and /l/ has been well documented (Goto, 1971; MacKain, Best, & Strange, 1981; Miyawaki et al., 1975; Mochizuki, 1981; Sheldon & Strange, 1982; Strange & Dittmann, 1984). Many studies have shown that even with extensive training, Japanese adults' discrimination of /r/ and /l/ improves very little and appears not to generalize strongly to new contexts or speakers (Logan, Lively, & Pisoni, 1991; MacKain et al., 1981; Mochizuki, 1981; Sheldon & Strange, 1982). If the boundaries of speech categories are sensory in nature, why do adult listeners from different cultures behave so differently in tests of speech perception? What is the nature of the change that is brought about by exposure to a specific language? Has language experience affected the basic sensory capabilities of listeners, or has it caused cognitive changes that affect perception?[5] To date, the psychoacoustic approach of Macmillan et al. (1977) has not been used to examine the effects of linguistic experience on the perception of speech. Nor have "cross-language" experiments been undertaken by those studying animals (who could rear animals listening to different kinds of signals) or those taking the nonspeech approach (who could test the perception of nonspeech signals in listeners whose phonetic inventories do not include sounds varying in the nonspeech dimension under test). Nonetheless, the cross-language differences that result from experience with a particular

[5]Data on the perception of musical intervals suggests that categorical-like results are shown in individuals who have had musical training; in the case of musical intervals, this is ascribed to training rather than the existence of natural boundaries (Burns & Ward, 1978). Thus for both music and speech there is a question as to how learning affects perception, both in the presence and in the absence of natural boundaries.

language are real-world phenomena and must be accounted for in any theory of speech perception.

A Focus on the Role of Memory in Speech Perception

The fact that listeners' long-term listening histories play such a potent role in speech perception implies that memory for speech sounds plays a critical role in listeners' performance. Formulations from a number of theoretical perspectives, which differ substantially in detail, are in agreement that there are two distinct memory modes operative in speech perception.

Studies on speech perception by Ades (1977), Pisoni (1973, 1975), Fujisaki and Kawashima's (1969, 1970), and Macmillan et al. (1988) lead to the conclusion that speech perception is the result of the combined operations of two memory mechanisms. One form of memory is based on the sensory trace of the stimulus in immediate memory ("trace" or "auditory" memory). The other is a more long-term memory code ("context" memory in Macmillan et al.'s terminology and "phonetic" memory in Fujisaki and Kawashima's as well as Pisoni's terminology). Trace or auditory memory is "echoic" memory that is subject to immediate decay over time and can be influenced by other sounds that occur in close temporal proximity to it. Phonetic or context memory is more robust and is not subject to immediate time decay. Phonetic memory constitutes the labeling process in which incoming stimuli are compared against stored reference points. The revised version of intensity resolution offered by Braida et al. (1984), in which the operation of context memory is described, fits into this scheme (see Macmillan et al., 1988 for discussion). The theory of intensity resolution asserts that listeners use "perceptual anchors" as referents for comparison with other stimuli in a discrimination task. In intensity perception, the anchors are the endpoint values of intensity used in the experiment, the highest and lowest intensities. The relationship between these experimenter-given perceptual anchors and those posited as phonetic entities stored in long-term memory for speech sounds is unclear, but the notion that perceptual anchors could in fact be ones established by a subject's long-term listening history has been mentioned (Macmillan et al., 1988; Macmillan et al., 1977).

This burgeoning interest in the role of long-term memory in speech dovetails with work on general categorization processes in cognition. In the cognitive literature, the ability to categorize objects and events is accounted for by positing the existence in long-term memory of some kind of cognitive reference point, or "prototype," to which incoming stimuli are compared (see Medin & Barsalou, 1987, for general review), and this approach has been adopted by speech researchers (Kuhl, 1991; Massaro, 1987; J. L. Miller & Volaitis, 1989; Samuel, 1982). A working hypothesis for these investigators is that listeners have developed referents for phonemes that are stored in long-term memory, and that when the techniques used to test subjects allow long-term memory to be tapped, the effects of language experience can be clearly shown. Thus psychoacousticians, speech scientists, and cognitive psychologists have recently shown increased interest in the memory codes used in the categorization of speech events. Researchers are currently very interested in how these memory modes function in speech perception, and whether they reflect general or specialized processes (Rosen & Howell, 1987; Schouten, 1987).

A Shift From Category Boundaries to Category Centers: Internal Standards, Prototypes, and Categorization

Research on speech in the 1950s, 1960s, and 1970s focused on the boundaries between speech categories as the key to categorization. This emphasis on the boundaries between categories has gradually given way to a focus on the *centers* of speech categories—the cognitive referent points, internal standards, or prototypes of speech categories—the mental representations that allow one to categorize a new instance of a category as being a member of an established category. Implicit in the shift in researchers' attention from boundaries to centers is the notion that linguistic experience is not altering the sensory thresholds of listeners from different cultures, but altering something else, namely, the listeners' definition of what constitutes an instance of the category.

Research on category centers began with an exploration of the nature of a "good instance" of a category. Unlike the original conceptions of categorical perception, in which within-category stimuli were considered virtually indistinguishable, this approach took the opposite view. Category members were distinguishable and category "goodness" was considered a matter of degree, where some members were perceived as better exemplars—more representative or prototypic—than others (Rosch, 1975). Studies on good exemplars of visual categories demonstrated that they have privileged status; they are more quickly encoded, they are more durably remembered, and they are often preferred over other members of the category (Garner, 1974; Goldman & Homa, 1977; Mervis & Rosch, 1981; Rosch, 1975, 1977).

Work in my own laboratory, and in others, was conducted to develop this approach for speech. For example, studies showed that when listeners were asked to rate the category goodness of individual members, the members differed in the degree to which they were perceived as good exemplars of the category (Grieser & Kuhl, 1989; Kuhl, 1986a; J. L. Miller & Volaitis, 1989). Moreover, it was demonstrated that certain stimuli were more effective adaptors in selective adaptation experiments (J. L. Miller, Connine, Schermer, & Kluender, 1983; Samuel, 1982) and were more effective competitors in dichotic competition experiments (J. L. Miller, 1977; Repp, 1977). This finding suggested that members of a phonetic category differed in perceptual potency. Taken together, the work supported the view that speech stimuli from a particular category varied, both qualitatively (certain stimuli are better exemplars than others) and quantitatively (certain members are more effective than others), and this in turn supported the view that speech sounds are *graded* in the degree to which they represent a given category. Correspondingly, the claim that speech categories have psychological centers (stimuli that best represent the category as a whole) was supported (Grieser & Kuhl, 1989; Kuhl, 1990, 1991; J. L. Miller, 1977; Oden & Massaro, 1978; Samuel, 1982).

The Seattle Work on Speech Prototypes

The work on speech categorization in my lab began 15 years ago. My work focused on models and theories of developmental speech perception. The question was: How do infants learn to identify speech sounds as members of phonetic categories? I argued that two abilities were essential. First, infants had to be able to discern differences between the sounds. That is, they had to resolve the acoustic differences that distinguished between minimal pairs of sounds, those that differed in just one critical feature. All of the work on categorical perception in infants had established that fact, for the sounds used were synthesized such that the speech sounds differed minimally. Infants' abilities to discriminate these sounds demonstrated their keen sensitivities for the perception of the acoustic differences used to differentiate speech sounds.

I argued, however, that the perception of differences was not sufficient for speech perception (Kuhl, 1976, 1979b, 1980, 1985a). In order to perceive speech, infants had to detect similarities between stimuli that differed greatly, and identify those diverse instances as members of the same category. My studies focused on this ability and demonstrated that infants at 6 months of age could perceptually classify stimuli differing in vowel quality (/a/ and /i/), pitch contour (rising and falling), and talker (man, woman, and child) into categories based on the identity of the vowel (Kuhl, 1979b, 1980, 1983; see Kuhl, 1985a, for review). Moreover, data from my lab showed that 6-month-old infants could sort syllables whose initial consonants differed (/s/ versus /ʃ/) when the consonants appeared in three different vowel contexts (/a/, /i/, or /u/) and were spoken by four different talkers (2 men and 2 woman) (Kuhl, 1980; see also Hillenbrand, 1983, 1984). The important difference between this work on categorization and categorical perception was that in my studies, infants had to classify into two groups an array of sounds that differed on many dimensions. All of the sounds were *discriminably different*. The task did not focus on the discrimination of *differences*, but on the perception of *similarities*. It mimicked "sorting," the classification of real stimuli into classes. We showed, for example, that when infants were trained to treat two single exemplars—each representing a separate category—as different, their responses immediately generalized to novel instances of both categories (Kuhl, 1979b, 1980, 1983). These category experiments established that infants were very good at recognizing the *similarities* among perceptually diverse instances representing the same phonetic category. They appeared to solve the "invariance" problem (see Kuhl, 1985a, for discussion).

It was my opinion that these studies on categorization examined what listeners—both adults and infants—had to do when listening to real speech. It seemed unlikely that these abilities would be explained by a simple sensory boundary, because the stimuli were multidimensional and could be categorized on any one of the dimensions. What was needed was an explanation for listeners' abilities to assign stimuli to categories.

A New Phenomenon: Vowel Prototypes

The series of experiments undertaken next were motivated by the assumption that adult listeners had some kind of mental representation (referred to here as a category prototype, even though the representations may not be based on a stored statistical average but instead a series of exemplars experienced by the listener) for each of the phonemes used in their language. The questions addressed were: Is there evidence that prototypes exist in adults and infants; and if so, do prototypes play a role in perception? Data will be presented here that suggest that both these questions can be answered affirmatively. The data suggest that adult listeners do have mental representations—prototypes—that define vowel categories. Cross-language data suggest that infants do as well. Finally, we have data suggesting that prototypes play a special role in speech perception.

The prototype phenomenon is new, and although there are considerable data, there is also much to be done before it is fully explained. Experiments that take a psychophysical approach to the phenomenon have not yet been completed.[6] Instead, I took a developmental, cross-language, and comparative approach to the phenomenon. Developmental data gathered in my laboratory (Grieser & Kuhl, 1989; Kuhl, 1990, 1991) have shown that the effect exists in infants very early in life. Cross-cultural experiments show that the effect is altered by early listening experience (Kuhl, Williams, Lacerda, Stevens, & Lindblom, 1992), and comparative tests show that the effect is not exhibited by monkeys (Kuhl, 1991). These findings will be used to address questions about the nature and origins of the effect.

Experiments on Internal Standards: Goodness Ratings for Vowel Stimuli

The rationale behind these studies was that if listeners of a particular language have internal representations or standards for the phonemes of their language and use these standards to assess whether an incoming stimulus is one contained in their language, then they must be able to judge the "goodness" or "adequacy" of a particular instance from the category as a member of that category. The first goal was to assess listeners' abilities to do this.

Stimuli. This series of studies began with vowels, specifically, the "point" vowel /i/, as in "peep." The choice of vowels over consonants was motivated by the fact that the perceived goodness of vowels could be altered by varying fewer dimensions (just two, F1 and F2) than would be true for consonants. Also, point vowels such as /i/, /a/, and /u/, are articulatory and acoustic extremes and are used universally in the world's languages (Jakobson, Fant, & Halle, 1969). K. N. Stevens (1981) believes that point vowels are special in the sense that they appear to

[6]The psychoacoustic approach would be to conduct discrimination tests using the fixed 2-interval, forced-choice (2IFC) procedure recommended by Macmillan et al. (1988). However, selection of a discrimination procedure to use in the initial studies was constrained by a different goal, which was to test adults, infants, and animals with the identical procedure. Because procedures such as 2IFC cannot be used with infants and animals, a Same–Different task was chosen. Experiments that fully explore the effects of psychoacoustic task on the prototype effect are currently under way with adults.

resist perceptual change. If prototypes exist for speech stimuli, point vowels seemed likely candidates.

Grieser and Kuhl (1989) synthesized a large set of /i/ vowels and selected an /i/ vowel that was consistently judged by adult speakers of the language as the best /i/. It was designated as the "prototype" /i/ (P). A second /i/ vowel was consistently judged by adults as a relatively poor exemplar of an /i/ vowel and was designated the "nonprototype" /i/ (NP). It is of fundamental importance to the logic of these studies that this relatively poor exemplar was always judged as /i/ rather than as some other vowel by adults; both the P and the NP were easily identified as exemplars of the /i/ category.

Grieser and Kuhl (1989) and Kuhl (1991) created category variants for P and NP by manipulating the first and second formants of the vowels. In Grieser and Kuhl, 16 variants were used; they formed semicircles around each of the two stimuli. In Kuhl, 32 variants were used and they fully orbited the two stimuli (Figure 1). The results of the experiments using the two sets of stimuli were identical; the results of Kuhl (1991) will be the focus here.

The 32 variants used by Kuhl (1991) formed four orbits (O_1–O_4) around the two vowel stimuli, with eight stimuli located on each orbit. The distance between the four orbits and the P (or the NP) vowel was equated in psychophysical terms using the mel scale (S. S. Stevens, Volkmann, & Newman, 1937). This allowed the creation of stimuli that differed from the P and the NP in uniform steps. Thus, the variants around the P and the NP were scaled in a common metric, and this was used to equate distance between the four orbits and their respective vowel targets. O_1 stimuli were located 30 mels from the target vowel; O_2 through O_4 stimuli were located at 60, 90, and 120 mels from the target vowel, respectively. The variants were created by manipulating the values of the first and second formants; the values of the third, fourth, and fifth formants remained constant for all vowels at 3010 Hz, 3300 Hz, and 3850 Hz, respectively (see Kuhl, 1991, for further details).

Adult Goodness Ratings. Quantitative ratings of category goodness (prototypicality) of each variant were obtained using a 7-point rating scale ranging from *7* (a good exemplar), one representative of the /i/ vowel category as a whole; to *1* (a poor exemplar), one not representative of the category as a whole. No auditory referent for a good exemplar of the /i/ vowel was provided to listeners. Instead, subjects were shown a card on which the word "peep" was written and told to

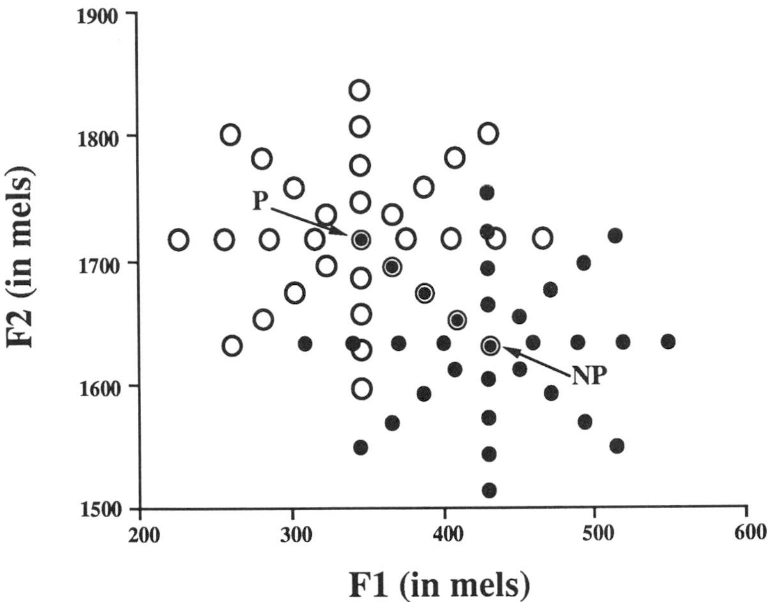

FIGURE 1 Formant frequency values in mels for variants surrounding the P and NP stimuli. The stimuli form four orbits (eight stimuli each) around the center stimulus. The stimuli on each orbit are a specified distance in mels from the center vowel (30, 60, 90, or 120 mels, starting from the first orbit). The stimuli on one vector were common to both sets. From Kuhl (1991). Copyright 1991 by the Psychonomic Society. Reprinted by permission.

rate the perceived goodness of each stimulus as an exemplar of the vowel contained in the word on the card.

Average ratings for the stimuli are plotted in Figure 2; the size of the circles represents the relative goodness, or typicality, of each stimulus. As shown, the P was given an average rating of 6.7[7] and the NP was given an average rating of 2.0. The ratings for the stimuli nearest the P tended to be highest, and the ratings consistently decreased with increases in distance from P. Conversely, stimuli in the orbits around NP received relatively low ratings, with an increase

[7]Data from a subsequent experiment (Kuhl et al., 1992) in which the adult listeners had less experience with synthetic speech showed that the prototype /i/ was judged less favorably; it received an average rating of 5.4, as opposed to the 6.7 it had received when individuals with more experience in listening to synthetic speech had been tested (Kuhl, 1991). Ratings given the nonprototype were similarly depressed; it received a rating of 1.2 as opposed to the 2.0 it had received earlier. Thus, while experience with synthesized utterances affects ratings, the difference between the prototype and the nonprototype remains substantial.

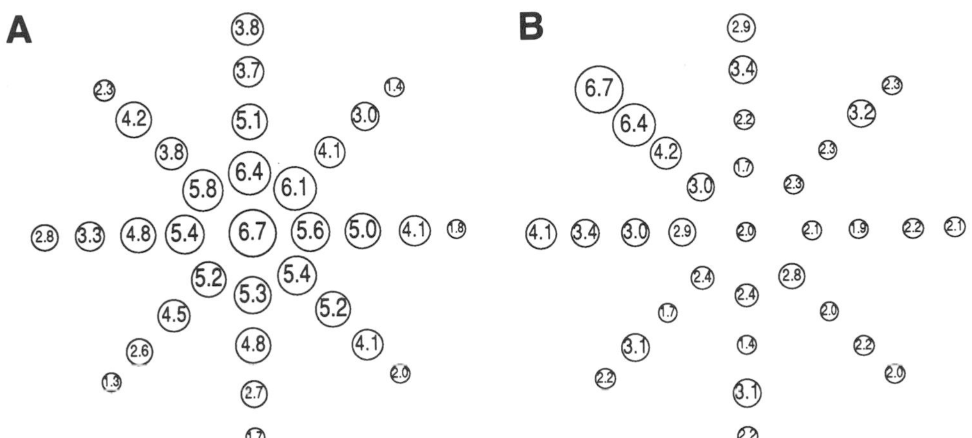

FIGURE 2 Category goodness (prototypicality) ratings for (*A*) the American English /i/ prototype, (*B*) the nonprototype /i/ vowel, and the variants surrounding each of the two vowels. Prototypicality was judged by adults using a scale from *1* (a poor exemplar) to *7* (a good exemplar). The size of the circles correlates with the degree of goodness, with larger circles indicating better exemplars. From Kuhl (1991). Copyright 1991 by the Psychonomic Society. Reprinted by permission.

in ratings as they neared the region of the vowel space occupied by P. The results thus showed that all /i/ vowels were not perceived to be equal by adults—some were perceived as better exemplars of the category than others. Stimuli in a particular region of the vowel space stood out as the best exemplars of the category; moreover, the ratings declined evenly and symmetrically around the best instances. The ratings were highly consistent across listeners.

Adult Goodness Ratings for Foreign-Language Categories. The data had shown that when adult speakers listen to variants of a vowel contained in their native language, they can reliably assign ratings to reflect the degree to which they consider it a good instance of the category. Our next question was whether adults from a different language environment would assign similar ratings to these stimuli. Swedish adults were asked to rate the set of American English /i/ vowels. Swedish contains a number of high-front vowels whose formant frequency patterns are similar, but not identical, to the American English /i/. The American English /i/ exemplars were presented to native speakers of Swedish, and they were asked three questions about each vowel: (a) whether it was a sound used in their language, (b) if yes, the category it belonged to, and (c) its representativeness as a member of that category using the same rating scale (*1* = poor and *7* = good). Not all Swedish adults considered the American English /i/ as "in their language." Only about half of the subjects considered it a Swedish vowel. Listeners who did consider it a Swedish vowel judged it to be a member of either the Swedish /e/ or Swedish /i/ category. The ratings of the American /i/ vowels as members of the Swedish /e/ are shown in Figure 3. As shown, Swedish adults gave the American English /i/ prototype a 2.6 on average as a member of the

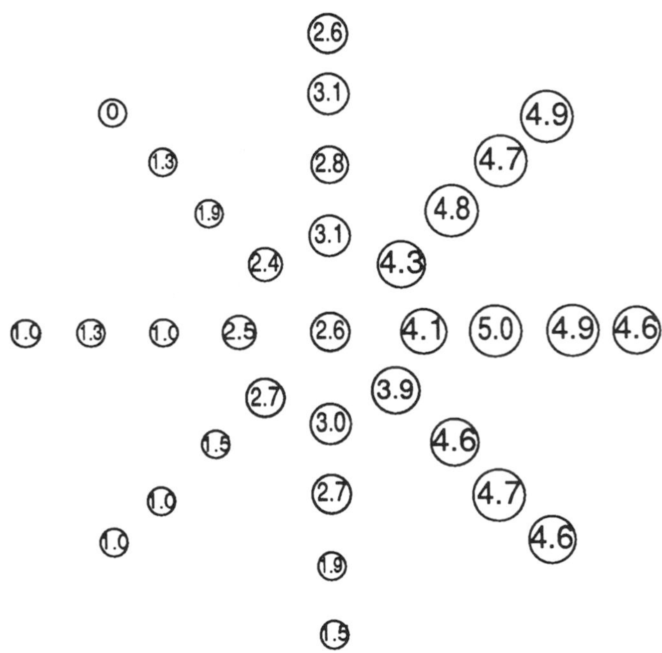

FIGURE 3 Category goodness (prototypicality) ratings for the American English /i/ stimuli by Swedish adults. Swedish adults judged the American English /i/ vowels to be members of the Swedish /e/ vowel category, and rated the stimuli as members of that category. Prototypicality was judged by adults using a scale from *1* (a poor exemplar) to *7* (a good exemplar). The size of the circles correlates with the degree of goodness, with larger circles indicating better exemplars. The American English /i/ prototype was given an average rating of 2.8 as a Swedish /e/. Thus American /i/ is a native-language nonprototypic for Swedish adults. The ratings also indicate that the best Swedish /e/ has a higher first formant than the American English /i/.

Swedish /e/ category. The ratings make it clear that the center of the /e/ vowel category is located to the right of the American English /i/ prototype.

A comparison of the ratings of the American /i/ stimuli by the American adults (Figure 2) and the Swedish adults (Figure 3) shows that adults from different countries rate the same stimuli differently, suggesting that adults use internal standards of the vowels of their native language when judging the goodness or adequacy of a new stimulus. The fact that the same stimuli are rated differently reinforces the view that the perception of vowels is determined not only by the stimulus but by something in the listener's head—a mental representation that defines the category.

Experiments on the Role of Prototypes in Speech Perception

The goodness ratings suggested that listeners had internal standards stored in memory for phonemes contained in their native language and that particularly good or prototypic instances of each category tapped that representation. The next series of experiments examined whether the instances that listeners had identified as prototypes played a special role in perception. The hypothesis was that adults' perception of members of a speech category would be affected by prototypicality. Specifically, the prediction was that the prototype would be perceived as more similar to other members of the category than was the case for a nonprototype.

The American English /i/ P and the NP vowels, along with their respective sets of 32 variants, were used to test adults in a same–different discrimination task. Adults listened to either the P or the NP as a standard sound to which its variants were compared. The standard (either P or NP) was repeated continuously over a loudspeaker, and listeners pressed a button when they heard the sound change. Two kinds of trials were run, each with a probability of .5. During *test* trials, the standard vowel was changed to a comparison stimulus (one of the variants surrounding P or NP) during a 4.5s interval. During *control* trials, the standard vowel was not changed, but responses were monitored to assess the probability of false-positive responses. Subjects were informed that all of the stimuli belonged to the same phonetic category and that they were to respond to any change that they heard in the stimulus.

The results strongly supported the hypothesis that prototypicality of the standard affected discrimination performance. Overall, adults were highly accurate at detecting these within-category vowel differences. Across both conditions, overall percent-correct scores were above 75% correct. However, discrimination performance varied significantly, $p < .001$, depending on the prototypicality of the standard. When P was the standard, overall percent-correct scores were significantly lower (Figure 4), indicating that the prototype was more difficult to discriminate from its variants than was true for the nonprototype.

The number of trials in which adults failed to detect a change from the standard to the comparison stimulus ("miss" responses) at each distance for the P and NP condition (Figure 5) were calculated. The results indicated that adults produced significantly higher numbers of miss responses when attempting to discriminate the prototype from its surrounding variants when compared to the nonprototype in relation to its surrounding variants. Statistical analyses of the results revealed a highly significant effect of condition, $F(1, 14) = 34.8, p < .001$, reflecting the fact that at each distance, miss responses were higher for the prototype condition. As expected, the effect of distance was also highly significant, $F(3, 42) = 15.3, p < .001$, indicating that for both groups, miss responses decreased as the comparison stimulus moved farther away from the standard vowel and became physically less similar to the standard vowel. The Condition $\times$ Distance interaction was also significant, $F(3, 42) = 8.3, p < .001$. Follow-up tests for simple effects showed that the effect of distance was highly significant for each group considered individually ($p < .001$ in both cases).

One of the goals of the experiment was to examine the effects of the P and the NP on the perception of identical stimuli. The P and NP conditions had included a subset of identical stimuli, those located on the vector that was shared by the two groups (Figure 2), but there were only three stimuli between the P and the NP. A stimulus series was constructed that varied in 10-mel steps; it consisted of 13 stimuli, 11 located between the P and the NP. The tests on adults were then replicated using the same technique previously described. The only difference between subjects tested in the two conditions was that subjects in the P condition heard the prototype stimulus as the referent and compared it to the 12 stimuli in the direction of the nonprototype stimulus, whereas subjects in the NP condition heard the nonprototype stimulus as the referent and compared it to the 12 stimuli in the direction of the prototype. In essence, the only difference was the direction of stimulus change—the stimuli themselves were identical.

The results are shown in Figure 6. As shown, the effect was reproduced in adults for the identical stimuli. Adult subjects tested in the P condition had to go

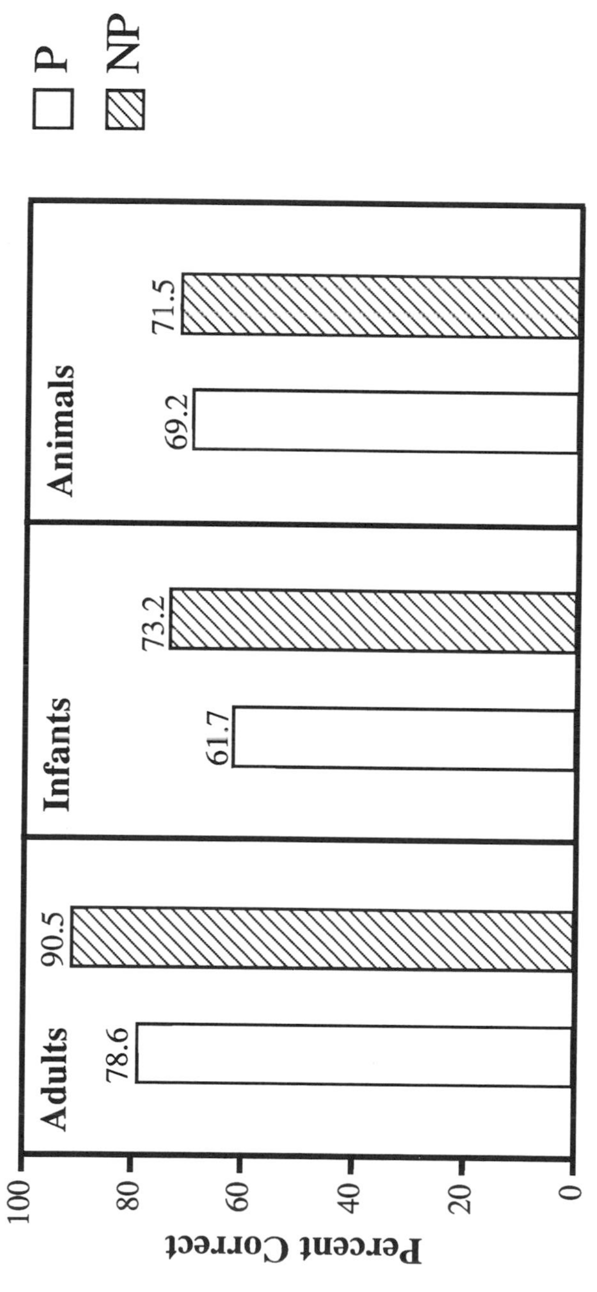

FIGURE 4 Average overall percent-correct scores achieved by adults, infants, and animals in the prototype (P) and the nonprototype (NP) conditions. For adults and infants (but not animals), there is a statistically significant difference between scores in the two conditions, with overall percent-correct scores being higher in the nonprototype condition. From Kuhl (1991). Copyright 1991 by The Psychonomic Society. Reprinted by permission.

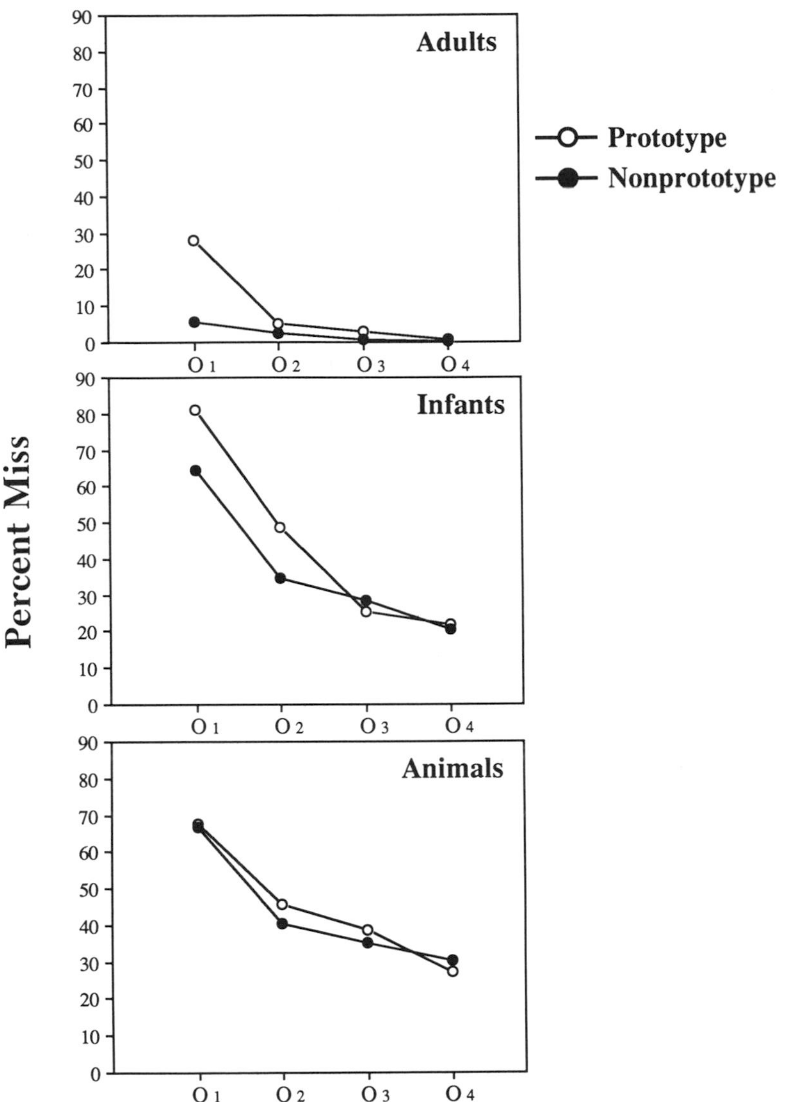

FIGURE 5 Average miss scores shown for stimuli surrounding the prototype and the nonprototype by adults, infants, and animals. For adults and infants (but not animals), there is a statistically significant difference between miss scores in the two conditions, with scores being higher in the prototype condition. From Kuhl (1991). Copyright 1991 by The Psychonomic Society. Reprinted by permission.

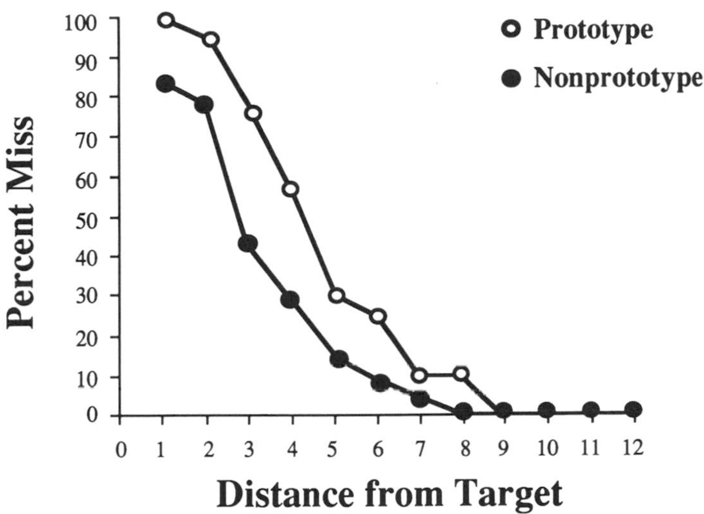

FIGURE 6 Average miss scores for American adults listening to /i/ stimuli on the vector that was common to the prototype (P) and nonprototype (NP) stimulus sets (see Figure 1). For both groups, a referent sound (either the P or the NP) was to be discriminated from stimuli in the direction of the opposite sound (either the P or the NP). Adults whose referent sound was the prototype had to go further in the direction of the nonprototype before they responded to the stimuli as different.

farther in the direction of the NP before they indicated hearing a difference than was true for adults tested in the NP condition.

The tests on adults demonstrated that when a "good" (prototypic), as opposed to a "poor" (nonprototypic), exemplar of the phonetic category served as the referent stimulus to which other stimuli from the category were compared, adults' perception was strongly affected by prototypicality. The findings on adults had suggested two things. First, members of phonetic categories are graded with regard to their representativeness or typicality. And second, best instances of a phonetic category play a special role in perception. The perceived distance between the prototype and surrounding members is effectively decreased (shrunk) in comparison to a nonprototype of the category (Kuhl, 1991). The directional asymmetry seen in the perception of the stimuli on the common vector underscores the prototype's effect on perception. It suggests that the prototype provides cohesion for the category; it pulls other stimuli toward it, effectively shortening the perceptual distance between stimuli at the outskirts of the category and the prototype center. This is why I have referred to the prototype as a "perceptual magnet" (Kuhl, 1991).

Theoretical Basis of the Perceptual Magnet Effect

What is the origin of the perceptual magnet effect for vowels? I can identify three theoretically possible bases for the perceptual magnet effect: (a) Vowel magnets are psychoacoustic in nature; (b) vowel magnets are specified as part of the specialized speech module; or (c) vowel magnets are learned through exposure to speech.

Consider the first of these three possibilities. It might be the case that the set of vowels used in the languages of the world represent locations in the vowel quadrangle where the perception of stimulus differences is inherently minimized due to psychoacoustic constraints. Such an idea is embodied in the "quantal theory" of vowel perception (K. N. Stevens, 1972). In other words, certain vowels might produce this pattern of results due solely to auditory factors, rather than factors related to perceptual learning and memory, or specialized processing. The psychoacoustic explanation would be supported if (a) the magnet effect were present at birth or in very young infants in the absence of experience with vowels, (b) if animals demonstrated the effect, and (c) if the effects were present under conditions of "fixed" discrimination, wherein memory demands are limited. If the perceptual magnet effect has a psychoacoustic basis, it would in some respects mirror the situation in color vision, where it has been reported that regardless of culture, adults and infants respond to certain hues as "focal" wavelengths for the four basic color categories (Bornstein, 1981).

The second possibility is that the magnet effect derives from specialized speech processing mechanisms—from a "speech module" (Fodor, 1983). According to this view, the effect is not attributable to psychoacoustic factors, nor to learning, but to a speech processing subsystem that is innately present in humans. The specialized processing alternative requires that the effect be present innately, for some and perhaps all vowels used in the languages of the world, and then that it be modified by experience. The specialized processing account is not supported if animals show the effect.

The third possibility is that the perceptual magnet effect is the result of learning—that is, of exposure to language. This model holds that linguistic experience results in the development of mental representations that are based on the stimuli that occur in the language environment of the child. This account requires that the perceptual magnet effect be absent at birth and that it develop only in the presence of experience with specific sounds. According to this view, the effect should be observed only for native-language sounds. The learning account is not supported if animals, who are not raised listening to speech, show the effect.

To provide data that address these theoretical alternatives, tests on the basis of the magnet effect therefore involved (a) testing the magnet effect in infants, (b) testing the magnet effect in animals, and (c) examining the magnet effect's sensitivity to linguistic experience.

Experiments on the Development of the Perceptual Magnet Effect

I initially reasoned that if prototypes were "built-in," as required by both the psychoacoustic and special mechanism accounts, then young infants should show the magnet effect. Alternatively, if prototypes are "built-up" through experience with language, then infants at 6 months might not show the effect.

Infants who were 6 months old were tested with only minor changes in the same–different discrimination procedure that had been used with adults. Using a head-turn conditioning procedure, a technique commonly used in tests of infant speech perception (see Kuhl, 1985b for review), infants were trained to produce a head-turn response when they heard a change in the standard vowel stimulus (either P or NP). The procedure involved conditioning an infant to produce a head-turn response for a visual reinforcer when the continuously repeated referent sound was changed. The visual reinforcer consisted of a toy animal that moves when activated (a bear pounds a drum, a monkey claps symbols). The animal is housed in a box made of darkened Plexiglas that is normally opaque; when the reinforcer is activated, the lights in the box are lit and the animated toy becomes visible.

Infants were tested in each of two conditions, the P condition and the NP condition. For the P group, the prototype /i/ served as the standard vowel and the 32 variants surrounding it served as the comparison stimuli; for the NP group, the nonprototype /i/ vowel served as the standard vowel and the 32 variants surrounding it served as the comparison stimuli. The training phase involved two stages: conditioning (C) and discrimination (D). During C, only test trials were presented until infants learned to produce the head-turn response. During these initial test trials, a single comparison stimulus (one of the eight stimuli located on O_4, counterbalanced across infants) was used for each infant. Criterion performance during the C phase was three test trials in a row in which the infant produced a head-turn response before the end of the trial, which had to occur before the end of 35 trials in order to progress to the next stage of training. In the D phase of training, two changes occurred. First, test and control trials were run, and second, the comparison stimuli presented on test trials now included all of the eight stimuli on O_4. Criterion performance was seven-out-of-eight consecutive correct responses within the first two sessions. Infants failing to meet this criterion were not tested further (see Kuhl, 1991, for further details).

The trials of theoretical interest were run during the generalization (G) phase. During G, each infant was tested with all of the 32 /i/ variants surrounding the standard vowel (either P or NP). The primary question of interest was whether infants' responses mirrored those of adults. The same two measures used to assess adult performance were used to assess infant performance. First, the overall percent-correct measure was calculated. Both the P and the NP groups achieved overall percent-correct scores that were significantly above chance (50% correct), $t(15) > 4.5$ in both cases, $p < .001$. As was the case for the adult data, the overall percent-correct measure revealed a significant difference between performance in the P and the NP group, with the NP group discriminating surrounding variants more accurately (73.2% correct) than did infants in the P group (61.7% correct), $t(30) = 3.87$, $p < .001$. In the measure of overall percent correct, therefore, infants replicated the result obtained with adults (Figure 4).

Infants' miss scores at each distance are shown in Figure 5. At each distance infants in the P group produced higher miss scores than those produced by infants in the NP group. Statistical comparisons showed that the condition effect was highly significant, $F(1,30) = 46.3$, $p < .001$, as was the effect of distance, $F(3,90) = 1069.9$, $p < .001$. The Group $\times$ Distance interaction was also significant, $F(3,90) = 37.3$, $p < .001$. Simple effects tests revealed that the effect of distance was significant for each group ($p < .001$ in both cases).

Infants' responses to the stimuli located on the vector that was common to the two stimulus sets—those located on the vector that was shared by the two groups (Figure 1)—were also examined. The only difference between subjects tested in the two conditions was that subjects in the P condition heard the prototype stimulus as the background and compared it to stimuli in the direction of the nonprototype stimulus, whereas subjects in the NP condition heard the non-prototype stimulus as the background and compared it to stimuli in the direction of the prototype. The results showed that infants tested in the P condition had to go farther away from the prototype before they indicated hearing a difference in the stimuli when compared to infants tested in the NP condition. A polynomial trend analysis revealed that the response profiles of infants tested in the two conditions differed significantly, $F(1,30) = 6.82, p < .05$.

In summary, the tests on infants provided strong support for the hypothesis that infants' perception of speech categories was affected by prototypicality. Moreover, the direction of the effect mirrored that shown by adult speakers of the language: Stimuli defined by adult speakers of the language as better exemplars of the phonetic category, prototypes of the category, resulted in poorer discrimination of nearby members of the category in infants. In other words, the prototype appeared to function like a perceptual magnet even for infants only 6 months old.

The data showed that the effect was present very early in life. By 6 months of age, infants responded as though they distinguished prototypes from nonprototypes. The question was: How did infants do this? Was the magnet effect "built-in"? And if so, was it the result of general psychoacoustic processing or a specialized speech module?

Experiments on Monkeys: Do Animals Show the Magnet Effect?

As previously noted, my early data demonstrated that categorical perception was demonstrated in monkeys (Kuhl, 1986b, 1988), indicating that the perceptual discontinuities that define the boundaries on speech–sound continua are not unique to man. I therefore wanted to know whether the centers of categories were also determined by basic psychoacoustic abilities.

Rhesus macaques were tested in an experiment that mirrored the one conducted with human infants (Kuhl, 1991). The procedure used to test monkeys was the same as that used in previous experiments of animals' perception of speech stimuli in this laboratory and have been described in detail (Kuhl & Padden, 1982, 1983). Briefly, the animal initiated trials by depressing a telegraph key. As soon as the animal depressed the key, the presentation of the standard stimulus began. Animals indicated detection of a sound change by releasing the response key rather than turning their heads and were reinforced with applesauce rather than with the visual stimulus of a dancing toy animal. The trial structure was the same as in the previous tests on adults and infants, and the training phase, consisting of conditioning (C) and discrimination (D) and the generalization (G) phase, was nearly identical to that used in the tests on human infants.

The results showed that animals behaved very differently from human adults and human infants. Animals in each of the two conditions achieved overall percent-correct scores that were significantly above chance (50% correct), $t(5) > 4.5$ in both cases, $p < .001$. However, unlike the case for human adults and infants, the overall percent-correct measure for animals revealed no difference between performance in the P and NP conditions (Figure 4). When tested on the P stimuli, animals performed nearly as accurately (69.2% correct) as they did when tested in the NP group (71.5% correct), $t(10) = -.908$, $p > .40$. In the measure of overall percent correct, therefore, animals did not replicate the results obtained with human adults and infants.

Animals' miss scores also revealed a very different pattern of results from those seen with adults and infants (Figure 5). As expected, the effect of distance was highly significant for animals. However, animal performance was also affected by the direction of formant frequency change (a "vector" effect; see Kuhl, 1991 for details), which had played no role in either the adult nor the infant data. Statistical tests revealed that only the distance and the vector effects were significant, $p < .001$ in both cases. Of main interest was the effect of condition (P vs. NP) and the Condition × Distance interaction. Both were significant in the adult and infant data, but neither of the two was significant for animals, $F < 2.5$, $p > .10$, in both cases. Thus, animals' perception of speech sounds was *not affected* by prototypicality. Discrimination of stimuli surrounding the prototype and the nonprototype was equal.

This difference is of interest in light of previous research demonstrating the commonalities between young infants and animals in tests of the categorical perception of consonants (Kuhl, 1981; Kuhl & J. D. Miller, 1975, 1978; Kuhl & Padden, 1982, 1983; Morse & Snowdon, 1975; Waters & Wilson, 1976). The present work thus established a point of dissociation between infants and animals in tests of speech perception. Unlike the tests on categorical perception, tests on the magnet effect in animals did not replicate the effects seen in humans. Thus, the results did not allow us to assert that the magnet effect was due to a basic psychoacoustic process that was common to man and monkey. Nonetheless, the psychoacoustic explanation has not been ruled out; further tests that will help resolve this issue are those currently under way on adults using a fixed discrimination procedure.

Experiments on the Effects of Early Linguistic Experience on the Magnet Effect

The specialized mechanism account predicted that animals would not show the effect, and animals' failure to exhibit the effect confirmed this prediction. The specialized mechanism account also predicted that linguistic experience was not necessary for the effect. The next experiment was designed to determine whether infants demonstrated the effect in the absence of linguistic experience.

American 6-month-old infants had shown the magnet effect for an American English vowel. But I did not know whether the magnet effect as seen in 6-month-olds occurred independently of language experience or whether exposure to a specific language was necessary. If infants showed the effect for vowels they had never heard, and animals failed to show the effect, that would provide evidence consistent with the specialized module account. On the other hand, if infants from two different language environments showed the effect only for vowels of their native language to which they had been exposed, it would provide evidence in support of a language-experience hypothesis.

To address these issues, I conducted a cross-language experiment (Kuhl et al., 1992). In that study, infants from the United States and Sweden were tested with both the American English /i/ vowel prototype used previously and with a prototype of the Swedish front-rounded /y/ vowel (Figure 7). The Swedish /y/ does not occur at all in American English, so American infants' responses to the Swedish /y/ prototype would reveal how infants responded in the total absence of linguistic experience. As seen in the ratings of American /i/ by Swedish adults, a sound resembling the American /i/ occurs in Swedish; however, the American English /i/ is not a good exemplar of any Swedish vowel category. It was a nonprototype sound in the Swedish language and would be expected to produce results typical of a nonprototype if linguistic experience played a critical role in the magnet effect (Kuhl, 1991).

If experience with language in the first 6 months affects phonetic perception, a specific pattern is predicted in which the two groups of infants would

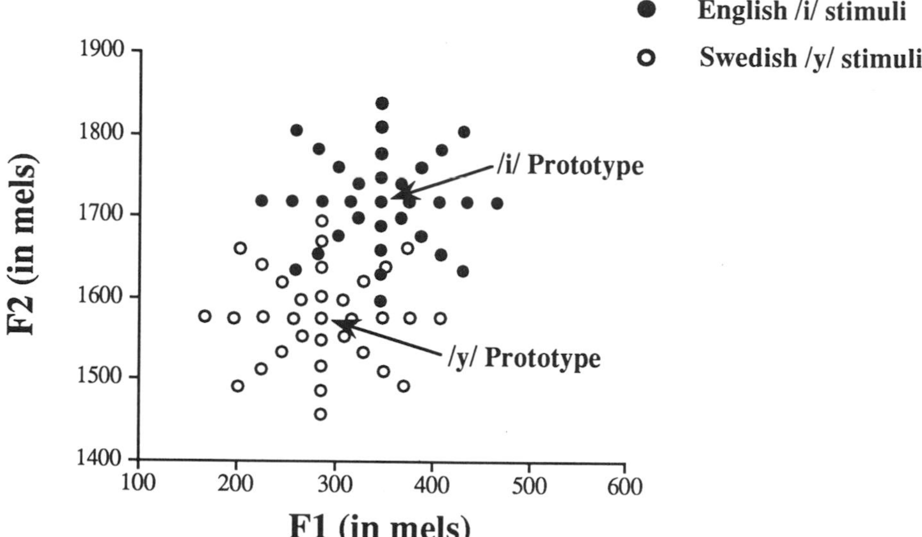

FIGURE 7 The two sets of vowel stimuli, American English /i/ and Swedish /y/, used in the cross-language tests on infants from the United States and Sweden. Each set included an exceptionally good instance of the vowel (the prototype, P) and a set of 32 variants that were acoustically similar, but not identical, to the prototype. From Kuhl, Williams, Lacerda, Stevens, and Lindblom (1992). Copyright 1992 by the American Association for the Advancement of Science. Reprinted by permission.

differ: (a) American infants would treat the American English /i/ as a prototype and the Swedish /y/ as a nonprototype, exhibiting a stronger magnet effect for American English /i/; and (b) Swedish infants would treat the Swedish /y/ as a prototype and the American English /i/ as a nonprototype, exhibiting a stronger magnet effect for Swedish /y/. However, if the results showed any other pattern (e.g., if both groups of infants exhibited the magnet effect equally for both vowels, or more strongly for the same one of the two vowels), then we would have no evidence that linguistic experience played a role in the appearance of the magnet effect in 6-month-old infants.

A "good instance" or prototype of the Swedish /y/ vowel was synthesized and cross-language comparisons of the perceived goodness of the Swedish /y/ were conducted. Adult native speakers were asked three questions about the two prototypes used in the present experiment: (a) whether it was a sound used in their language; (b) if yes, which category it belonged to; and (c) its representativeness as a member of that category using a scale from *1* (poor) to *7* (good) (Kuhl et al., 1992). American listeners unanimously judged the /i/ prototype as an American English vowel, giving it an average rating of 5.4 as a member of the English /i/ category. They unanimously rated the Swedish /y/ prototype as not in their language. Swedish adults unanimously judged the /y/ prototype as a Swedish vowel, giving it an average rating of 4.7 as a member of the category /y/. As shown in Figure 3, they often rated the American English /i/ prototype as present in the language but judged it to be a poor exemplar of the Swedish /e/ category.

To conduct the developmental cross-language comparison, the entire laboratory (computer, loudspeaker, cables, reinforcers, everything used to conduct the experiment) and three experimenters were moved from Seattle to Stockholm. The methods and procedures used to conduct the study in the two countries were identical. Only the critical variable changed—the language experience of the 6-month-old infants.

The results demonstrated that linguistic experience in the first half-year of life alters infants' perception of speech sounds (Kuhl et al., 1992). Infants from both countries showed a significantly stronger magnet effect for their native-language prototype (Figure 8). American infants perceived the American English /i/ prototype as identical to its variants on 66.9% of all trials; in contrast, they perceived the Swedish /y/ prototype as identical to its variants on only 50.6% of the trials. Swedish infants perceived the Swedish /y/ prototype as identical to its variants on 66.2% of all trials; in contrast, they treated the American English /i/ prototype as identical to its variants on only 55.9% of the trials. Statistical analysis of the effects of infants' language environment (American English vs. Swedish) and the prototype vowel tested (American English /i/ vs. Swedish /y/) showed that only the interaction between the two factors was highly significant $F(1, 60) = 20.107, p < .0001$). Neither of the main effects was significant: language environment, $F(1, 60) = .526, p > .40$; vowel, $F(1, 60) = .978, p > .30$.

The findings demonstrated that by 6 months, infants exhibit a strong magnet effect only for native-language phonetic prototypes. By this age, foreign-language prototypes have begun to function like nonprototypes in the native lan-

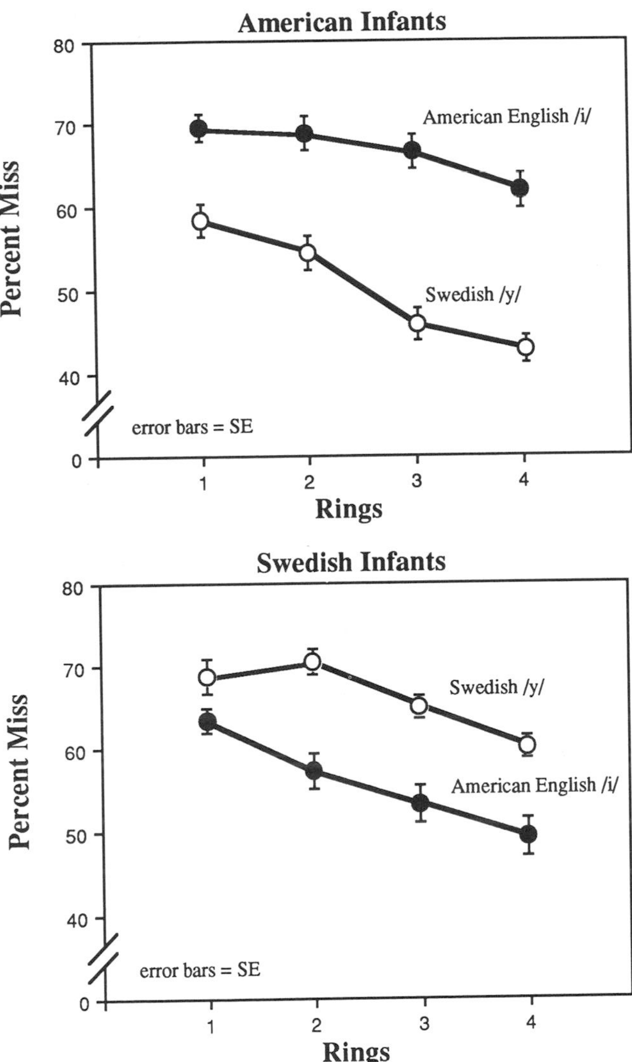

FIGURE 8 Results showing an effect of language experience on young infants' perception of speech. Two groups of 6-month-old infants (American and Swedish) were tested with two different vowel prototypes, American English /i/ and Swedish /y/. Plotted are the mean number of trials in which variants were equated to the prototype (% miss on change trials). Infants from both countries produced a stronger magnet effect (equated variants to the prototype more often) for the native-language vowel prototype when compared to the foreign-language vowel prototype. From Kuhl, Williams, Lacerda, Stevens, and Lindblom (1992). Copyright 1992 by the American Association for the Advancement of Science. Reprinted by permission.

guage. This is the earliest age at which language experience has been shown to have a measurable effect on infants.[8]

Summary of Experiments and Implications of the Results

Speech Categories are Internally Structured. The results of these experiments strongly suggest that phonetic categories are internally structured. Adults from two countries have shown that they are able to provide subjective ratings of the overall adequacy or quality of a speech stimulus. Adults' ratings are uniformly symmetrical around a particular location in vowel space. Vowels exhibit a kind of "hot spot" that receives consistently high ratings across listeners. These data support those of J. L. Miller and Volaitis (1989), who also show that the perception of category goodness is graded and that goodness ratings change with factors such as the rate of speech.

Adults Have Internal Standards for Speech Categories. The results of the goodness-ratings experiments on adults suggest that speech categories are somehow mentally represented in adults. Adults were not provided with a model on which to base their judgments of category goodness; they had to rely on an internal standard of the "ideal" /i/ vowel. Adults' internal standards appear to be based on a good stimulus or prototype of the category. The fact that adults' ratings were so consistent suggests that adult listeners—at least those who speak the same dialect of a particular language—have internal standards for vowels that are quite similar.

The cross-language adult data suggest that adult listeners can rate the goodness of vowels present only in their own native language. They cannot judge the goodness of a vowel that is not contained in their own native language. Even when they are provided with an exemplar to use in making the judgments, adult

[8]Previous studies had suggested that the effects of linguistic experience on phonetic perception occur at about 1 year of age (Werker, 1991), coinciding with the age at which children begin to acquire word meanings. It was thus proposed that the change from a language-universal pattern of phonetic perception to one that is language-specific was brought about by the emergence of a milestone in the child's linguistic development, namely, the child's understanding that phonetic units are used contrastively to specify different word meanings. These results show that the initial appearance of a language-specific pattern of phonetic perception does not depend on the emergence of contrastive phonology and an understanding of word meaning. Rather, infants' language-specific phonetic categories may initially emerge from an underlying cognitive capacity and proclivity to store in memory biologically important stimuli, such as faces, voices, and speech (Barrera & Maurer, 1981; DeCasper & Fifer, 1980; Mehler et al., 1988), and the ability to store representations of complex information in some form (shown here for speech; see Bomba & Siqueland, 1983, and Strauss, 1979, for faces and visual patterns).

listeners of English cannot, for example, judge the goodness of a Swedish front-rounded vowel—one not contained in their own native language. This suggests that the speech representations stored in long-term memory are those of the native language only. When listeners rate a vowel from a foreign language, they either declare it "out of their language" (as American adults listening to the Swedish /y/ were forced to do because it was insufficiently close to any stored representation in their vowel system) or, in the case in which the foreign vowel is close to one in their own language, reference it to one or more of the stored representations of the vowels in their own language (as Swedish adults did when they listened to the American English /i/).

Prototypes Function Like Perceptual Magnets. These experiments addressed the effects of a prototypic stimulus on the perception of other members of the category. The results showed that adults' perception of speech stimuli was strongly affected by prototypicality: When the prototype of the category served as the referent, the other members of the category were perceived as very similar to it. The prototype perceptually assimilated near neighbors in the category, effectively reducing the perceptual distance between it and the other members of the category. The nonprototype of the category did not function in this way. Thus, the prototype of a speech category plays a special role in perception: It functions like a perceptual magnet.

The magnet effect can be summarized in this way: The perceptual space underlying speech categories is modified such that the perceptual distance around the prototype is reduced in relation to the perceptual space around the nonprototype. Outlying members of a speech category are thus perceptually pulled toward the center of the category. This "warping" of the perceptual space underlying vowels may be due to attentional mechanisms (e.g., Nosofsky, 1986, 1987).

The magnet effect may help account for other results in adult and infant speech perception such as those related to the perception of sounds from a foreign language, and specific results on adults' attempts to learn a second language. These studies suggest that a speech sound from a foreign language that is similar, but not identical, to one in the subject's own native language is perceptually assimilated to the native language sound (Best, McRoberts, & Sithole, 1988; Flege, 1987). Moreover, the magnet effect may help explain why Japanese adults have such difficulty with the English /r/ and /l/. These two sounds are both members of the same phonetic category in Japanese and may both be assimilated to the Japanese adults' native language prototype. Finally, research shows that infants tested at 10 to 12 months of age fail to detect the difference between two foreign-language sounds that they could discriminate earlier in life (Werker, Gilbert, Humphrey, & Tees, 1981). This may be the result of native-language representations that assimilate both of the foreign-language sounds. In other words, the hypothesis may be advanced that the results of these cross-language tests in adults and infants are themselves attributable to the representation's perceptual magnet effect.

Native-Language Speech Prototypes Exist in Infants at 6 Months of Age. The results of the initial tests here in America and the cross-language tests both here and in Sweden suggest that speech is, at least in some primitive form, mentally represented by infants at a very early age. The infants tested in the cross-language experiment conducted in America and Sweden were only 6 months of age. Yet they already show the effects of linguistic experience when tested on the perceptual magnet effect. For each language group, the perceptual magnet effect was greatest for the native language sound. Foreign language sounds have, by 6 months, begun to function like nonprototypes in the native language. The inference is that infants have had sufficient exposure to the ambient language to form some primitive representation in long-term memory of at least some of the vowels of their native language.

Speech Prototypes Do Not Exist in Monkeys. The data provided here show that the phonetic categories of young infants are structured in a way that diverges from that of monkeys. The present results thus differ from those obtained previously when comparing infants' and animals' reactions to speech signals (see Kuhl, 1987, for review). The present experiments tapped the internal structure and the psychological organization of speech categories—the centers of speech categories—whereas previous tests focused on the boundaries between speech categories. The suggestion provided here is that certain boundaries of speech continua may be inherent to basic auditory processing but that the centers providing internal organization to speech categories may require more than this. Isolating the particular level at which differences exist between species helps clarify both the evolutionary foundation and the subsequent emergence of the speech system. The study of speech prototypes may thus provide a particularly fruitful way to examine the "initial state" of the speech code and reveal how this, in conjunction with exposure to the ambient language, leads to the adult's mature species-specific representation of speech.

Future Experiments and a Return to Theory

Are Speech Prototypes Innate?

How do prototypes get into the mind of a 6-month-old infant? By 6 months of age, infants tested in the cross-language experiment demonstrated a significantly stronger perceptual magnet effect for vowels contained in the ambient language (Kuhl et al., 1992). This could be interpreted to mean that infants develop speech prototypes in response to language input, thus supporting the learning account. However, it is also possible that infants at birth will show the perceptual magnet effect for vowels (some, if not all vowels) and that these innate tendencies have already been altered by linguistic experience. We are currently involved in tests on younger infants in order to test whether the perceptual magnet effect exists in infants who are younger than 6 months. These tests will inform us as to the "initial state" of infants' responses to prototypic vowels, both native and foreign vowels, and compare their responses to prototypes as opposed to nonprototypes (stimuli that are not prototypic of a vowel in any language). If the prototypes of all vowels (native- and foreign-language) initially show the magnet effect, and prototypes always show a greater magnet effect than nonprototypes, then prototypes for speech are not learned entities. They are either the result of inherent psychoacoustic or specialized speech processing that exists at birth. However, if native- and foreign-language prototypes initially show the effect to the same degree as nonprototypes, then that would provide strong support for the idea that prototypes are learned. Regardless of the outcomes of these experiments, however, these new cross-language results support the hypothesis that by 6 months of age, infants have had sufficient experience with the ambient language to show a measurable effect of language input on perception. That 6 months of listening experience is sufficient is quite remarkable.

What Makes a Vowel a Prototype?

Left to be determined in future experiments is the underlying nature of speech representations. Are they psychoacoustic entities, entities innately specified by a speech module, or learned entities? And what form do these representations take? Are they statistical averages restructured by listeners, or lists of real exemplars experienced by listeners? One cannot say, at this point, which is the most apt description. Two kinds of experiments are critical. Experiments on younger infants, described earlier, which compare their responses to native-language prototypes, native-language nonprototypes, and foreign-language prototypes are important. They will clarify the initial state of infants' responses to speech prototypes, and this will help determine whether certain speech sounds have special status at birth. Experiments on adults from different language backgrounds in which psychoacoustic task factors are manipulated will reveal the degree to which prototypes are psychoacoustically special. At present, a variety of discrimination designs are being used to assess the degree to which the magnet effect can be attributed to sensory as opposed to long-term memory factors. Additional experiments are under way that will examine the form that speech representations take.

Psychoacoustics and Speech Revisited

Psychoacoustics can and has contributed powerful methods and theories to the study of speech perception. It has been extremely helpful to have converging evidence showing that speech perception capitalizes on sensory thresholds that exist at birth, independent of experience. What is now necessary is for psychoacousticians to take the next step and tackle the issue that gives the area of speech perception its greatest current challenge—the fact that speech perception is profoundly altered by linguistic experience. Humans' perception of speech is alterable by language input early in life, presumably due to a cognitively powerful memory system that is affected by early listening experience. Both the psychoacoustic and higher-order processes involved in this change have to be understood in order to develop a comprehensive account of both the sensory and cognitive processes involved in speech perception. Such an account would constitute a *general* sensory and cognitive theory of speech perception rather than a *specialized* module account.

References

Abramson, A. S., & Lisker, L. (1970). Discriminability along the voicing continuum: Cross-language tests. *Proceedings of the Sixth International Congress of Phonetic Sciences: Prague, 1967* (pp. 569–573). Prague: Academia.

Ades, A. E. (1977). Theoretical notes: Vowels, consonants, speech, and non-speech. *Psychological Review*, *84*, 524–530.

Barrera, M. E., & Maurer, D. (1981). Recognition of mother's photographed face by the three-month-old infant. *Child Development*, *52*, 714–716.

Best, C. T., McRoberts, G. W., & Sithole, N. M. (1988). Examination of perceptual reorganization for nonnative speech contrasts: Zulu click discrimination by English-speaking adults and infants. *Journal of Experimental Psychology: Human Perception and Performance*, *14*, 345–360.

Bomba, P. C., & Siqueland, E. R. (1983). The nature and structure of infant form categories. *Journal of Experimental Child Psychology*, *35*, 294–328.

Bornstein, M. H. (1981). Two kinds of perceptual organization near the beginning of life. In W. A. Collins (Ed.), *The Minnesota Symposia on Child Psychology: Vol. 14. Aspects of the development of competence* (pp. 39–91). Hillsdale, NJ: Erlbaum.

Braida, L. D., Lim, J. S., Berliner, J. E., Durlach, N. I., Rabinowitz, W. M., & Purks, S. R. (1984). Intensity perception. XIII. Perceptual anchor model of context-coding. *Journal of the Acoustical Society of America*, *76*, 722–731.

Burns, E. M., & Ward, W. D. (1978). Categorical perception—phenomenon or epiphenomenon: Evidence from experiments in the perception of melodic musical intervals. *Journal of the Acoustical Society of America*, *63*, 456–468.

Cutting, J. E., & Rosner, B. S. (1974). Categories and boundaries in speech and music. *Perception & Psychophysics*, *16*, 564–570.

DeCasper, A. J., & Fifer, W. P. (1980). Of human bonding: Newborns prefer their mothers' voices. *Science*, *208*, 1174–1176.

Diehl, R. L., & Walsh, M. A. (1989). An auditory basis for the stimulus-length effect in the perception of stops and glides. *Journal of the Acoustical Society of America*, *85*, 2154–2164.

Durlach, N. I., & Braida, L. D. (1969). Intensity perception. I. Preliminary theory of intensity resolution. *Journal of the Acoustical Society of America*, *46*, 372–383.

Eimas, P. D., Miller, J. L., & Jusczyk, P. W. (1987). On infant speech perception and the acquisition of language. In S. Harnad (Ed.), *Categorical perception: The groundwork of cognition* (pp. 161–195). Cambridge, England: Cambridge University Press.

Flege, J. E. (1987). The production of "new" and "similar" phones in a foreign language: Evidence for the effect of equivalence classification. *Journal of Phonetics*, *15*, 47–65.

Fodor, J. A. (1983). *The modularity of mind: An essay on faculty psychology*. Cambridge, MA: MIT Press.

Fujisaki, H., & Kawashima, T. (1969). *On the modes and mechanisms of speech perception*. Annual Report of the Engineering Research Institute, Faculty of Engineering, University of Tokyo.

Fujisaki, H., & Kawashima, T. (1970). *Some experiments on speech perception and a model for the perceptual mechanism*. Annual Report of the Engineering Research Institute, Faculty of Engineering, University of Tokyo.

Garner, W. R. (1974). *The processing of information and structure*. Potomac, MD: Erlbaum.

Goldman, D., & Homa, D. (1977). Integrative and metric properties of abstracted information as a function of category discriminability, instance variability, and experience. *Journal of Experimental Psychology: Human Learning and Memory*, *3*, 375–385.

Goto, H. (1971). Auditory perception by normal Japanese adults of the sounds "l" and "r". *Neuropsychologia*, *9*, 317–323.

Green, D. M., & Swets, J. A. (1966). *Signal detection theory and psychophysics*. New York: Wiley.

Grieser, D., & Kuhl, P. K. (1989). Categorization of speech by infants: Support for speech-sound prototypes. *Developmental Psychology*, *25*, 577–588.

Hillenbrand, J. (1983). Perceptual organization of speech sounds by infants. *Journal of Speech and Hearing Research*, *26*, 268–282.

Hillenbrand, J. (1984). Speech perception by infants: Categorization based on nasal consonant place of articulation. *Journal of the Acoustical Society of America*, *75*, 1613–1622.

Jakobson, R., Fant, C. G. M., & Halle, M. (1969). *Preliminaries to speech analysis: The distinctive features and their correlates*. Cambridge, MA: MIT Press.

Kuhl, P. K. (1976). Speech perception in early infancy: The acquisition of speech-sound categories. In S. K. Hirsh, D. H. Eldredge, I. J. Hirsh, & S. R. Silverman (Eds.), *Hearing and Davis: Essays honoring Hallowell Davis* (pp. 265–280). St. Louis, MO: Washington University Press.

Kuhl, P. K. (1979a). Models and mechanisms in speech perception: Species comparisons provide further contributions. *Brain, Behavior and Evolution*, *16*, 374–408.

Kuhl, P. K. (1979b). Speech perception in early infancy: Perceptual constancy for spectrally dissimilar vowel categories. *Journal of the Acoustical Society of America*, *66*, 1668–1679.

Kuhl, P. K. (1980). Perceptual constancy for speech-sound categories in early infancy. In G. H. Yeni-Komshian, J. F. Kavanagh, & C. A. Ferguson (Eds.), *Child phonology: Vol. 2. Perception* (pp. 41–66). New York: Academic Press.

Kuhl, P. K. (1981). Discrimination of speech by nonhuman animals: Basic auditory sensitivities conducive to the perception of speech-sound categories. *Journal of the Acoustical Society of America*, *70*, 340–349.

Kuhl, P. K. (1983). Perception of auditory equivalence classes for speech in early infancy. *Infant Behavior and Development*, *6*, 263–285.

Kuhl, P. K. (1985a). Categorization of speech by infants. In J. Mehler & R. Fox (Eds.), *Neonate cognition: Beyond the blooming buzzing confusion* (pp. 231–262). Hillsdale, NJ: Erlbaum.

Kuhl, P. K. (1985b). Methods in the study of infant speech perception. In G. Gottlieb & N. Krasnegor (Eds.), *Measurement of audition and vision in the first year of postnatal life: A methodological overview* (pp. 223–251). Norwood, NJ: Ablex.

Kuhl, P. K. (1986a). Reflections on infants' perception and representation of speech. In J. S. Perkell & D. H. Klatt (Eds.), *Invariance and variability in speech processes* (pp. 19–30). Hillsdale, NJ: Erlbaum.

Kuhl, P. K. (1986b). Theoretical contributions of tests on animals to the special-mechanisms debate in speech. *Experimental Biology*, *45*, 233–265.

Kuhl, P. K. (1987). The special-mechanisms debate in speech research: Categorization tests on animals and infants. In S. Harnad (Ed.), *Categorical perception: The groundwork of cognition* (pp. 355–386). Cambridge, England: Cambridge University Press.

Kuhl, P. K. (1988). Auditory perception and the evolution of speech. *Human Evolution*, *3*, 19–43.

Kuhl, P. K. (1990). Towards a new theory of the development of speech perception. In H. Fujisaki (Ed.), *Proceedings of the International Conference on Spoken Language Processing* (pp. 745–748). Tokyo: The Acoustical Society of Japan.

Kuhl, P. K. (1991). Human adults and human infants show a "perceptual magnet effect" for the prototypes of speech categories, monkeys do not. *Perception & Psychophysics*, *50*, 93–107.

Kuhl, P. K., & Miller, J. D. (1975). Speech perception by the chinchilla: Voiced-voiceless distinction in alveolar plosive consonants. *Science*, *190*, 69–72.

Kuhl, P. K., & Miller, J. D. (1978). Speech perception by the chinchilla: Identification functions for synthetic VOT stimuli. *Journal of the Acoustical Society of America*, *63*, 905–917.

Kuhl, P. K., & Padden, D. M. (1982). Enhanced discriminability at the phonetic boundaries for the voicing feature in macaques. *Perception & Psychophysics*, *32*, 542–550.

Kuhl, P. K., & Padden, D. M. (1983). Enhanced discriminability at the phonetic boundaries for the place feature in macaques. *Journal of the Acoustical Society of America*, *73*, 1003–1010.

Kuhl, P. K., Williams, K. A., Lacerda, F., Stevens, K. N., & Lindblom, B. (1992). Linguistic experience alters phonetic perception in infants by 6 months of age. *Science*, *255*, 606–608.

Liberman, A. M., Cooper, F. S., Shankweiler, D. P., & Studdert-Kennedy, M. (1967). Perception of the speech code. *Psychological Review*, *74*, 431–461.

Liberman, A. M., Harris, K. S., Hoffman, H. S., & Griffith, B. C. (1957). The discrimination of speech sounds within and across phoneme boundaries. *Journal of Experimental Psychology*, *54*, 358–368.

Lieberman, P. (1991). *Uniquely human: Speech, thought, and selfless behavior*. Cambridge, MA: Harvard University Press.

Logan, J. S., Lively, S. E., & Pisoni, D. B. (1991). Training Japanese listeners to identify English /r/ and /l/: A first report. *Journal of the Acoustical Society of America*, *89*, 874–886.

MacKain, K. S., Best, C. T., & Strange, W. (1981). Categorical perception of English /r/ and /l/ by Japanese bilinguals. *Applied Psycholinguistics*, *2*, 369–390.

Macmillan, N. A., Goldberg, R. F., & Braida, L. D. (1988). Resolution for speech sounds: Basic sensitivity and context memory on vowel and consonant continua. *Journal of the Acoustical Society of America*, *84*, 1262–1280.

Macmillan, N. A., Kaplan, H. L., & Creelman, C. D. (1977). The psychophysics of categorical perception. *Psychological Review*, *84*, 452–471.

Massaro, D. W. (1987). *Speech perception by ear and eye: A paradigm for psychological inquiry*. Hillsdale, NJ: Erlbaum.

Medin, D. L., & Barsalou, L. W. (1987). Categorization processes and categorical perception. In S. Harnad (Ed.), *Categorical perception: The groundwork of cognition* (pp. 455–490). New York: Cambridge University Press.

Mehler, J., Jusczyk, P., Lambertz, G., Halsted, N., Bertoncini, J., & Amiel-Tison, C. (1988). A precursor of language acquisition in young infants. *Cognition*, *29*, 143–178.

Mervis, C. B., & Rosch, E. (1981). Categorization of natural objects. *Annual Review of Psychology*, *32*, 89–115.

Miller, G. A. (1956). The magical number seven, plus or minus two: Some limits on our capacity for processing information. *Psychological Review*, *63*, 81–97.

Miller, J. D., Wier, C. C., Pastore, R. E., Kelly, W. J., & Dooling, R. J. (1976). Discrimination and labeling of noise-buzz sequences with varying noise-lead times: An example of categorical perception. *Journal of the Acoustical Society of America*, *60*, 410–417.

Miller, J. L. (1977). Properties of feature detectors for VOT: The voiceless channel of analysis. *Journal of the Acoustical Society of America*, *62*, 641–648.

Miller, J. L., Connine, C. M., Schermer, T. M., & Kluender, K. R. (1983). A possible auditory basis for internal structure of phonetic categories. *Journal of the Acoustical Society of America*, *73*, 2124–2133.

Miller, J. L., & Liberman, A. M. (1979). Some effects of later-occurring information on the perception of stop consonant and semivowel. *Perception & Psychophysics*, *25*, 457–465.

Miller, J. L., & Volaitis, L. E. (1989). Effect of speaking rate on the perceptual structure of a phonetic category. *Perception & Psychophysics*, *46*, 505–512.

Miyawaki, K., Strange, W., Verbrugge, R., Liberman, A. M., Jenkins, J. J., & Fujimura, O. (1975). An effect of linguistic experience: The discrimination of [r] and [l] by native speakers of Japanese and English. *Perception & Psychophysics*, *18*, 331–340.

Mochizuki, M. (1981). The identification of /r/ and /l/ in natural and synthesized speech. *Journal of Phonetics*, *9*, 283–303.

Morse, P. A., & Snowdon, C. T. (1975). An investigation of categorical speech discrimination by rhesus monkeys. *Perception & Psychophysics*, *17*, 9–16.

Nosofsky, R. M. (1986). Attention, similarity, and the identification-categorization relationship. *Journal of Experimental Psychology: General*, *115*, 39–57.

Nosofsky, R. (1987). Attention and learning processes in the identification and categorization of integral stimuli. *Journal of Experimental Psychology: Learning, Memory and Cognition*, *15*, 700–708.

Oden, G. C., & Massaro, D. W. (1978). Integration of featural information in speech perception. *Psychological Review*, *85*, 172–191.

Pastore, R. E., Ahroon, W. A., Baffuto, K. J., Friedman, C., Puleo, J. S., & Fink, E. A. (1977). Common-factor model of categorical perception. *Journal of Experimental Psychology: Human Perception and Performance*, *3*, 686–696.

Pisoni, D. B. (1973). Auditory and phonetic codes in the discrimination of consonants and vowels. *Perception & Psychophysics*, *13*, 253–260.

Pisoni, D. B. (1975). Auditory short-term memory and vowel perception. *Memory and Cognition*, *3*, 7–18.

Pisoni, D. B. (1977). Identification and discrimination of the relative onset time of two component tones: Implications for voicing perception in stops. *Journal of the Acoustical Society of America*, *61*, 1352–1361.

Pisoni, D. B., Carrell, T. D., & Gans, S. J. (1983). Perception of the duration of rapid spectrum changes in speech and nonspeech signals. *Perception & Psychophysics*, *34*, 314–322.

Repp, B. H. (1977). Dichotic competition of speech sounds: The role of acoustic stimulus structure. *Journal of Experimental Psychology: Human Perception and Performance*, *3*, 37–50.

Repp, B. (1984). Categorical perception: Issues, methods, findings. In N. J. Lass (Ed.), *Speech and language: Vol. 10. Advances in basic research and practice* (pp. 243–335). New York: Academic Press.

Rosch, E. (1975). Cognitive reference points. *Cognitive Psychology*, *7*, 532–547.

Rosch, E. H. (1977). Human categorization. In N. Warren (Ed.), *Studies in cross-cultural psychology: Vol. 1* (pp. 1–49). San Francisco: Academic Press.

Rosen, S., & Howell, P. (1987). Auditory, articulatory and learning explanations of categorical perception in speech. In S. Harnad (Ed.), *Categorical perception: The groundwork of cognition* (pp. 113–160). Cambridge, England: Cambridge University Press.

Samuel, A. G. (1982). Phonetic prototypes. *Perception & Psychophysics*, *31*, 307–314.

Schouten, M. E. H. (1987). Speech perception and the role of long-term memory. In M. E. H. Schouten (Ed.), *The psychophysics of speech perception* (pp. 66–79). Boston: Nijhoff.

Sheldon, A., & Strange, W. (1982). The acquisition of /r/ and /l/ by Japanese learners of English: Evidence that speech production can precede speech perception. *Applied Psycholinguistics*, *3*, 243–261.

Stevens, E. B., Kuhl, P. K., & Padden, D. M. (1988). *Macaques show context effects in speech perception*. Paper presented at the 116th meeting of the Acoustical Society of America, Honolulu, HI.

Stevens, K. N. (1972). The quantal nature of speech: Evidence from articulatory-acoustic data. In E. E. David & P. B. Denes (Eds.), *Human communication: A unified view* (pp. 51–66). New York: McGraw-Hill.

Stevens, K. N. (1981). Constraints imposed by the auditory system on the properties used to classify speech sounds: Data from phonology, acoustics and psychoacoustics. In T. F. Myers, J. Laver, & J. Anderson (Eds.), *The cognitive representation of speech* (pp. 61–74). Amsterdam: North Holland.

Stevens, S. S., Volkmann, J., & Newman, E. B. (1937). A scale for the measurement of the psychological magnitude pitch. *Journal of the Acoustical Society of America*, *8*, 185–190.

Strange, W., & Dittmann, S. (1984). Effects of discrimination training on the perception of /r-l/ by Japanese adults learning English. *Perception & Psychophysics*, *36*, 131–145.

Strauss, M. S. (1979). Abstraction of prototypical information by adults and 10-month-old infants. *Journal of Experimental Psychology: Human Learning and Memory*, *5*, 618–632.

Waters, R. S., & Wilson, W. A., Jr. (1976). Speech perception by rhesus monkeys: The voicing distinction in synthesized labial and velar stop consonants. *Perception & Psychophysics*, *19*, 285–289.

Werker, J. (1991). The ontogeny of speech perception. In I. G. Mattingly & M. Studdert-Kennedy (Eds.), *Modularity and the motor theory of speech perception* (pp. 91–109). Hillsdale, NJ: Erlbaum.

Werker, J. F., Gilbert, J. H. V., Humphrey, K., & Tees, R. C. (1981). Developmental aspects of cross-language speech perception. *Child Development*, *52*, 349–355.

Werker, J. F., & Logan, J. S. (1985). Cross-language evidence for three factors in speech perception. *Perception & Psychophysics*, *37*, 35–44.

CHAPTER 13

Bridging the Gap Between Developmental Psychoacoustics and Pediatric Audiology

Arlene Earley Carney

This volume focuses on developmental psychoacoustics in a number of contexts, including those of anatomical and physiological correlates, results from adult studies, speech perception, and other sensory systems. In this chapter, a new context is explored, that of pediatric audiology. In effect, attention will turn to the application of the information acquired from developmental psychoacoustics to the actual assessment and management of hearing-impaired infants and children.

A fundamental difference between psychoacoustics and audiology is in their primary focuses. The focus of psychoacoustics is to define the perceptual capacity of a given population. In contrast, the focus of audiology is to define the perceptual capacity of a particular listener. Furthermore, having identified this individual perceptual capacity and its deficit, the audiologist must try to maximize it for the listener.

The preparation of this chapter was partially supported by NIH-NIDCD P60 DC00982.

The basic link between the two fields is the audiologist's use of the normative data provided by psychoacoustics. Specifically, audiologists determine how the perceptual capacity of a particular listener differs from that of the normal population. Pediatric audiologists must consider both how normally hearing infants and children differ from adults with normal hearing, and how hearing-impaired children subsequently differ from children with normal hearing.

The purpose of this chapter is to discuss how the fields of developmental psychoacoustics and pediatric audiology are related currently and how their relationship should grow in the future. For the purposes of this discussion, I will include both research and clinical practice as integral parts of pediatric audiology. I hope that, as a result of this discussion, developmental psychoacousticians might see further questions to intrigue them concerning hearing-impaired children and that audiologists might attempt to broaden their applications of techniques and results from developmental psychoacoustics.

In its most generic sense, psychoacoustics is the study of auditory function in listeners. In its purest form as a basic science, psychoacoustics may be regarded as the study of auditory function in adults with normal hearing. However, there has already been an extensive application of psychoacoustic paradigms to the study of listeners with hearing losses—once again, primarily in hearing-impaired adults. These studies have focused on how hearing-impaired listeners differ from normal listeners in areas such as frequency resolution, temporal coding, and binaural processing, (e.g., Carney & Nelson, 1983; Fitzgibbons & Wightman, 1982; Florentine, Buus, Scharf, & Zwicker, 1980; Jesteadt, Bilger, Green, & Patterson, 1976; Smoski & Trahiotis, 1986; Wightman, McGee, & Kramer, 1977). As discussed by McFadden and Wightman (1983), these studies of hearing-impaired listeners have had to deal with a number of problematic issues, such as stimulus level (either in sound pressure level or sensation level) and large inter- and intrasubject variability. These authors concluded that, in contrast to the field of vision in which studies of pathology contributed new information about normal vision, investigations of listeners with auditory pathologies have not provided many new insights into normal auditory processing.

Recently, a great deal has been said about the extension of psychoacoustics in a developmental direction in order to consider auditory function in infants and children with normal hearing. This extension has brought its own problematic issues, discussed in previous papers in this volume in some detail, including nonsensory and/or nonauditory factors such as memory, attention, habituation, and fatigue on the part of the subjects. What is missing to a great extent is data for those infants and children for whom hearing loss and development are combined, along with all their problematic sensory and nonsensory issues.

Whether there will be a growth of investigation by developmental psychoacousticians for this hearing-impaired population is not clear. However, because audiology is the discipline in which auditory pathology is treated as a communication disorder, it is true that hearing-impaired children, the potential subjects of these studies, will fall to pediatric audiology for assessment, management, and research for the present time.

There are three main focuses in this chapter: (a) subject samples, (b) testing procedures, and (c) priorities for future research in both fields as they relate to hearing-impaired infants and children. With these three topics, researchers can examine who is and is not being studied now; how infants and children are being tested, and how those approaches might be altered; and finally, what the broader questions are that emerge in the areas of developmental psychoacoustics and pediatric audiology.

Subject Samples

There is an interesting uniformity in subject selection in all of the developmental psychoacoustics literature, despite the wide variety of procedures, stimuli, and tasks used. The criteria for exclusion of subjects, as compiled from the work of Werner and her associates (Olsho, 1984, 1985; Olsho, Koch, Carter, Halpin, & Spetner, 1988; Olsho, Koch, Halpin, & Carter, 1987; Spetner & Olsho, 1990); Trehub, Schneider, and associates (Schneider, Trehub, & Thorpe, 1991; Trehub, 1987; Trehub, Schneider, & Endman, 1980), Sinnott, Pisoni, and Aslin (1983); Sinnott and Aslin (1985); Clarkson and Clifton (1985); Clarkson, Clifton, and Perris (1988); and others are given later.

The exclusion criteria include: (a) indication of hearing loss, (b) family history of hearing loss, (c) active middle ear pathology, (d) presence of other handicapping conditions, and (e) prenatal and perinatal abnormalities, including preterm birth. As a result, despite other differences between investigations, the samples of infants chosen for study in developmental psychoacoustics are remarkably homogeneous. In effect, they represent an elite sample of normal infant listeners. Interestingly, these exclusionary criteria include many of the risk factors listed in the High Risk Register from the Joint Committee on Infant Hearing (1991). Consequently, the very children who are excluded from developmental studies of hearing are those referred to audiologists for the evaluation of their auditory abilities. It is clear that the populations to be tested to date in studies of developmental psychoacoustics and pediatric audiology (as well as in clinical practice) are generally mutually exclusive. This difference in subject samples is likely to be an important factor in choosing appropriate test procedures and in making interpretations of results, as I will discuss later.

An examination of these investigations cited above also shows an interesting pattern of subject retention. Even for these selected normal subjects, a substantial percentage (up to approximately 30–50% in some investigations, e.g., Nozza, 1987; Spetner & Olsho, 1990) did not complete the target experiment. Subjects did not complete the studies because of fussiness, crying, inattention, sleepiness, or failure to meet the training criterion. It seems likely that these factors that terminate test sessions for normal infants will occur at least as frequently and may have an even higher incidence in the population of infants with hearing losses, actual or suspected. Yet infants and children suspected of having a hearing loss cannot be excluded from testing or any follow-up procedures, regardless of their level of cooperation and attention.

One concern expressed frequently in the developmental psychoacoustics literature is the interference of nonsensory (in this case, nonauditory) factors with the measurement of hearing. Such nonsensory factors will clearly have an even greater impact in a population of children with multiple handicaps.

Boys Town National Research Hospital, in cooperation with local area school districts, has established a special, longstanding program for early intervention with hearing-impaired infants, called the Diagnostic Early Intervention Program (DEIP). In this program, infants are followed by a multidisciplinary team of professionals who evaluate a large number of factors, including degree of hearing loss, age at identification, age of amplification, speech and language development, family system, and medical status (Moeller, Coufal, & Hixon, 1990). In an analysis of the hearing-impaired infants enrolled in this program, 38% of them had at least one other handicapping condition (Brookhouser & Moeller, 1986). These included visual, intellectual, and motor deficits that were often detected during the first 6 months of follow-up. This percentage of multiple handicaps is representative of that found across other parts of the country. Consequently, expectations for training these infants and children to come under stimulus control and to finish a test protocol in an assessment paradigm may have to be altered.

In contrast to the homogeneity of the normally hearing infant and child subjects in studies of developmental psychoacoustics, the population of hearing-impaired infants and children is extremely heterogeneous and is becoming more so over time (Matkin, 1988). This heterogeneity includes range and etiology of hearing loss, fluctuating hearing loss, as well as the presence of other handicapping conditions mentioned earlier. It is very likely that studies of hearing-impaired children will demonstrate the same intra- and intersubject variability problems seen in the hearing-impaired adult studies. These studies will also contain the developmental variability seen in studies of infants and children with normal hearing. This compound variability will make generalizations to the hearing-impaired pediatric population as a whole difficult.

Nevertheless, an important outcome of studies of developmental psychoacoustics for application to pediatric audiology will be the definition of "normal threshold" for infants and children. Clearly, there is consensus among investigators that detection thresholds of infants and children obtained behaviorally improve with age until they reach adult values (Berg & Smith, 1983; Elliott & Katz, 1980; Nozza & Wilson, 1984; Olsho et al., 1988; Schneider et al., 1991; Sinnott, et al., 1983; Trehub & Schneider, 1983; Trehub, Schneider, Morrongiello, & Thorpe, 1988). However, the specific adult–child threshold differences vary from study to study, depending upon the stimuli, procedure, and condition (i.e., soundfield or headphone). Similarly, there are differences in these same parameters in clinical pediatric testing (Diefendorf, 1988; Wilson & Gerber, 1983). At the present time, there does not appear to be a recommended correction factor to be applied to infant and child data relative to normal adult thresholds calibrated in either sound pressure level or hearing level. The question is: Should such a correction be made, and if so, how much should it be at different frequencies or for what different stimuli? These questions are particularly important in determining whether an infant or child patient has passed or failed some screening level that separates normal hearing from mild hearing loss.

Testing Procedures

Because of all the differences noted between children with normal and impaired hearing, there are a number of procedural variables to be considered for assessing hearing-impaired infants and children, either in psychoacoustic studies or in the clinical practice of audiology. Some of these are global and vary across paradigms; others are specific to individual paradigms. Both types of issues are addressed in the following section.

General Procedural Differences

Training

Despite the variety of procedures for testing hearing in infants and children, another uniform aspect of these investigations is the training of subjects prior to the start of a study. This is a particularly crucial aspect of the work, and its outcome determines whether the infant or child remains in the study. Regardless of the particular psychoacoustic paradigm to be used or the auditory ability to be measured, infants are presented with a suprathreshold stimulus at sensation levels that vary from approximately 30–50 dB (e.g., Sinnott et al., 1983; Trehub et al., 1980). Infants are trained at levels that are comfortably loud (as judged by adult listeners) and well within their dynamic range (Nozza & Wilson, 1984; Olsho et al., 1988; Schneider et al., 1991; Trehub & Schneider, 1983).

It is in the area of training that the problem of stimulus level first appears in testing hearing-impaired children. When a very young infant is suspected of having a hearing loss, electrophysiological testing (i.e., assessing the click-evoked auditory brainstem response [ABR]) is frequently done before behavioral testing is attempted. These electrophysiological results can then be compared to clinical norms established for normally developing and premature infants (Gorga, Kaminski, Beauchaine, Jesteadt, & Neely, 1989; Gorga, Reiland, Beauchaine, Worthington, & Jesteadt, 1987). As a result of this testing, the audiologist has some notion of the starting level necessary for training for behavioral testing. In cases where profound hearing loss is suspected, there may only be a limited dynamic range between detection and the limits of the test equipment. Consequently, training may be started, inadvertently or by necessity, near or even at threshold, rather than at the sensation levels used in studies of developmental psychoacoustics. Thus, it may be difficult or impossible to bring some young profoundly hearing-impaired infants under stimulus control during the first few test sessions. For these children, alternative stimuli and sensory systems (e.g., vibrotactile stimuli delivered through a bone vibrator) may be used to establish stimulus control with training. When such approaches are necessary, or when the starting stimulus level has to be established in multiple trials, response variability, as well as deviation from protocols established in studies of developmental psychoacoustics, is quickly evident.

Measurement of Psychometric Functions

Across studies of developmental sensitivity changes, investigators have measured psychometric functions (the proportion of hits as a function of level; Berg & Smith, 1983; Olsho et al., 1988; Trehub & Schneider, 1983). Once again, in studies of hearing-impaired children and infants, it is likely that the psychometric function may be compressed dramatically and shifted to the right because of hearing loss. In addition, there may well be no 100% point on the curve (previously observed for some normally hearing infants, for example, by Olsho et al., 1988) due to both developmental level and elevated threshold.

As a rule in clinical testing, audiologists do not make specific estimates of psychometric functions for detection, although they may note levels at which infants or children respond 100% or 0% of the time, as well as a 50–75% point estimated as threshold. At the present time, there are no data to suggest the potential differences in psychometric functions between infants and children with different degrees of auditory sensitivity. Thus, it is not clear whether audiologists should change their approach and specifically measure psychometric functions in routine pediatric assessments. It is unlikely that the information provided in such functions will affect management decisions for that hearing-impaired infant or child, including type of amplification or intervention program.

False-Alarm Rates

In studies of developmental psychoacoustics, false-alarm rates are measured routinely and are used as exclusionary criteria. In the clinical practice of audiology, false-alarm behavior is noted qualitatively more often than quantitatively. Thus, it is unclear whether hearing-impaired infants and children have higher false-alarm rates than their normally hearing peers or whether their behavior changes over time with development. Such comparisons are even more complicated because normally hearing infants with false-alarm rates higher than about 25% are already excluded from the basic studies of auditory sensitivity in infants (e.g., Olsho et al., 1988). In investigations of hearing-impaired infants and children, using a high false-alarm rate as an exclusionary factor would seriously reduce the available subject pool and compromise any generalization to the population as a whole.

In clinical situations, there is a high likelihood of interaction between false-alarm rates and the training that precedes testing. If training level has not been previously established with ABR results, the tester may actually enhance the pediatric patient's false-alarm rate. Further, higher false-alarm rates may be observed in infants who are highly motivated by the visual reinforcer in procedures such as visual reinforcement audiometry (VRA) or in children who are highly motivated to please the tester.

It is useful, however, to keep track of false-alarm rates as descriptive data for an individual subject, particularly for longitudinal follow-up. In a study of speech discrimination in profoundly hearing-impaired children who received cochlear implants or tactile devices as sensory aids, Carney, Osberger, Robbins, Renshaw, and Miyamoto (1989) measured both hit rates and false-alarm rates in a change/no-change task. Subjects ranged between age 7 and 11 years of age and were all prelingually deafened. The test consisted of nine subtests addressing suprasegmental and segmental speech contrasts. Each subtest had 15 trials, 5 of which were no-change trials. Subjects were asked whether stimuli were all the same or different, or were trained to make a motor response for a change trial. False-alarm rates for individual subjects across subtests ranged from 0–100%, with a modal false-alarm rate of approximately 40% (i.e., a false-alarm response on 2 out of 5 no-change trials). These rates represent a relatively high occurrence of false alarms, far exceeding the rates accepted by investigators in infant studies of hearing. For this study, d' was calculated to determine performance with a particular type of device, a two-channel tactile aid, a single-channel cochlear implant, or a multichannel cochlear implant. Results indicated highest mean d' values for hearing-impaired children with a multichannel cochlear implant, although within group intersubject variability was quite high.

These same children with high false-alarm rates who had received multichannel cochlear implants were followed longitudinally (along with a larger set of children) by Osberger et al., (1991). These investigators reported that many of these same children with high false-alarm rates had achieved perfect performance on a number of subtests over time, indicating zero or near zero false-alarm rates. This provides some evidence for clear change in hearing-impaired children's false-alarm rates over time in discrimination tasks that have become easier as auditory skills increase. To date, most studies that examine change in performance in hearing-impaired children with cochlear implants have focused only on hit rates. Because the measurement of false-alarm data provides new information, it is important to examine them over time, rather than to exclude children with initial high false-alarm rates from investigation. Such studies also provide an impetus for the development of routine clinical measures of detection or speech perception that assess false-alarm rate along with hit rate or percent correct.

Testing of Individual Subjects

The fourth important procedural variable to consider is that of individual subject testing. The majority of data from normal infant auditory testing is a composite of group data. It is not always the case that each subject is tested at each detection frequency or masking condition, for example. Repeated measures appear to be more the exception than the norm. In pediatric audiology, a complete (or nearly complete) audiogram is expected for each patient. Moreover, serial audiograms are collected to determine changes in hearing over time, either in a positive or negative direction. To make more precise comparisons between results from infants with normal and impaired hearing, it would be useful to have detection data collected longitudinally from a group of infants. In addition, data from infants with normal hearing collected over repeated test sessions at different ages would provide further background comparison information for clinicians.

Change in threshold is an important factor for follow-up of hearing-impaired infants and children to determine progression of hearing loss, either from auditory pathology or overamplification. Even for children with mild conductive losses, monitoring changes in hearing loss is important. In a study of hearing aid use and overamplification in hearing-impaired children, Binnie et al. (1983) studied potential changes in detection threshold as a result of use of high-gain hearing aids. For this investigation, children with bilateral hearing impairment were amplified monaurally for the duration of the study (approximately 3 years) to provide a control non-aided hearing-impaired ear. Binnie et al. formulated the following criteria to determine a true change in threshold in an individual child: (a) Threshold shift had to occur in the presence of normal immittance results; (b) the change had to be greater than the standard test step size, 5 dB for clinical purposes; (c) the change had to be greater than two standard deviations from the mean of 10 baseline threshold measures at that test frequency; and (d) the threshold shift had to occur in the ear with a hearing aid and not in the unaided ear. The use of such criteria presumed that extensive baseline testing had been done for each child. However, it did permit the examination of significant changes in detection over time. No significant changes in detection threshold were observed for this group of subjects, nor for any individual subjects participating in the study. Continued formulation of such criteria, based on data, would be useful to pediatric audiologists, particularly for infants and young children.

Normative data from developmental psychoacoustic studies would permit audiologists to see how a hearing-impaired infant's possible improvement in threshold over time may reflect normal changes in auditory or nonsensory factors also observed in normally hearing infants. It would also allow a tester to determine if an infant's hearing impairment was progressive.

In a study of frequency resolution with normally hearing preschool and school-aged children, Allen, Wightman, Kistler, and Dolan (1989) provided a very interesting analysis of trial-by-trial data from subjects. They were able to demonstrate that memory was not a factor in children's performance on a three-alternative, forced-choice task. Through such analysis they were also able to show greater intrasubject variability for younger subjects (age 3–4 years). Such information about normal development in auditory tasks is particularly helpful in analyzing the behavior of young hearing-impaired children and in separating the variability produced by development from that produced by hearing loss.

Specific Procedural Differences

The final procedural issue is concerned with application of particular paradigms for use with hearing-impaired children. It is clear that the VRA procedure has received the most widespread application clinically for testing infants in detection tasks. In addition to the initial work of investigators at University of Washington (Moore, Wilson, & Thompson, 1977; Wilson & Moore, 1978; Wilson & Thompson, 1984) describing the procedure and its application, there have been a number of reports of the application of VRA to clinical research studies. Primus (1987, 1988) has examined aspects of reinforcement and attention in VRA. Gravel and associates (Gravel, 1989) have used VRA with follow-up of infants with high-risk developmental histories. Widen (1990) has described a successful automated VRA screening procedure for following high-risk infants longitudinally. Talbott (1987) has provided both VRA and play audiometry data on the same hearing-impaired children, demonstrating that the technique is an appropriate one for long-term use with hearing-impaired children. In addition, VRA has been successfully applied to children with Down syndrome and general low intellectual function for assessing detection (Greenberg, Wilson, Moore, & Thompson, 1978; Thompson, Wilson, & Moore, 1979).

A particularly interesting application of VRA testing has been described by Eilers and colleagues (Eilers, Miskiel, Ozdamar, Urbano, & Widen, 1991; Eilers, Widen, Urbano, Hudson, & Gonzales, 1991). These investigators described automated VRA procedures for clinical use to reduce the tremendous variability introduced into the clinical testing of infant hearing by different testers and their individual decision rules for accepting responses and providing reinforcement. Eilers, Miskiel, et al. (1991) first demonstrated the applicability of an automated VRA approach through computer simulations of infant performance, using the decision rules they had created. Subsequently, Eilers, Widen, et al. (1991) showed the validity of the approach by comparing simulation results with those from testing real infants with the same set of decision rules. Such automated procedures have the potential to reduce the variability of test results for infants both within and across clinical settings by reducing the variability of one important controllable factor, tester decisions.

In contrast to the frequent use of the VRA paradigm in clinical research and practice, the two-alternative, forced-choice (2AFC) approach described by Trehub, Schneider, and associates (Schneider et al., 1991; Trehub et al., 1980) and the Observer-based Psychoacoustic Procedure (OPP) described by Werner and associates (Olsho et al., 1987) have not yet received widespread acceptance.

The 2AFC approach carries with it the inherent problem of allowing an infant or child listener the possibility of obtaining multiple looks at a given signal because of the nature of the paradigm. Specifically, the signal remains on in this procedure until the infant or child has signaled either a left or right response. This ability to obtain multiple looks may affect the overall shape of the psychometric function (see chapter 7 in this volume) by changing its slope or its asymptote. However, this very factor that affects the shape of the psychometric function may enhance performance for hearing-impaired children on this task. In other words, providing multiple looks for hearing-impaired listeners may reduce variability of performance. This question remains unanswered, because the procedure has not as yet been used with hearing-impaired subjects on a large scale (Trehub, personal communication, 1991). This 2AFC procedure also has promise in the assessment of children with unilateral impairment to address issues of localization and speech discrimination with and without amplification systems, including FM auditory trainers. It is difficult to show the benefit of FM system amplification for children with unilateral hearing impairment in controlled sound-field environments. It would be particularly appropriate to carry out studies of masked speech discrimination for these children to determine how FM units might aid them in difficult listening situations.

The OPP paradigm (Olsho et al., 1987) holds a great deal of promise for clinical testing because of its applicability to infants as young as 3 months of age. The results of studies of normally hearing infants carried out with OPP suggest that multiply handicapped children with developmental levels as low as 3 months might become more reasonable candidates for behavioral testing. Because OPP does not require a head turn, as such, nor any other specific motor response to be observed, it can be adapted for low-functioning children. Even now, these children most frequently receive a combination of electrophysiological testing combined with modified VRA or behavioral observation procedures. Results of the latter are very unsatisfying for pediatric audiologists because of poor test reliability and poor threshold estimates. In a clinically modified OPP paradigm, trained observers could respond to a wide variety of behaviors during a signal trial. In the laboratory version of OPP, the blind observer, who is outside the test booth, indicates when a signal has been presented. The use of a blind observer is not always feasible in clinical practice. However, one could change the blinded observer to be the tester in the booth with the child and caregiver, and the signal could be presented by the tester outside the booth. When the observer in the booth indicates that a signal has been presented, the other tester could present the reinforcement on a signal trial. Although this is not optimal for research applications, it is similar to the modifications made in VRA in clinical practice. As indicated earlier, false-alarm rate could be monitored specifically in this manner, rather than being used as a factor for elimination of subjects. The use of OPP could extend testing to younger infants and those more developmentally disabled.

In addition, OPP can be modified to accommodate more informal testing of infants and young children. Moeller (1984) has described a series of tasks that she calls FAST—the Functional Auditory Skills Test. In this procedure, a number of environmental and speech stimuli are presented to children in detection, discrimination, and recognition tasks. These tasks involve auditory stimuli that may occur in the home or classroom environment to see how skills assessed formally in a test-booth condition transfer over to real situations. This approach is used during the parent/infant (age of identification up to approximately 2 years) management period in particular. Each stimulus is presented at least three and as many as five times. Hits on signal trials are counted. No reinforcement other than social is provided for responding. It is possible to add reinforcement (other than social) to the procedure along with a second observer to assess these functional skills. The use of the OPP is likely to increase the precision and reliability of the FAST.

Priorities for Future Research

I have already mentioned a number of areas where future research is indicated. Intrasubject variability, particularly in young normally hearing infants and children, is a concern. Earlier, I discussed this aspect of testing for detection threshold. It would be useful for pediatric audiologists in planning future assessment and management to know whether a particular child's performance was within expected variability ranges for his or her developmental age or whether this child's performance was more variable than expected.

Clinical audiology has not incorporated many psychoacoustic paradigms in testing hearing-impaired adults in areas of frequency resolution, temporal coding, or intensity discrimination. It is not likely that such areas will be probed for hearing-impaired children. However, clinical research with this population has interesting applications. Training studies with hearing-impaired children have the potential to address the time course of auditory learning in a plastic but disordered system. Historically, audiologists and teachers of the hearing impaired have used a variety of auditory training procedures with hearing-impaired children without necessarily keeping track of the variability of responses, false-alarm rates, or the type of task used.

There is a current and pressing need for developmental work in the area of loudness judgement for application to cochlear implant mapping. After receiving a Nucleus 22-channel cochlear implant, adults must make judgments of equal loudness across electrodes and loudness comfort overall (Skinner et al., 1991). To date, a number of cochlear implant centers for children use rather cognitively demanding tasks to assess loudness comfort, such as comparing the loudness of an electrically presented sound to a glass of water full, half full, and empty, or asking a child to move a sliding switch along a continuum of faces. The construction of paradigms to assess loudness comfort in children would have immediate clinical application for loudness discomfort as well. Several studies (Kawell,

Kopun, & Stelmachowicz, 1988; Macpherson, Elfenbein, Schum, & Bentler, 1991) have used facial drawings and stop and go lights, respectively, with children in these tasks. However, there is a clear need for further work in these more subjective tasks.

Finally, there is some need for combining paradigms and stimuli from developmental psychoacoustics and infant and child speech perception to use with hearing-impaired children. In testing hearing-impaired adults, audiologists generally use a combination of behavioral detection tasks along with word recognition and acoustic immittance tests and/or electrophysiological measures for evaluation. A similar battery is used with children, with varied speech recognition tasks employed. Some development has already taken place in this area. For example, Boothroyd, Springer, Smith, and Schulman (1988) have described the Three Alternative Forced Choice Task (THRIFT) for assessing speech perception in hearing-impaired children age 7 years and above. Researchers have used the change/no-change task for speech perception testing of hearing-impaired children both pre- and postcochlear implant down to age 4 years (Carney et al., 1989; Osberger et al., 1991). These approaches are rooted in both the areas of developmental psychoacoustics and speech perception.

In conclusion, a developmental metaphor is in order. It appears that the disciplines of developmental psychoacoustics and pediatric audiology have been engaged in "parallel play," observing what the other is doing, but not really interacting on a regular basis. In the mutual development of both fields, it appears appropriate to evolve to a level of "cooperative play" in which both disciplines grow as a result of interaction.

References

Allen, P., Wightman, F., Kistler, D., & Dolan, T. (1989). Frequency resolution in children. *Journal of Speech and Hearing Research*, *32*, 317–322.

Berg, K. M., & Smith, M. C. (1983). Behavioral thresholds for tones during infancy. *Journal of Experimental Child Psychology*, *35*, 409–425.

Binnie, C. A., Carney, A. E., Danz, A., Sessler, C. H., Cooper, W. A., Mason, C. R., Feth, L. L., & Klein, A. J. (1983). *The effects of amplification on the residual hearing of children*. Miniseminar presented at the meeting of the American Speech-Language-Hearing Association, Cincinnati, OH.

Boothroyd, A., Springer, N., Smith, L., & Schulman, J. (1988). Amplitude compression and profound hearing loss. *Journal of Speech and Hearing Research*, *31*, 362–376.

Brookhouser, P. E., & Moeller, M. P. (1986). Choosing the appropriate habilitative track for the newly identified hearing-impaired child. *Annals of Otology, Rhinology, & Laryngology*, *95*, 51–59.

Carney, A. E., & Nelson, D. A. (1983). An analysis of psychophysical tuning curves in normal and pathological ears. *Journal of the Acoustical Society of America*, *73*, 268–278.

Carney, A. E., Osberger, M. J., Robbins, A. M., Renshaw, J. J., & Miyamoto, R. T. (1989). A comparison of speech discrimination with cochlear implants and tactile aids. *Journal of the Acoustical Society of America*, *85*, S25(A).

Clarkson, M. G., & Clifton, R. K. (1985). Infant pitch perception: Evidence for responding to pitch categories and the missing fundamental. *Journal of the Acoustical Society of America*, *77*, 1521–1528.

Clarkson, M. G., Clifton, R. K., & Perris, E. E. (1988). Infant timbre perception: Discrimination of spectral envelopes. *Perception & Psychophysics*, *43*, 15–20.

Diefendorf, A. (1988). Behavioral evaluation of hearing-impaired children. In F. H. Bess (Ed.), *Hearing impairment in children* (pp. 133–151). Parkton, MD: York Press.

Eilers, R. E., Miskiel, E., Ozdamar, O., Urbano, R., & Widen, J. E. (1991). Optimization of automated hearing test algorithms: Simulations using an infant response model. *Ear and Hearing*, *12*, 191–198.

Eilers, R. E., Widen, J. E., Urbano, R., Hudson, T., & Gonzales, L. (1991). Optimization of automated hearing test algorithms: A comparison of data from simulations and young children. *Ear and Hearing*, *12*, 199–204.

Elliott, L. L., & Katz, D. R. (1980). Children's pure-tone detection. *Journal of the Acoustical Society of America*, *67*, 343–344.

Fitzgibbons, P., & Wightman, F. L. (1982). Gap detection in normal and hearing-impaired listeners. *Journal of the Acoustical Society of America*, *72*, 761–765.

Florentine, M., Buus, S., Scharf, B., & Zwicker, E. (1980). Frequency selectivity in normally-hearing and hearing-impaired observers. *Journal of Speech and Hearing Research*, *23*, 646–669.

Gorga, M. P., Kaminski, J. R., Beauchaine, K. L., Jesteadt, W., & Neely, S. T. (1989). Auditory brainstem responses from children three months to three years of age: Normal patterns of response II. *Journal of Speech and Hearing Research*, *32*, 281–288.

Gorga, M. P., Reiland, J. K., Beauchaine, K. L., Worthington, D. W., & Jesteadt, W. (1987). Auditory brainstem responses from graduates of an intensive care nursery: Normal patterns of response. *Journal of Speech and Hearing Research*, *30*, 311–318.

Gravel, J. S. (1989). Behavioral assessment of auditory function. *Seminars in Hearing*, *10*, 216–228.

Greenberg, D. B., Wilson, W. R., Moore, J. M., & Thompson, G. (1978). Visual reinforcement audiometry (VRA) with young Down's syndrome children. *Journal of Speech and Hearing Disorders*, *43*, 448–458.

Jesteadt, W., Bilger, R. C., Green, D. M., & Patterson, J. H. (1976). Temporal acuity in listeners with sensorineural hearing loss. *Journal of Speech and Hearing Research*, *19*, 357–360.

Joint Committee on Infant Hearing. (1991). 1990 position statement. *American Speech-Language-Hearing Association*, *33* (Suppl. 5), 3–6.

Kawell, M. E., Kopun, J. G., & Stelmachowicz, P. G. (1988). Loudness discomfort levels in children. *Ear and Hearing*, *9*, 133–136.

Macpherson, B., Elfenbein, J. L., Schum, R., & Bentler, R. A. (1991). Thresholds of discomfort in young children. *Ear and Hearing*, *12*, 184–190.

Matkin, N. D. (1988). Re-evaluating our approach to evaluation: Demographics are changing—Are we? In F. H. Bess (Ed.), *Hearing impairment in children* (pp. 101–111). Parkton, MD: York Press.

McFadden, D., & Wightman, F. L. (1983). Audition: Some relations between normal and pathological hearing. *Annual Review of Psychology*, *34*, 95–128.

Moeller, M. P. (1984). Assessing hearing and speechreading in hearing-impaired children. In D. Sims (Ed.), *Deafness and communication: Assessment and training* (pp. 127–140). Baltimore: Williams & Wilkins.

Moeller, M. P., Coufal, K., & Hixon, P. (1990). The efficacy of speech-language intervention: hearing-impaired children. *Seminars in Speech and Language*, *11*, 227–241.

Moore, J. M., Wilson, W. R., & Thompson, G. (1977). Visual reinforcement of head-turn responses in infants under 12 months of age. *Journal of Speech and Hearing Disorders*, *42*, 328–334.

Nozza, R. J. (1987). The binaural masking level difference in infants and adults: Developmental change in binaural hearing. *Infant Behavior and Development*, *10*, 105–110.

Nozza, R. J., & Wilson, W. R. (1984). Masked and unmasked thresholds of infants and adults: development of auditory frequency selectivity and sensitivity. *Journal of Speech and Hearing Research*, *27*, 613–622.

Olsho, L. W. (1984). Infant frequency discrimination. *Infant Behavior and Development*, *7*, 27–35.

Olsho, L. W. (1985). Infant auditory perception: Tonal masking. *Infant Behavior and Development*, *8*, 371–384.

Olsho, L. W., Koch, E. G., Carter, E. A., Halpin, C. F., & Spetner, N. B. (1988). Pure-tone sensitivity of human infants. *Journal of the Acoustical Society of America*, *84*, 1316–1324.

Olsho, L. W., Koch, E. G., Halpin, C. F., & Carter, E. A. (1987). An observer-based psychoacoustic procedure for use with young infants. *Developmental Psychology*, *5*, 627–640.

Osberger, M. J., Miyamoto, R. T., Zimmerman-Phillips, S., Kemink, J. L., Stroer, B. S., Firszt, J., & Novak, M. A. (1991). Independent evaluation of the speech perception abilities of children with the Nucleus 22-channel cochlear implant system. *Ear and Hearing*, *12*, (Suppl) 665–805.

Primus, M. A. (1987). Response and reinforcement in operant audiometry. *Journal of Speech and Hearing Disorders*, *52*, 294–298.

Primus, M. A. (1988). Infant thresholds with enhanced attention to the signal in visual reinforcement audiometry. *Journal of Speech and Hearing Research*, *31*, 480–485.

Schneider, B. A., Trehub, S. E., and Thorpe L. (1991). Developmental perspectives on the localization and detection of auditory signals. *Perception & Psychophysics*, *49*, 10–20.

Sinnott, J. M., & Aslin, R. N. (1985). Frequency and intensity discrimination in human infants and adults. *Journal of the Acoustical Society of America*, *78*, 1986–1992.

Sinnott, J. M., Pisoni, D. B., & Aslin, R. N. (1983). A comparison of pure tone auditory thresholds in human infants and adults. *Infant Behavior and Development*, *6*, 3–17.

Skinner, M. W., Holden, L. K., Holden, T. A., Dowell, R. C., Seligman, P. M., Brimacombe, J. A., & Beiter, A. L. (1991). Performance of postlinguistically deaf adults with the Wearable Speech Processor (WSP III) and Mini Speech processor (MSP) of the Nucleus multi-electrode cochlear implant. *Ear and Hearing*, *12*, 3–22.

Smoski, W., & Trahiotis, C. (1986). Discrimination of interaural temporal disparities by normal-hearing listeners and listeners with high-frequency sensorineural hearing loss. *Journal of the Acoustical Society of America*, *79*, 1541–1547.

Spetner, N. B., & Olsho, L. W. (1990). Auditory frequency resolution in human infancy. *Child Development*, *61*, 632–652.

Talbott, C. B. (1987). A longitudinal study comparing responses of hearing-impaired infants to pure tones using visual reinforcement and play audiometry. *Ear and Hearing*, *8*, 175–179.

Thompson, G., Wilson, W. R., & Moore, J. M. (1979). Application of visual reinforcement audiometry to low-functioning children. *Journal of Speech and Hearing Disorders*, *44*, 80–90.

Trehub, S. E. (1987). Infants' perception of musical patterns. *Perception & Psychophysics*, *41*, 635–641.

Trehub, S. E., & Schneider, B. A. (1983). Recent advances in the behavioral study of infant audition. In S. E. Gerber & G. T. Mencher (Eds.), *The development of auditory behavior* (pp. 167–186). New York: Grune & Stratton.

Trehub, S. E., Schneider, B. A., & Endman, M. (1980). Developmental changes in infants' sensitivity to octave-band noises. *Journal of Experimental Child Psychology*, *29*, 282–293.

Trehub, S. E., Schneider, B. A., Morrongiello, B. A., & Thorpe, L. A. (1988). Auditory sensitivity in school-age children. *Journal of Experimental Child Psychology*, *46*, 273–285.

Widen, J. E. (1990). Behavioral screening of high-risk infants using visual reinforcement audiometry. *Seminars in Hearing*, *11*, 342–356.

Wightman, F. L., McGee, T., & Kramer, M. (1977). Factors influencing frequency selectivity in normal and hearing-impaired listeners. In E. F. Evans & J. P. Wilson (Eds.), *Psychophysics and physiology of hearing* (pp. 295–306). London: Academic Press.

Wilson, W. R., & Gerber, S. E. (1983). Auditory behavior in infancy. In S. E. Gerber & G. T. Mencher (Eds.), *The development of auditory behavior* (pp. 167–186). New York: Grune & Stratton.

Wilson, W. R., & Moore, J. M. (1978). *Pure-tone earphone thresholds of infants utilizing visual reinforcement audiometry (VRA)*. Paper presented at the meeting of the American Speech-Language-Hearing Association, San Francisco, CA.

Wilson, W. R., & Thompson, G. (1984). Behavioral audiometry. In J. Jerger (Ed.), *Pediatric audiology* (pp. 1–44). San Diego: College Hill Press.

Index